Contents

ii

Other titles in the BSAVA Manuals series:

Manual of Advanced Veterinary Nursing
Manual of Canine and Feline Behavioural Medicine
Manual of Canine and Feline Emergency and Critical Care
Manual of Canine and Feline Gastroenterology
Manual of Canine and Feline Haematology and Transfusion Medicine
Manual of Canine and Feline Nephrology and Urology
Manual of Companion Animal Nutrition and Feeding
Manual of Canine and Feline Infectious Diseases
Manual of Exotic Pets
Manual of Ornamental Fish
Manual of Psittacine Birds
Manual of Rabbit Medicine and Surgery
Manual of Raptors, Pigeons and Waterfowl
Manual of Reptiles
Manual of Small Animal Anaesthesia and Analgesia
Manual of Small Animal Arthrology
Manual of Small Animal Clinical Pathology
Manual of Small Animal Dentistry
Manual of Small Animal Dermatology
Manual of Small Animal Diagnostic Imaging
Manual of Small Animal Endocrinology
Manual of Small Animal Fracture Repair and Management
Manual of Small Animal Neurology
Manual of Small Animal Oncology
Manual of Small Animal Ophthalmology
Manual of Small Animal Reproduction and Neonatology
Manual of Veterinary Care
Manual of Veterinary Nursing
Manual of Wildlife Casualties

For information on these and all BSAVA publications please visit our website: www.bsava.com

BSAVA Manual of Small Animal Dermatology

Second edition

Editors:

Aiden P. Foster
Diplomate ACVD MRCVS

...ience, University of Bristol,
...angford, Bristol BS40 5DU

and

Carol S. Foil
MS DVM Diplomate ACVD

...hool of Veterinary Medicine,
...ton Rouge, LA 70803, USA

Published by:

British Small Animal Vete...
Woodrow House, 1 Telford...
Business Park, Quedgeley,...

A Company Limited by Gua...
Registered Company No. 2...
Registered as a Charity.

Figures 35.1, 35.2, 35.3 ar...
and are printed with her pe...

A catalogue record for this book is available from the British Library.

ISBN 0 905214 58 7

The publishers and contributors cannot take responsibility for information
provided on dosages and methods of application of drugs mentioned in
this publication. Details of this kind must be verified by individual users
from the appropriate literature.

Typeset by: Fusion Design, Wareham, Dorset, UK

Printed by: Grafos, Barcelona, Spain

Contributors

Zeineb Alhaidari DrVet Diplomate ECVD
Clinique Vétérinaire, Cedex 248, RN 85, F – 06330, Roquefort-les-Pins, France

Emmanuel Bensignor DrVet Diplomate ECVD
Clinique Vétérinaire, 6 rue Mare Pavée, 35510 Cesson Sevigne, France

Mandy Burrows BVMS FACVSc
Veterinary Dermatologist, Murdoch University Veterinary Hospital, Division of Veterinary & Biomedical Sciences,
Murdoch Drive, Murdoch, Perth, WA 6150, Australia

Kevin Byrne DVM MS Diplomate ACVD
Allergy, Ear and Skin Care for Animals LLC, 120 E. Montgomery Ave. Suite 203, Ardmore, PA 19003-2431, USA

Rosario Cerundolo DVM CertVD Diplomate ECVD MRCVS
Department of Clinical Studies, The School of Veterinary Medicine, University of Pennsylvania, Room 1119 VHUP,
3900 Delancey Street, Philadelphia, PA 19104-6010, USA

Sarah Colombini DVM Diplomate ACVD
Gulf Coast Veterinary Dermatology & Allergy, 1111 West Loop South, Suite 120, Houston TX 77072, USA

Mark Craig BVSc CertSAD MRCVS
31 Porchester Rd, Newbury, Berks RG14 7QH

Cathy Curtis BVetMed DVD Diplomate ECVIM-CA MRCVS
7 Chadwell, Ware, Herts SG12 9JX

Jane Dobson MA DVetMed Diplomate ECVIM-CA MRCVS
RCVS Specialist in Veterinary Oncology, Queens Veterinary School Hospital, University of Cambridge, Madingley Road,
Cambridge CB3 0ES

Ewan A. Ferguson BVM&S DVD MRCVS
16 Tennyson Avenue, Wanstead, London, E11 2QN

Carol S. Foil MS DVM Diplomate ACVD
Professor, Veterinary Clinical Sciences, School of Veterinary Medicine, Louisiana State University, Baton Rouge, LA 70803, USA

Neil A. Forbes BVetMed CBiol MIBiol Diplomate ECAMS FRCVS
RCVS Specialist in Zoo Animal and Wildlife Medicine (Avian); European Veterinary Specialist Avian Medicine and Surgery,
Avian and Exotic Animal Department, Lansdown Veterinary Surgeons, Clockhouse Veterinary Hospital, Wallbridge, Stroud GL5 3JD
e-mail: drhawk@lansdown-vets.co.uk

Aiden P. Foster PhD Diplomate ACVD MRCVS
23 Tennyson Avenue, Clevedon, North Somerset BS21 7UJ

Linda A. Frank MS DVM Diplomate ACVD
Associate Professor of Dermatology, University of Tennessee, Department of Small Animal Clinical Sciences,
C247 Veterinary Teaching Hospital, Knoxville, TN 37996-4544, USA

Richard Halliwell MA VetMB PhD MRCVS
Emeritus Professor, University of Edinburgh, Royal (Dick) School of Veterinary Studies, Easter Bush Veterinary Centre,
Easter Bush, Roslin, Midlothian, EH25 9RG

Julie Henfrey BVM&S CertSAD MRCVS
Dermatology Referral Services, Sheriff's Highway Veterinary Hospital, 94 Sheriff's Highway, Gateshead, Tyne & Wear NE9 5SD

Hilary Jackson BVM&S DVD MRCVS Diplomate ACVD
Assistant Professor, Dermatology, College of Veterinary Medicine, North Carolina State University, 4700 Hillsborough St.,
Raleigh, NC 27502, USA

Soraya Juarbe-Diaz DVM Diplomate ACVB
Florida Veterinary Specialists, 3000 Busch Lake Boulevard, Tampa, FL 33614, USA

Gail Kunkle DVM Diplomate ACVD
Department of Small Animal Clinical Sciences, College of Veterinary Medicine, University of Florida, Box 100126, Gainesville,
FL 32610-0126, USA

Kenneth W. Kwochka DVM Diplomate ACVD
Animal Dermatology Specialty Clinic, 13286 Fiji Way, Marina del Rey, CA 90292, USA

Stephen L. Lemarié MS DVM Diplomate ACVD
Southeast Veterinary Specialists, 400 N. Causeway Boulevard, Metairie, LA 70001, USA

Janet D. Littlewood MA PhD BVSc (Hons) DVR DVD MRCVS
Veterinary Dermatology Referrals, Providence Cottage, 11 High Street, Landbeach, Cambridge CB4 8DR

David Lloyd PhD BVetMed Diplomate ECVD FRCVS
Royal Veterinary College, University of London, Hawkshead Lane, North Mymms, Hatfield, Herts AL9 7TA

Dawn Logas DVM Diplomate ACVD
4846 NE 60th Terrace, Silver Springs, FL 34488, USA

Sandra Merchant DVM Diplomate ACVD
Veterinary Clinical Sciences, School of Veterinary Medicine, Louisiana State University, Baton Rouge, LA 70803, USA

Mark A. Mitchell DVM MS PhD
Assistant Professor, Zoological Medicine, Department of Veterinary Clinical Sciences, School of Veterinary Medicine, Louisiana State University, Baton Rouge, LA 70803, USA

Karen A. Moriello DVM Diplomate ACVD
Clinical Professor of Dermatology, School of Veterinary Medicine, University of Wisconsin – Madison, 2015 Linden Drive West, Madison WI 53706-1102, USA

Ralf Mueller DrMedVet FACVSc Diplomate ACVD
Department of Clinical Sciences, College of Veterinary Medicine, Colorado State University, Fort Collins, CO 80523, USA

Chiara Noli DVM Diplomate ECVD
Strada Madonna 58, 12016 Peveragno (CN), Italy

Tim Nuttall BSc(Hons) BVSc CertVD CBiol MIBiol MRCVS
Lecturer in Veterinary Dermatology, University of Liverpool, Small Animal Hospital, Crown Street, Liverpool L7 7EX

Manon Paradis DMV MVSc Diplomate ACVD
Department of Clinical Sciences, Faculté de Medecine Vetérinaire, CP 5000, St-Hyacinthe, Québec, Canada, J2S 7C6

Anita Patel BVM DVD MRCVS
23 Searchwood Road, Warlingham, Surrey CR6 9BB

Sue Paterson MA VetMB DVD Diplomate ECVD MRCVS
Rutland House Veterinary Hospital, Cowley Hill Lane, St Helens, Merseyside WA10 2AW

Ron Rees Davies BVSc CertZooMed MRCVS
Exotic Animal Centre, 12 Fitzilian Avenue, Harold Wood, Romford, Essex RM3 0QS

Petra J. Roosje DVM PhD Diplomate ECVD
Interdisciplinary Dermatology Unit, Department of Clinical Veterinary Medicine, University of Berne, Länggasstrasse 128, CH-3012 Berne, Switzerland

Karen Rosenthal DVM MS Diplomate ABVP-Avian
Director of Special Species Medicine, University of Pennsylvania, School of Veterinary Medicine, 3900 Delancey Street, Philadelphia, PA19104-6010, USA

David H. Scarff BVetMed CertSAD MRCVS
2 Highlands, Old Costessey, Norwich, Norfolk NR8 5EA

Danny Scott DVM Diplomate ACVD
Department of Clinical Sciences – Box 34, College of Veterinary Medicine, Cornell University, Ithaca, NY 14853-6401, USA

Kevin Shanley DVM Diplomate ACVD
209 Hunting Hill Lane, Westchester, PA 19382, USA

David H. Shearer BVetMed CertSAD PhD MRCVS
Vetcutis, Holly House, Station Road, Pulham St Mary, Diss, Norfolk IP21 4QQ

David M. Vail DVM MS Diplomate ACVIM (Oncology)
Associate Professor of Oncology, Chief, Clinical Oncology Service, Department of Medical Sciences, School of Veterinary Medicine and The Comprehensive Cancer Center, University of Wisconsin–Madison, 2015 Linden Drive, Madison, WI 53706, USA

Stephen D. White DVM Diplomate ACVD
Department of Medicine and Epidemiology, School of Veterinary Medicine, University of California, Davis, CA 95616, USA

David Williams MA VetMB CertVOphthal PhD MRCVS
Department of Clinical Veterinary Medicine, University of Cambridge, Madingley Road, Cambridge CB3 0ES

Foreword

This is the second edition of the *BSAVA Manual of Dermatology* and it is my pleasure, as an editor of the first edition, and President of BSAVA, to congratulate the editors and authors for producing a Manual in the mould we have come to expect – authoritative, relevant and practitioner-friendly.

Dermatological complaints account for a large proportion of first-opinion consultations and an up-to-date, readable and approachable text is mandatory. The editors have drawn contributions from leading veterinary dermatologists in the UK, Europe and North America, covering all aspects of canine and feline dermatology. There are chapters covering structure, lesions (e.g. papules, pustules, alopecia), clinical signs (e.g. pruritus, otitis, nail diseases) and specific disease (e.g. atopy, *Malassezia* dermatitis, pemphigus, mast cell neoplasia). In addition there are chapters on the dermatological problems of rabbits and rodents, ferrets, birds, reptiles, amphibians and ornamental fish.

I would like to thank the editors, authors and members of BSAVA Publications Committee, for producing yet another high quality BSAVA Manual of which we can be justifiably proud.

Richard G Harvey BVSc PhD DVD MRCVS
BSAVA President 2002–2003

Preface

Veterinary dermatology is a rapidly maturing specialty and it also enjoys ever-increasing numbers of practitioners who devote themselves part-time or full-time to the practice and advancement of dermatology. The 4th World Congress of Veterinary Dermatology, held in San Francisco in September of 2000, had over 1000 attendees from 42 countries, attesting to the international scope of veterinarians' growing interest in dermatology.

The second edition of the BSAVA *Manual of Small Animal Dermatology* truly incorporates the new international scope of knowledge in the field. The co-editors are British and American, and the authors include experts from both sides of the Atlantic and Australia. This new edition has been completely rewritten, reflecting the rapid advances in our understanding of long-described diseases and in characterizations of newly named skin diseases in small animals since the first edition was published. It has also been redesigned with the increasingly busy and increasingly web-oriented veterinary surgeon in mind. The information provided is concise and readily accessible to the busy practitioner, and the book is generously illustrated with colour figures, practical tables and useful diagrams.

The *Manual* has been organized into four sections. The first provides the practitioner a thorough survey of the basics of dermatological practice, from structure and function of mammalian skin to a practical coverage of dermatopathology as it interfaces with the practice of clinical dermatology. The second section provides a problem-oriented approach to the common dermatological presentations. Each chapter in this section presents a differential diagnosis to a common skin problem, suggests a database of diagnostic tests and, in many instances, includes an algorithmic approach for working toward a diagnosis. Some representative diseases that are not covered in the third section are presented in brief. The third section is disease-based, incorporating complete chapters on the commonest skin diseases of dogs and cats. The final section is devoted to skin disease of small animals other than dogs and cats, and includes chapters on rabbits and rodents, ferrets, birds, reptiles, amphibians and fish.

We do hope that this *Manual,* with its international approach, will provide veterinarians in the many countries in which they practice a well-rounded, thorough, yet very accessible coverage of skin diseases of small animals.

We are very grateful for the support provided by the BSAVA Publications Committee, and particularly for the expertise and hard work of the Publishing Manager, Marion Jowett.

Aiden Foster
Carol Foil
November 2002

Structure and function of the skin

David H. Lloyd and Anita P. Patel

The skin is the largest of the organs and performs a wide variety of functions vital to maintenance of the homeostatic status of the body (Figure 1.1). In addition, different regions of the skin such as the ear, eyelids, lips, prepuce, footpads and nails have specialized functions and differ structurally from the skin covering the general body surface. A consideration of all of these topics is beyond the scope of this chapter. Attention will be concentrated on the anatomy and physiology of the unspecialized skin and its role in body defence, with the aim of providing a basis for understanding the pathogenesis of cutaneous disease.

Function	Range of activities
Barrier	Controls loss of water, electrolytes etc. Excludes chemical, physical, biological agents
Sensation	Heat, cold, pain, itch, pressure
Temperature regulation	Insulation, variable blood flow, sweating
Haemodynamic control	Peripheral vascular changes
Secretion, excretion	Glandular function, hair and epidermal growth. Percutaneous loss of gases, liquids and solutes
Synthesis	Vitamin D
Immune function	Surveillance, response

1.1 Skin activities associated with homeostasis.

The epidermis

The epidermis forms the superficial layer of the skin and is thus subjected to a wide variety of chemical, physical and biological stresses. It is not, in itself, physically strong but preserves its integrity by continually secreting protective components. These include the hair coat, the keratinized cells of the stratum corneum and the secretions of the skin glands. The epidermis rests on the basement membrane, which provides not only the firm attachment of the epidermis to the dermis but also allows the passage of molecules between the two structures. In canine skin, the stratum corneum is 12–15 μm in thickness and is composed of 45–52 layers. The living epidermis has 3–4 layers and is 8–12 μm thick over the general body surface.

Epidermal structure and function

The epidermis is a stratified squamous epithelium and is normally composed of four layers (Figure 1.2), which are, from the inside out:

- Basal layer (stratum basale)
- Spinous layer (stratum spinosum)
- Granular layer (stratum granulosum)
- Horny layer (stratum corneum).

Each layer is one to several cells thick depending on the anatomical site. The keratinocyte is the principal cell of the epidermis (~85%), the remainder being resident epidermal dendritic cells, Langerhans' cells (~5–8%), melanocytes (~5%) and Merkel cells (~3–5%). Other cells such as lymphocytes, eosinophils and neutrophils may also be present in the epidermis but are not resident. The origins and functions of cells in the skin are summarized in Figure 1.3.

Basal layer
The keratinocytes of the basal layer are tightly packed columnar cells. They are daughter cells produced by mitosis of a small number of more primitive cells known as stem cells. This process is called epidermal proliferation. The daughter keratinocytes are also transiently able to divide and gradually migrate outwards to replace the cells shed from the skin surface.

The cytoskeleton of the keratinocyte is composed of actin filaments, keratin intermediate filaments and microtubules, which provide it with structural strength. The cell's ability to produce pro- and anti-inflammatory cytokines and interferons, and to function as a phagocytic cell, allow it to perform an important role in inflammation and immunity.

Spinous layer
The spinous layer is largely composed of polygonal keratinocytes that undergo biochemical and structural changes as they migrate towards the surface. They are called spinous cells because in conventional histological sections they appear to have spines when examined microscopically. The spines are in fact the desmosomes, intercellular bridges that allow cell-to-cell adhesion. These are important structures, which allow firm attachment between cells and which also allow communication between cells. The molecular structure of desmosomes has been defined. They are composed of transmembrane proteins (desmogleins

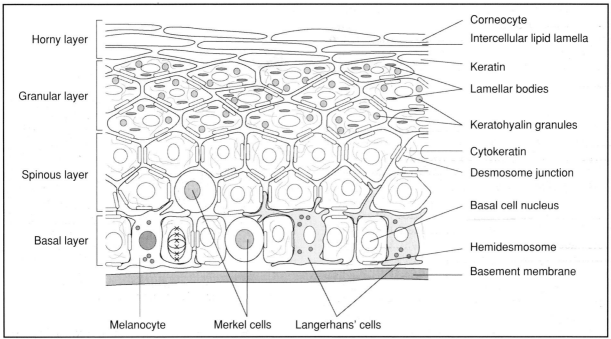

Horny layer

Granular layer

Spinous layer

Basal layer

Corneocyte
Intercellular lipid lamella

Keratin
Lamellar bodies

Keratohyalin granules

Cytokeratin
Desmosome junction

Basal cell nucleus

Hemidesmosome
Basement membrane

Melanocyte   Merkel cells   Langerhans' cells

1.2 Diagrammatic representation of the epidermis, illustrating the organization of the cells and their maturation into fully cornified cells. © Anita Patel.

Skin structure	Cell type	Origin	Function
Epidermis	Keratinocyte	Ectoderm	Barrier due to structure Immune response via production of cytokines and phagocytosis
	Langerhans' cell	Haematopoietic progenitor cells	Immune surveillance
	Melanocyte	Neural crest	Production of pigment, which protects from UV light, provides camouflage and allows sexual display in some species
	Merkel cell	Primitive epidermal cells	Slow adapting mechanoreceptors
Dermis	Fibroblast	Mesenchyme	Synthesis of extracellular matrix components Wound healing Production of degrading enzymes
	Dermal dendrocyte	Bone marrow-derived	Antigen presentation Haemostasis Wound healing
	T lymphocytes	Bone marrow-derived	Promote cell-mediated and humoral immune response Generally CD3, $\alpha\beta$ positive
	Mast cell	Bone marrow-derived	Involved in early immune response by releasing preformed granules and initiation of the process of inflammation
	Microvascular endothelial cells	Haematopoietic progenitor cells	Involved in immune response via the adhesion of effector cells such as neutrophils, eosinophils, basophils and monocytes

1.3 Origin and functions of the cells found in the epidermis and the dermis.

(Dsg) 1, 2, 3 and desmocollins) and plaque proteins (plakoglobin, plakophillin, desmoplakin, desmocalmin and intermediate filament associated protein (IFAP) 300). These molecules form attachments to corresponding molecules on adjacent cells.

The structural and biochemical change, which occurs as the keratinocyte migrates through the epidermis, is referred to as differentiation. This process involves formation of keratin and the cornified envelope. The formation of intermediate keratin filaments accelerates in this layer; as the keratinocytes migrate towards the surface the filaments are aggre-

gated into keratin bundles. The keratinocytes of the spinous layer also commence synthesis of lamellar bodies. Both proliferation and differentiation are highly regulated by a complex chain of events controlled by growth factors, interleukins, arachidonic acid and its metabolites, vitamin D_3, calcium and retinoids.

Granular layer
The cells of the granular layer are fusiform in shape and are characterized by the presence of keratohyalin granules. The granules contain a precursor protein, profilaggrin which, when dephosphorylated to filaggrin,

is involved in the aggregation of the keratin bundles. The lamellar bodies containing lipid and hydrolytic enzymes are extruded into the intercellular spaces where they are reorganized to form the outer layer of the cornified cell envelope and the intercellular lamellae. Both play an important role in barrier function.

Horny layer

The stratum corneum is the outermost layer of the epidermis and is in direct contact with the external environment. The flattened polyhedral cells, that form this compact layer (Figure 1.4) have undergone structural and biochemical changes and are composed mainly of aggregated keratin bundles and filaggrin within a cornified envelope that replaces the plasma membrane. The latter is composed of an inner proteinaceous portion composed of envelope proteins (involucrin, cystatin A, loricrin, trichohyalin, filaggrin and others), which are cross-linked by transglutaminase enzymes to form the insoluble envelope. The outer lipid portion of the cornified cell envelope is a continuous layer of hydroxyceramide that is covalently bonded to the inner portion of the cornified envelope.

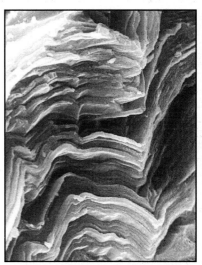

1.4

Scanning electron micrograph of frozen hydrated canine stratum corneum, showing the compact layered arrangement of the squames. (Courtesy of IS Mason and DH Lloyd)

The cells of the stratum corneum are continually shed from the skin surface by a process called desquamation. In the looser outer layer of the corneum, the intercellular spaces are permeated by sweat and sebum (Figure 1.5). The shedding of cells in healthy skin is in equilibrium with the processes of proliferation and differentiation. All three processes are influenced by the epidermal lipids. The interaction between the lipid portion of the cornified cell envelope and the intercellular lamellae is important for normal cohesion and epidermal permeability barrier function. The structure of the stratum corneum is likened to a brick and mortar structure where the keratins and the inner portion of the cornified envelope form the bricks and the lipid forms the mortar, which holds the corneocytes together and provides a hydrophobic barrier.

Resident and transient cells

The protective functions of skin are further enhanced by the resident and transient cells found within the epidermis (see Figure 1.3).

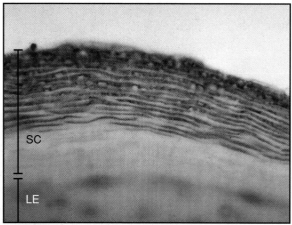

1.5 Frozen section of bovine skin after treatment with alkaline buffer, swelling the stratum corneum. Red-staining lipid (Sudan IV stain) can be seen in the distal intercellular layers of the corneum. The stratum corneum is somewhat thinner in dogs and cats. LE, living epidermis; SC, stratum corneum.

Langerhans' cells: These are antigen-presenting cells which are capable of phagocytosing and presenting processed native antigen to naïve T lymphocytes, which can mount a primary immune response, and also to memory T cells. By performing this task, the Langerhans' cells protect an individual from superficial infections. They are also thought to play a role in preventing cancer by responding to new tumour antigens.

Melanocytes: Melanocytes are melanin-producing dendritic cells found mainly in the basal layer. Mammalian melanocytes produce two main types of melanin: eumelanin (black) and phaeomelanin (yellow to reddish-brown). Melanins absorb ultraviolet light but also serve as free radical scavengers, bind to drugs and provide camouflage, thus protecting the individual in several ways.

Merkel cells: The Merkel cells are slow-adapting type 1 mechanoreceptors that are located in the basal layer or just below it. They occur mainly in the tylotrich pads and the hair epithelium and are able to respond to tactile stimuli.

Hair and its associated structures

Hair is a characteristic of mammals and protects the individual in several ways. It provides physical, microbial and chemical barriers and aids in camouflage and in signalling between animals. The length and density of the hair coat provides thermal insulation, whilst colour and glossiness play thermoregulatory roles. Specialized tactile hairs (sinus and tylotrich hairs) have been modified structurally to be able to perceive sensory stimuli.

Hair follicle structure and function

The hair follicle and hair cycle

Hair is formed by the hair follicle in a growth cycle (Figure 1.6) that is controlled by both internal and external factors (Figure 1.7). Hair follicles are formed

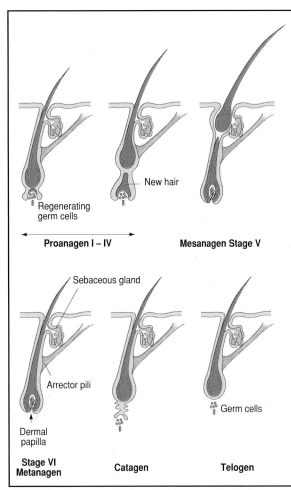

Proanagen I – IV

Mesanagen Stage V

New hair

Regenerating
germ cells

Sebaceous gland

Arrector pili

Dermal
papilla

Germ cells

Stage VI
Metanagen

Catagen

Telogen

1.6 The hair growth cycle. Anagen, the active growth phase, is divided into 6 stages. Proanagen stages I–IV, mesanagen stage V and metanagen stage VI. During these stages, the hair follicle undergoes differentiation, rapid growth and hair elongation. Telogen represents the resting phase of the hair follicle and catagen is the transitional period between the growth and resting phases. © Anita Patel.

Factors	Effect on hair growth
Intrinsic:	
Cytokines	Either inhibit or stimulate hair growth
Adhesion molecules	Found in dermal papilla during anagen
Oncogenes and tumour suppressor genes	Influence mRNA synthesis and control cell death (apoptosis)
Extrinsic:	
Environmental (photoperiod and temperature)	Stimulates or inhibits
Hormonal (melatonin, prolactin, sex hormones, glucocorticoids, growth hormone)	Varying effect on the hair cycle i.e. hair growth and differentiation depending on body location
Nutrition	
General health status	
Genetics	

1.7 Intrinsic and extrinsic factors that control the hair cycle.

during embryonic development by complex interactions between the mesenchymal and ectodermal cells. Their task is to produce hair in clearly defined growth cycles, to replace hair lost by moulting or pathological conditions. Hair in cats and dogs is replaced in a mosaic pattern with peaks in the spring and autumn and replacement is influenced by the photoperiod, temperature and nutritional status. Other replacement patterns include seasonal and wave patterns.

Anatomically the hair follicle is divided into three segments, the infundibulum, the isthmus and the inferior segment (Figures 1.8 and 1.9). Each primary follicle is associated with an arrector pili muscle, a sweat gland and a sebaceous gland, which jointly form the hair follicle unit. Grouped follicles, as found in dogs and cats, are referred to as compound follicles in which a primary hair is associated with several smaller secondary hairs, all of which leave the epidermis through the same opening. The ratio of primary to secondary hairs determines the different types of hair coats seen in different species and breeds of mammal. Compound hair follicles are grouped into follicular units usually comprising three compound follicles.

Hairs

Figure 1.10 shows the surface ultrastructure of a canine hair. Sinus hairs, known as vibrissae or whiskers, are found on the face and throat of domestic animals and in the cat on the palmar carpal pad. These are stiff hairs, which are associated with a blood-lined endothelial sinus in close association with Pacinian corpuscles. They act as slow-adapting mechanoreceptors. Tylotrich hairs are large stout single hairs, that have a neurovascular complex at the level of the sebaceous gland and are scattered throughout the skin surface in close association with the tylotrich pads. They act as rapidly adapting mechanoreceptors.

Sebaceous glands

The sebaceous glands are simple alveolar glands with ducts opening directly on to the skin surface or into the infundibulum. The former are referred to as free sebaceous glands and the latter as pilosebaceous glands. Their density and size depend on their anatomical site. They are most abundant around mucocutaneous junctions, interdigital spaces, on the dorsal neck, rump and tail, and the chin. They are absent on the nasal planum and footpads. Figure 1.11 lists the types and location of exocrine glands.

Sebum has both protective and behavioural roles. Combined with sweat it forms a waxy emulsion that provides a protective barrier against pathogenic organisms. Sebum is rich in wax esters and, by coating the surface of the skin and hair, controls wetting and provides the animal with a glossy coat which may assist in reflection of heat. Specialized sebaceous glands are able to produce pheromones and thus play a role in behaviour. In recent years, the sebaceous gland has been used in modulating the distribution of topical medicaments such as flea control products.

Sebaceous lipids are actively synthesized by sebaceous glands and secreted as products of cell death

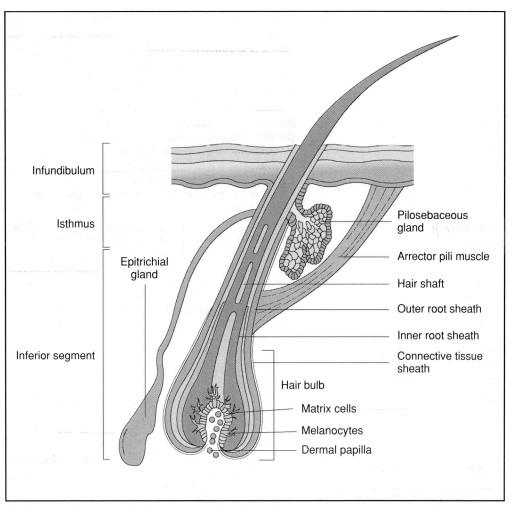

Infundibulum

Isthmus

Epitrichial gland

Inferior segment

Pilosebaceous gland

Arrector pili muscle

Hair shaft

Outer root sheath

Inner root sheath

Connective tissue sheath

Hair bulb

Matrix cells

Melanocytes

Dermal papilla

1.8 The hair follicle and its associated structures. © Anita Patel.

Structure	Characteristic	Function
Dermal papilla	Dermal fibrocytes embedded in extracellular matrix and containing nervous and vascular supplies	Induces follicular development Nourishes hair matrix
Hair matrix	Proliferative epithelial cells. Melanocytes visible and active during anagen	Produce inner and outer root sheaths and hair shaft. Produce and transfer pigment to hair shaft
Hair shaft: 　　Medulla 　　Cortex 　　Cuticle	Consists of cuboidal cells absent in secondary hairs Pigment-containing cornified cells Outermost overlapping cornified cells	Insulation Bulk and strength of hair, hair colour Protects the cortex, provides glossiness or reflexivity
Inner root sheath (IRS): 　　Cuticle 　　Huxley's layer 　　Henley's layer	Flat overlapping cells interlocking with hair cuticle One to three nucleated cells containing trichohyalin granules Single layer of non-nucleated cells also containing trichohyalin	Protects and supports the growing hair
Outer root sheath (ORS)	Covered by IRS below the isthmus. Cells contain glycogen vacuoles. Does not undergo keratinization At isthmus undergoes tricholemmal keratinization In infundibulum undergoes normal keratinization and is characterized by keratohyaline granules	Provides continuity with the epidermis
Basement membrane zone	Surrounds ORS, composed of a fibrous tissue and glassy membrane	

1.9 Hair follicle structural components and their functions.

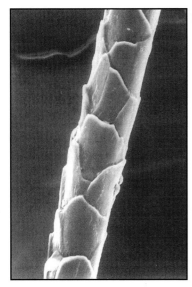

1.10 Scanning electron micrograph of a normal canine hair. The surface is tiled with cells of the cuticle which point away from the base of the hair.

known as atrichial (formerly 'eccrine') (Figure 1.12). In some species, specialized sweat glands are involved in scent production.

Whilst sweat does not have a universal function, it protects the skin and its specialized structures, such as the eyelids and footpads, from frictional damage, maintains skin pliability and provides microbial defence through the presence of immunoglobulins, cytokines, the iron-binding protein transferrin and inorganic ions such as sodium chloride. Sweat does not play a significant role in thermoregulation in cats and dogs.

Sweat secretion varies with species and several different modes have been described. They include cell death, paracellular transport, exocytosis, microapocrine blebbing and transcellular ion and water transport.

It has been postulated that sympathetic nerves control sweat gland activity in some species, such as dog, cat, cow, sheep and goat. It is thought that production of epinephrine (adrenaline) and norepinephrine (noradrenaline) by adrenergic and cholinergic sympathetic nerve endings on the cutaneous blood vessels, or dopamine released by mast cells, transfers neurotransmitter substances such as epinephrine and norepinephrine to the gland. In man and horses, and in the footpads of cats and dogs, it has been suggested that sweating is controlled directly by acetylcholine and catecholamines produced by sympathetic nerve endings located next to the fibrocyte sheaths of the glands.

	Specialized gland	Type	Species
Skin	Atrichial/epitrichial	Sweat	Dog, cat, cow, horse, pig, man
	Free and pilosebaceous	Sebaceous	As above
Eyelids	Moll's gland	Sweat	As above
	Meibomian (tarsal)	Sebaceous	As above
	Glands of Zeis (cilia)	Sebaceous	As above
Ears	Ceruminous	Sweat	As above
Perineum	Hepatoid (circumanal)	Sebaceous	Dog
	Anal sac gland	Combined	Cat, dog
Tail	Tail gland	Sebaceous	Cat, dog
Prepuce	Preputial glands	Sweat	Dog, cat, cow, horse, pig, man
Muzzle	Nasolabial glands	Muco-serous	Cattle, sheep, goat, pig
Footpads	Atrichial	Sweat	Cat, dog

1.11 Occurrence and distribution of cutaneous exocrine glands in mammalian skin.

(holocrine). However, recent studies have suggested that the passage of ionic components into sebum results from paracellular transport. Sebum is stored in the sebaceous glands, which are controlled by both endocrine and non-endocrine factors. In general, androgens stimulate glandular activity by increasing mitotic rate and sebum output. Oestrogens and glucocorticoids tend to have the opposite effect.

Sweat glands

The sweat glands are simple or coiled tubular glands of the skin. Those with a duct opening into the infundibulum are referred to as epitrichial (formerly 'apocrine') glands, while those which have ducts opening directly on to the skin surface are

The dermoepidermal junction

The dermoepidermal junction (DEJ) is the interface between the epidermis and the dermis. It is composed of the plasma membrane on the basal aspect of the basal cell and the basement membrane. The latter is subdivided ultrastructurally into the lamina lucida, lamina densa and sublamina densa (Figure 1.13).

The basal keratinocytes are firmly attached to anchoring filament proteins found in the lamina lucida, mainly by hemidesmosomes. These cell-substrate attachments are composed of plaque proteins (bullous pemphigoid antigen type 1) and transmembrane proteins (bullous pemphigoid antigen type 2 and α6β4 integrin). Focal adhesions are located along the basal aspect of cultured keratinocytes and are thought to mediate adhesion during cell migration.

The lamina densa is composed of collagen IV, laminin, nidogen and perlecan, forming a tight network which acts as a filter restricting the passage of molecules from the dermis to the epidermis and vice versa, but allowing the movement of immune cells between the two.

The sublamina densa is located below the lamina densa and is formed by anchoring fibrils, composed of collagen VII, which insert on to anchoring plaques in the superficial dermis. This intricate network of molecules provides the overall basis of the firm attachment between the dermis and the epidermis.

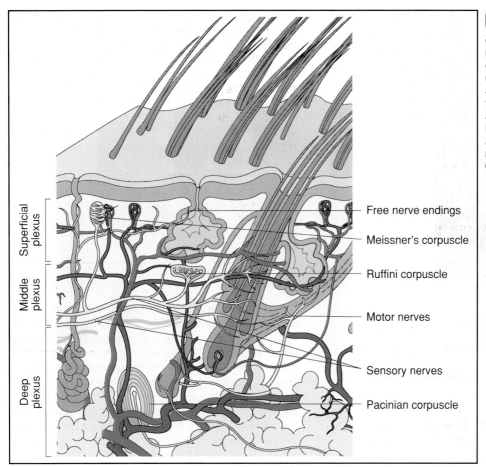

1.12 Diagrammatic representation of components of mammalian skin including epidermal structures (compound hair follicle and adnexal structures, free sebaceous gland, atrichial sweat gland), blood supply, nerves and associated mechanoreceptors. © Anita Patel.

Superficial plexus

Middle plexus

Deep plexus

Free nerve endings

Meissner's corpuscle

Ruffini corpuscle

Motor nerves

Sensory nerves

Pacinian corpuscle

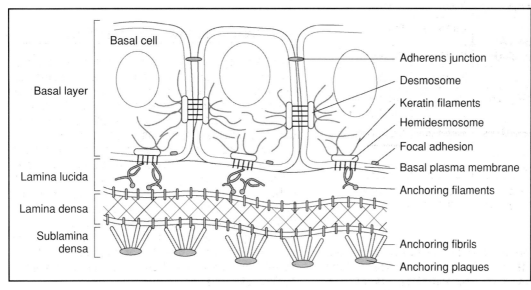

1.13 Diagrammatic representation of structural components of the dermoepidermal junction. © Anita Patel.

Basal cell

Basal layer

Lamina lucida

Lamina densa

Sublamina densa

Adherens junction

Desmosome

Keratin filaments

Hemidesmosome

Focal adhesion

Basal plasma membrane

Anchoring filaments

Anchoring fibrils

Anchoring plaques

The dermis

The dermis is the major structural component of the skin. It provides a matrix of supporting structures and secretions which maintain and interact with the epidermis and its adnexae. These include the connective tissue, blood and lymphatic vessels, nerves and receptors, and cellular components. It is an important thermoregulatory and sensory structure and also contributes significantly to body water storage.

Connective tissue

The dermal connective tissue matrix consists mainly of collagen and elastic fibres organized in a coherent pattern, principally bundles of collagen bordered by the elastic fibres. The non-fibrous component consists of the proteoglycan ground substance and certain glycoproteins. The superficial dermis is composed of fine irregularly distributed, loose, collagen fibres and a network of fine elastin fibres. Deeper in the dermis the collagen is thicker and

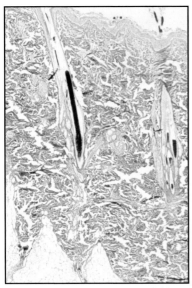

1.14 Section through canine skin, illustrating the dermal connective tissue structure. The deep dermis is characterized by thicker and denser collagen. (Silver stain)

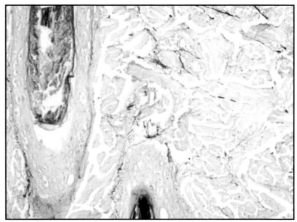

1.15 Section through canine skin, illustrating the dermal connective tissue structure. This high-power view shows elastin fibres surrounding a hair follicle. (Gomori's aldehyde fuchsin with light green stain: collagen, green; elastin fibres, mauve)

denser (Figure 1.14) and the fibres tend to run parallel to the skin surface; the elastin fibres are also thicker but less numerous.

Collagen

Collagen is the major extracellular protein of the dermis and forms about 80% of the extracellular matrix. The fibres provide strength and elasticity but are also involved in cell migration, adhesion and chemotaxis. They are secreted by the skin fibroblasts. The fibres are very resistant to animal proteases but are broken down by collagenases that are secreted chiefly by fibroblasts. The collagenases are neutral metalloendoproteases which require calcium as an activator and zinc as the intrinsic metal ion; they are uniquely able to break down the native collagen triple helix.

Collagen turnover in the dermis is slow. It is controlled by dermal cellular components, particularly fibroblasts but also inflammatory cells (macrophages, neutrophils, eosinophils, keratinocytes) which are able to respond to particular demands such as skin damage and wound healing. Hydroxyproline, an amino acid which is an abundant and vital component of collagen, is released during collagen breakdown. Urinary hydroxyproline levels can be used as an indicator of this *in vivo*.

In mature individuals, the majority of dermal collagen is formed by types I (87%) and III (10%) which align into relatively large fibrils. Types IV, V and VII are found in basement membranes. Type V collagen, which represents about 3% of dermal collagen, is found in nearly all connective tissues.

Elastic fibres

Elastic fibres form a network throughout the dermis and are also present in sheaths of hair follicles and in the walls of the blood and lymphatic vessels (Figure 1.15). They are composed of two components, elastin and microfibrillar protein. The elastin is amorphous and, in fully mature elastic fibres, forms the core, surrounded by an envelope of microfibrils. Microfibrillar material in the absence of elastin is called oxytalan. When small amounts of elastin are present it is called elaunin.

Elastin is a covalently cross-linked polypeptide with a very characteristic amino acid composition (rich in valine and alanine, low in cystine, absence of histidine and methionine). Like collagen, it possesses much glycine and also contains hydroxyproline. It is synthesized by fibroblasts and smooth muscle cells. Metabolic turnover is slow but continuous. Degradation is by a variety of elastases including some calcium-dependent metalloenzymes. The microfibrils are composed of type VI collagen and fibrillin.

Glycosaminoglycans and proteoglycans

These substances are secreted by fibroblasts. Originally called mucopolysaccharides (viscous polysaccharides), the term glycosaminoglycan was then introduced (glycan = polysaccharide; glycosamino = containing hexosamines). However, the polysaccharides are normally linked to protein and are thus called proteoglycans.

The glycosaminoglycans and proteoglycans form the ground substance, a viscous sol–gel which encompasses and supports the other dermal components. The ground substance is composed chiefly of hyaluronic acid and dermatan sulphate with heparin, chondroitin 4 and chondroitin 6 sulphates. Its degradation and turnover is not well understood but half-lives of 2–5 days and 7–14 days have been demonstrated for dermal hyaluronic acid and chondroitin sulphate. Hyaluronidase has been demonstrated in skin wounds and also in normal rat skin.

The ground substance appears to be involved in salt and water balance and can bind over 100 times its weight of water. It may also play a part in promoting growth, differentiation and cellular migration.

Blood supply and lymphatic drainage

Blood supply

The skin has a well developed vascular supply in keeping with its role in thermoregulation and in haemodynamics; blood flow through the skin substantially exceeds that required merely to supply oxygen and metabolites. The cutaneous arteries (see Figures 1.12 and 1.16) ascend from the subcutaneous region and branch to form three networks. These are located:

- At the base of the dermis, supplying the hair papillae and sweat glands
- At the level of the follicular isthmus, supplying the sebaceous glands, arrector pili and mid-portion of the hair follicle
- Just below the epidermis (superficial plexus), giving rise to the superficial capillary network supplying the epidermis which is, itself, avascular.

The veins draining the skin run parallel to the arteries. Arteriovenous anastomoses, which enable the capillary beds to be bypassed and are associated with thermoregulation, are concentrated in the deeper parts of the dermis and are particularly common in the extremities. They vary in form from the complex glomus to simple coiled structures. Control of blood flow in the capillaries is regulated by the contractile, fusiform pericytes which are aligned parallel to them.

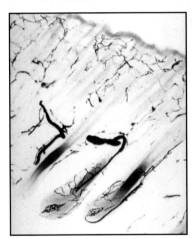

1.16 A section of bovine skin stained with haematoxylin following arterial perfusion with Indian ink. Note that the thin, superficial epidermal tissue is avascular.

Lymphatic drainage
The lymph vessels provide drainage for tissue fluid from the dermis. This fluid is collected in lymphatic capillary networks in the more superficial layers of the dermis, associated with components of the hair follicle units. The lymph vessels also provide a channel by which cellular traffic can flow to the lymph nodes. They differ from blood vessels in being flatter and wider, with thinner and flatter endothelial cells and no contractile components.

Nerves
The general pattern of nerve distribution is similar to that of the blood vessels since they generally travel alongside one another (see Figure 1.12). A plexus of nerves is present beneath the epidermis and free nerve endings also penetrate the epidermis itself. Nerve networks are also associated with the hair follicle, sweat and sebaceous glands, and the arrector pili muscle. Encapsulated nerve endings are found in mechanoreceptors (Figure 1.17) such as the Pacinian corpuscles which are found deep in the dermis.

Receptor	Sensory end organ	Function
Mechanoreceptors (Corpuscular)	Pacinian corpuscle	Pressure and vibrations
	Merkel cells	Slow adapting changes in pressure
	Meissner's corpuscle	Rapidly adapting pressure and velocity changes
	Ruffini's end bulb	Skin movement
Nociceptor	Free nerve endings	Itch and pain
Thermoreceptors	Free nerve endings	Warm and cold

1.17 Sensory nerve endings and organs, and their functions.

Cellular components
A variety of cells is present in the normal dermis (see Figure 1.3) in addition to those of the glandular, muscular, nervous and vascular tissues. It is becoming clear that these cells are capable of performing a wide variety of different tasks and can interact with the dermal matrix and the other cellular components of the epidermis and dermis both by direct contact and by means of soluble mediators.

Fibroblasts
These are mesenchymal cells responsible for the synthesis and degradation of both fibrous and non-fibrous connective tissue matrix proteins. They are quite active and are capable of secreting multiple matrix components simultaneously. Attachment of fibroblasts to the fibrous matrix is mediated via fibronectin on the cell surface; collagen and fibronectin have complementary binding sites. Fibroblasts produce collagenase and gelatinase which degrade collagen. They migrate along the fibre bundles. Fibroblasts are also able to secrete a variety of cytokines and influence proliferative activity in the epidermis.

Mast cells
Mast cells are found throughout the dermis (rarely in the epidermis), particularly associated with the superficial vascular plexus and the epidermal adnexae. They contain abundant darkly staining secretory and lysosomal cytoplasmic granules. The secretory granules contain a predominance of histamine and heparin. The lysosomal granules contain acid hydrolases capable of degrading glycosaminoglycans, proteoglycans and glycolipids, as well as some enzymes also found in the secretory granules. The cell surfaces possess microvilli and a coating of fibronectin which may assist attachment to the connective tissue matrix. Skin mast cells belong to the connective tissue mast cell group and differ from mucosal mast cells both in morphology and staining reaction.

Mast cells are important mediators of immediate hypersensitivity reactions. In dog skin three subtypes are recognized, containing tryptase (T), chymase (C) or both tryptase and chymase (TC). TC mast cells form about 60% of the mast cell population in normal canine skin.

Dendritic cells

These include melanocytes and antigen-presenting dendritic cells that are often present in the perivascular spaces of the superficial dermal blood vessels. The latter are differentiated from Langerhans' cells because they are positive for CD4 and CD90 (Thy-1) antigens.

References and further reading

Dunstan RW, Credille KM and Walder EJ (1998) The light and the skin. In: *Advances in Veterinary Dermatology, Volume III*, ed. KW Kwochka *et al.*, pp. 3–35. Butterworth Heinemann, Oxford

Ebling JG, Hale PA and Randall VA (1991) Hormones and hair growth. In: *Physiology, Biochemistry and Molecular Biology of the Skin, 2nd edn*, ed. LA Goldsmith, pp. 660–696. Oxford University Press, New York

Garthwaite G, Lloyd DH and Thomsett LR (1982) Location of immunoglobulins and complement (C3) at the surface and within the skin of dogs. *Journal of Comparative Pathology* **93**, 185–193

Haake AR and Holbrook K (1999) The structure and development of skin. In: *Dermatology in General Medicine, 5th edn*, ed. IM Freedberg *et al.*, pp. 70–107. McGraw–Hill, New York

Jenkinson D McEwan (1990) Sweat and sebaceous glands and their function in domestic animals. In: *Advances in Veterinary Dermatology, Volume I*, eds. C von Tscharner and REW Halliwell, pp. 229–251. Baillière Tindall, London

Kwochka KW and Rademakers AM (1989) Cell proliferation of epidermis, hair follicles and sebaceous glands of Beagles and Cocker Spaniels with healthy skin. *American Journal of Veterinary Research* **50**, 587

Lavker RM, Bertolino AP, Freedberg IM *et al.* (1999) Biology of hair follicles. In: *Dermatology in General Medicine*, ed. IM Freedberg *et al.*, pp. 230–238. McGraw–Hill, New York

Lloyd DH and Garthwaite G (1982) Epidermal structure and surface topography of canine skin. R*esearch in Veterinary Science* **33**, 99–104

Mason IS and Lloyd DH (1993) Scanning electron microscopical studies of the living epidermis and stratum corneum in dogs. In: *Advances in Veterinary Dermatology 2*, ed. PJ Ihrke *et al.*, pp. 131–140. Pergamon Press, Oxford

Odland G (1991) Structure of skin. In: *Physiology, Biochemistry and Molecular Biology of the Skin, 2nd edn*, ed. LA Goldsmith, pp. 3–62. Oxford University Press, New York

Scott DW (1990) The biology of hair growth and its disturbances. In: *Advances in Veterinary Dermatology, Volume 1*, eds. C von Tscharner and REW Halliwell, pp. 3–33. Baillière Tindall, London

Scott DW, Miller WH and Griffin CE (2001). *Muller and Kirk's Small Animal Dermatology, 6th edn*. WB Saunders, Philadelphia

Suter M, Crameri FM, Olivry T *et al.* (1997) Keratinocyte biology and pathology. *Veterinary Dermatology* **8**, 67–100

White SD and Yager JA (1995) Resident dendritic cells in the epidermis: Langerhans' cells, Merkel cells and melanocytes. *Veterinary Dermatology* **6**, 1–8

2

History, examination and initial evaluation

Carol S. Foil

The first point to be made about any thorough dermatological evaluation is that it is a difficult procedure to achieve with the owner providing restraint (and also providing distraction from the business at hand). It is preferable that the initial evaluation be scheduled as a special procedure, just as one might schedule a set-aside time for a lameness evaluation. The only part of the procedure that should be incorporated into a routine appointment period is the decision between the owner and the veterinary surgeon that a thorough dermatological evaluation is indicated. Once that decision has been taken, the owner can be provided with suitable dermatological history forms (see Figure 2.3) and an appointment can be scheduled for the dermatological evaluation and minimum database. It is also advisable to utilize a problem-oriented approach to dermatological evaluations. A dermatological glossary is provided at the end of this Manual.

Dermatological evaluation

Signalment

Some skin diseases show strong associations with age, breed or sex. Accordingly, in making a list of differential diagnoses, the practitioner takes into account some diseases that are relatively specific to, or very common in, the category of patient being evaluated. It should be kept in mind though, that such considerations are fraught with the potential for error. One might, for example, fail to consider demodicosis, a disease prevalent in young dogs, when evaluating older dogs or cats. Figures 2.1 and 2.2 list some strong breed and age associations for skin diseases.

Congenital and hereditary dermatoses may not be clinically apparent at birth, but are always manifested within the first year of life. In addition to the conditions noted in Figure 2.2, aging animals will exhibit dryer, thinner skin and sparser haircoats.

Breed	Common skin diseases
Abyssinian cats	Psychogenic alopecia and dermatitis; follicle dysplasia
Afghan Hound	Hypothyroidism
Airedale Terrier	Flank alopecia
Akita Inu	Hypothyroidism; pemphigus; post-clipping alopecia; sebaceous adenitis; uveodermatological syndrome (VKH)
Alaskan Malamute	Eosinophilic granuloma – oral; post-clipping alopecia; woolly syndrome; zinc-responsive dermatopathy
American Bulldog	Actinic dermatitis; ichthyosis; squamous cell carcinoma (SCC)
Basset Hound	Hair follicle tumours; *Malassezia* dermatitis; seborrhoea
Bearded Collie	Black hair follicle dysplasia; flank alopecia; lupoid onychodystrophy; pemphigus
Beauceron	Epidermolysis bullosa
Belgian Shepherd	Vitiligo
Boston Terrier	Atopy; demodicosis; pattern baldness; mast cell tumour; pituitary-dependent hyperadrenocorticism (PDH)
Boxer	Atopy; demodicosis; flank alopecia; mast cell tumour; nodular dermatofibrosis; pattern baldness; urticaria
Bouvier de Flandres	Flank alopecia
Bull Mastiff	Callus and interdigital pyoderma; otitis externa; recurrent superficial pyoderma (RSP)
Bull Terrier	Atopy; demodicosis (severe, chronic); lethal acrodermatitis; solar dermatitis and furunculosis (white); tail chasing and mutilation (coloured)
Cavalier King Charles Spaniel	Arnold–Chiari Syndrome; eosinophilic granuloma (oral); ichthyosis

2.1 Breeds with strong skin disease predilection. (continues) ▶

Breed	Common skin diseases
Chihuahua	Pattern baldness; pinnal vasculopathy
Chow Chow	Alopecia X; atopy; demodicosis; food allergy; hypothyroidism; pemphigus; post-clipping alopecia
Cocker Spaniel	Hypothyroidism; lip fold dermatitis; otitis; spaniel seborrhoea; sebaceous nodular hyperplasia; vitamin-A responsive dermatosis
Rough Collie	Discoid lupus erythematosus; dermatomyositis; systemic lupus erythematosus; ulcerative dermatosis of collies and shelties
Curly-coated Retriever	Follicle dysplasia
Dachshund	Acanthosis nigricans; colour dilution alopecia; ear margin seborrhoea; interdigital dermatitis; juvenile cellulitis; *Malassezia* dermatitis; pemphigus foliaceus; pattern baldness; PDH; pinnal vasculopathy; RSP; sterile nodular panniculitis
Dalmatian	Actinic dermatitis; atopy; black spot necrosis; food allergy; RSP; SCC
Devon Rex cat	Familial hypotrichosis
Dobermann	Acral lick dermatitis; canine acne; colour dilution alopecia; flank sucking; follicular seborrhoea; hypothyroidism; ichthyosis; pemphigus foliaceus; sulphonamide hypersensitivity; vitiligo
Dogue de Bordeaux	Footpad hyperkeratosis
English Bulldog	Atopy; demodicosis; flank alopecia; fold and interdigital dermatitis
English Springer Spaniel	Adverse food reaction; ichthyosis; lichenoid-psoriasiform dermatitis; spaniel seborrhoea
Eskimo Spitz	Pemphigus; post-clipping alopecia; uveodermatological syndrome (VKH)
French Bulldog	Flank alopecia
German Shepherd Dog	Adverse food reaction; atopy; calcinosis circumscripta; DLE; familial cutaneous vasculopathy; focal metatarsal fistulae; German Shepherd Dog pyoderma; lupoid onychodystrophy; nodular dermatofibrosis; perianal fistula/anal furunculosis; seborrhoea; SLE
German Short-Haired Pointer	Acral mutilation syndrome; epidermolysis bullosa; flank alopecia; hereditary lupoid dermatosis; vitiligo
Golden Retriever	Acral lick dermatitis; atopy; histiocytosis; hot spots; hypothyroidism; ichthyosis; juvenile cellulitis; nodular dermatofibrosis
Great Dane	Acral lick dermatitis; calcinosis circumscripta; callus, chin and interdigital pyoderma; epidermolysis bullosa acquisita (EBA) ?
Greyhound	Actinic dermatitis; actinic haemangioma; haemolytic–uraemic syndrome; androgen-withdrawal alopecia; colour dilution alopecia; pattern baldness
Griffon Korthal	Flank alopecia
Himalayan cat	Dermatophytosis; granulomatous dermatophytosis; Ehlers–Danlos syndrome; seborrhoea
Irish Terrier	Footpad hyperkeratosis
Irish Setter	Acral lick dermatitis; atopy; hypothyroidism; ichthyosis; RSP
Irish Water Spaniel	Follicle dysplasia
Italian Greyhound	Actinic dermatitis; actinic haemangiomas; colour dilution alopecia; pattern baldness
Jack Russell Terrier	Atopy; familial vasculitis; ichthyosis
Keeshond	Alopecia X; keratoacanthoma – multiple; post-clipping alopecia
Kerry Blue Terrier	Spiculosis
Labrador Retriever	Acral lick dermatitis; adverse food reaction; atopy; interdigital furunculosis; juvenile cellulitis; lipomas; *Malassezia* dermatitis; mast cell tumour; nasal hyperkeratosis
Lhasa Apso	Atopy; *Malassezia* dermatitis; sebaceous adenitis
Manchester Terrier	Pattern baldness
Miniature Pinscher	Pattern baldness
Norwegian Elkhound	Keratoacanthomas – multiple; post-clipping alopecia
Papillon	Black hair follicle dysplasia
Persian cat	Dermatophytosis; granulomatous dermatophytosis; dirty face syndrome; seborrhoea (greasy cat syndrome)
Pit Bull – white	Actinic dermatitis with furunculosis; SCC; demodicosis; interdigital furunculosis; lick granuloma
Pomeranian	Alopecia X; *Malassezia* dermatitis

2.1 (continued) Breeds with strong skin disease predilection. (continues) ▶

Breed	Common skin diseases
Poodle (Standard)	Sebaceous adenitis
Portuguese Water Dog	Follicle dysplasia
Rhodesian Ridgeback	Acral lick dermatitis; dermoid cysts; flank alopecia; ichthyosis
Rottweiler	Acral lick dermatitis; callus and interdigital pyoderma; ichthyosis; lupoid onychodystrophy; vitiligo
Saluki	Black hair follicle dysplasia; colour dilution alopecia
Samoyed	Alopecia X; eosinophilic granuloma – oral; post-clipping alopecia; sebaceous adenitis; uveodermatological syndrome (VKH)
Schipperke	Pemphigus foliaceus
Schnauzer (all sizes)	Atopy; aurotrichia (Mini); flank alopecia; mast cell tumour; Schnauzer comedo syndrome
Scottish Terrier	Atopy; nasal vasculopathy
Shar Pei	Adverse food reaction; atopy; cutaneous mucinosis; demodicosis; fold dermatitis; histiocytomas – multiple; hypothyroidism; idiopathic seborrrhoea; IgA deficiency; otitis externa; pemphigus; Shar Pei fever; staphylococcal folliculitis
Shetland Sheepdog	Dermatomyositis; ulcerative dermatosis of collies and shelties
Shih Tzu	Atopy; *Malassezia* dermatitis; traction alopecia
Siamese cat	Mast cell tumour; pinnal alopecia; psychogenic alopecia; vitiligo
Siberian Husky	Alopecia X; eosinophilic granuloma – oral; post-clipping alopecia; zinc-responsive dermatopathy; VKH; woolly syndrome
Silky Terrier	Short-hair syndrome
Sphinx cats	Hereditary alopecia; urticaria pigmentosa
Viszla	Sebaceous adenitis
Weimaraner	Colour dilution alopecia; pattern baldness
West Highland White Terrier	Atopy; demodicosis; ichthyosis; *Malassezia* dermatitis; primary seborrhoea (epidermal dysplasia)
Whippet	Actinic dermatitis; actinic haemangioma; colour dilution alopecia
Yorkshire Terrier	Atopy; colour dilution alopecia; dermatophytosis; ichthyosis; melanoderma + alopecia; traction alopecia; short-hair syndrome

2.1 (continued) Breeds with strong skin disease predilection.

Birth to 6 months
Demodicosis
Dermatophytosis
Impetigo
Cutaneous asthenia
Congenital hypotrichosis
Black hair follicle dysplasia
Ichthyosis
Dermoid cyst
Bull Terrier lethal acrodermatitis

Before 3 years
Allergy
Follicular dysplasias
Keratinization defects
Colour dilution alopecia
Histiocytoma

After 6 years
Hypothyroidism
Hyperadrenocorticism
Neoplasia

2.2 Skin diseases with strong age predilection.

History

The collection of a thorough dermatological history may be facilitated by adopting a standardized dermatological history form (Figure 2.3) or a routine set of questions for the client. Features of the dermatological syndrome that should be ascertained include the age or time that the problem was first noted and whether location, appearance or distribution have changed since the outset. History taking should include collection of general husbandry and housing data, including exposure to other animals and routine flea control procedures. Also included should be information on other medical problems and medication and diagnostic test history. Records from previous veterinary evaluations should be sought. Finally, specific questions about involvement of other pets or family members with dermatological symptoms should always be posed.

For pruritic patients, especially allergy suspects, additional information should be sought about the nature and severity of pruritus, whether it is worse in association with any time of day or activity, and whether there is seasonality to the overall severity or occurrence. Also, a complete dietary history, including ingredient lists, should be sought, not overlooking treats and table food items.

Dermatology history

Date _____

Owner details

(Mr/Mrs/Miss/Ms) Surname/Family name_____ First name or Initials _____

Address _____

_____ Post Code/Zip _____

Phone (day) _____ (evening) _____
(mobile)_____ Fax _____
e-mail _____

Patient details

Name _____ Breed _____
Sex: [ ] Male   [ ] Female   [ ] Male neutered   [ ] Female spayed
Date of birth _____ Colour _____
Identifying marks _____

CHIEF COMPLAINT(S) _____

_____

_____

Date (age) problem first noticed _____ Onset: [ ] Sudden   [ ] Slow
Is there a seasonal influence?   [ ] No   [ ] Spring/Summer   [ ] Autumn   [ ] Winter
Where did the problem begin? _____
What did it look like then? _____
Does the animal itch?   [ ] Yes   [ ] No   When? [ ] Constant   [ ] Sporadic   [ ] Night
Is there any exposure to other animals (neighbours, etc.)? _____
Do other animals or people have skin problems, rash? _____
Describe the animal's indoor environment, time (%): _____

_____

Describe the animal's outdoor environment, time (%): _____

_____

What does the animal sleep on? _____
What diagnostic tests have been performed? _____
What local treatment has been used? Success? _____

_____

What systemic treatment has been used? Success? _____

_____

Does owner have an idea of the cause? What makes it worse? _____
When did the owner last see fleas? _____ Describe flea control _____
Animal's diet _____
Reproductive history: Age of neutering? _____ Date, duration of last oestrus _____
Breeding history (male or female) _____
Medical history: Previous diseases, treatments, results: _____

_____

Is animal on any medication at present? _____
What other facts does owner think would be helpful? _____

_____

_____

2.3 An example of a dermatological history form.

General physical examination

There are many systemic diseases with important dermatological manifestations (Figure 2.4 and see Chapter 25) that may themselves be the reason for presentation for examination. Detecting signs of systemic illness with a thorough physical examination is key to determining the correct diagnosis. In addition, the general health status of the dermatology patient may dictate the choice of therapy for skin disease in some instances. Finally, some dermatological therapies will cause systemic side effects, and these must be uncovered in the course of a thorough examination of patients under treatment.

Drug allergy
Alopecia; eczema; erosion; erythema; erythema multiforme; petechiation; pigmentary disturbance; pruritus; pustular/vesicular dermatitis; ulceration; urticaria
Feline leukaemia virus, feline immunodeficiency virus
Demodicosis; giant cell dermatosis; mucositis??; recurrent abscess; vasculitis
Superficial necrolytic dermatitis (NME; hepatocutaneous syndrome)
Acral and peri-orificial hyperkeratosis; crusting; erosion
Hypothyroidism
Demodicosis; hyperpigmentation; keratinization defects; myxoedema; poor wound healing; post-clipping alopecia; recurrent superficial pyoderma; symmetrical hypotrichosis
Hyperadrenocorticism
Calcinosis cutis; cutaneous atrophy; cutaneous telangiectasis; demodicosis; hyperpigmentation; keratinization defect; recurrent superficial pyoderma; skin fragility
Leishmaniasis
Acral and facial crusting; cutaneous nodules; erythema; hypotrichosis; keratinization defect; ulcers
Mast cell tumour
Cutaneous nodules; erythroderma; exfoliation; flushing; plaques
Cutaneous T cell lymphoma
Alopecia; erosion; erythema; exfoliation; nodules; oral mucositis (inflammation of the mucosa); plaques
Gonadal neoplasm
Keratinization defect; preputial linear erythema or hyperpigmentation; scrotal dermatitis; symmetrical alopecia; symmetrical hyperpigmentation

2.4 Systemic diseases with dermatological manifestations.

Thorough dermatological examination

Good lighting and proper restraint by a trained veterinary assistant, on an examination table, are prerequisites for a good examination. Uncooperative patients should be sedated as required to allow a complete and thorough examination in every case. Thick-coated animals may have to be clipped so that skin lesions can be visualized adequately; permission for this should be obtained prior to the scheduled examination time.

One of the barriers to performing a thorough dermatological examination is time constraint. The examination should be specifically scheduled as a diagnostic procedure if consultation time is limited by appointment scheduling.

- Examine mucous membranes, skin and hair coat thoroughly in a systematic fashion. Use a standardized approach to ensure that the examination is thorough. For example, always start at the nose and work backwards, first with the pet upright and then again with the pet restrained in lateral recumbency to examine the ventrum. Examine the interdigital spaces, ungual folds, claws and footpads while the animal is restrained in lateral recumbency. All mucous membranes should be inspected as they are encountered
- At regular intervals, the hair should be parted or the skin examined by rolling it up in folds to separate the hair in short-coated dogs
- Palpate lesions
- Identify primary skin lesions (Figure 2.5):
  - Macule
  - Papule
  - Pustule
  - Nodule
  - Tumour
  - Wheal
  - Vesicle
  - (Pruritus)
- Learn to recognize which secondary skin lesions are diagnostically significant*:
  - Scale, epidermal collarette* (Figure 2.6)

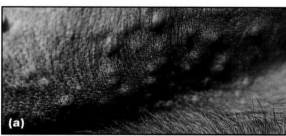

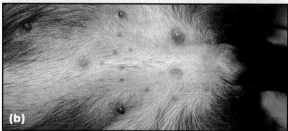

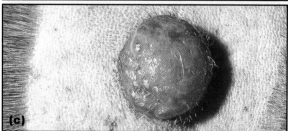

2.5 Some primary skin lesions. (a) Papules. (b) Pustules. (c) A tumour (histiocytoma).

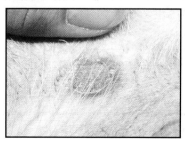

2.6 Scale in the form of an epidermal collarette (suggests antecedent pustule or, rarely, vesicle).

Dermatology examination

Date _____

Owner details

(Mr/Mrs/Miss/Ms) Surname/Family name _____   First name or Initials _____

Address _____

Post Code/Zip _____

Phone (day) _____   (evening) _____
(mobile) _____   Fax _____
e-mail _____

Patient details

Name _____   Breed _____
Sex: [ ] Male   [ ] Female   [ ] Male neutered   [ ] Female spayed
Date of birth _____   Colour _____
Identifying marks _____

EAR EXAM:

PRURITUS?   R:

PARASITES?   L:

DISTRIBUTION OF LESIONS

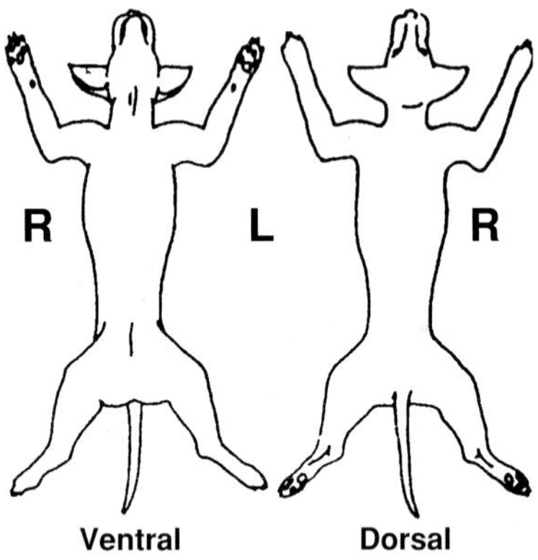

PRIMARY LESIONS (Circle)

1 Bulla	4 Papule	7 Pustule	9 Vesicle
2 Macule	5 Patch	8 Tumour	10 Wheal
3 Nodule	6 Plaque		

SECONDARY LESIONS (Circle)

11 Abscess	16 Cyst	21 Fissue	25 Lichenification
12 Alopecia	17 Epidermal collarette	22 Hyperkeratosis	26 Scale
13 Callus	18 Erosion	23 Hyperpigmentation	27 Scar
14 Comedone	19 Erythema	24 Hypopigmentation	28 Ulcer
15 Crust	20 Excoriation		

QUALITY OF HAIR COAT   OTHER FACTORS

Epilation: + −   Footpads
Pelage is: Dry,   Nails
    Brittle, Dull, Oily

R   L   R

Ventral   Dorsal

PROBLEM LIST:
_____
_____
_____
_____

LABORATORY TESTS

Ear swabs: R _____   L _____

Adhesive tape: _____   Wood's light + − _____

Skin scraping: _____   [ ] Survey form

KOH digestion: _____   *Malassezia* preps: 1– _____

Tzanck: _____   2– _____

DTM: [ ] _____   3– _____

Bacterial culture: _____   4– _____

Allergy: [ ] Flea only   [ ] Complete test

Endocrine: _____

Immune: _____

Other tests: _____

Biopsy: Site(s) _____

RESULTS: _____
_____
_____
_____
_____
_____
_____

DIFFERENTIAL DIAGNOSIS:
_____
_____
_____
_____
_____

COMMENTS:
_____
_____
_____
_____
_____
_____

SIGNED BY ATTENDING CLINICIAN
_____

2.7   A sample dermatological examination form.

- Crust*
- Scar
- Ulcer*
- Excoriation
- Lichenification
- Hyperpigmentation
- Hyperkeratosis
- Comedo

- Evaluate for inducible pruritus by attempting to elicit a scratch reflex, rubbing the pinnae and scratching the lateral thorax
- The evaluation should be completed with a thorough otoscopic examination of the ear canals.

In dogs and cats with allergic, parasitic or infectious diseases, macules, papules and pustules are often all seen together, along with secondary lesions. The characteristic grouping of erythematous macules, follicular papules, occasional pustules and numerous epidermal collarettes provides an association that is very characteristic of staphyloccal folliculitis in the dog.

Observations of lesions and distribution should be recorded thoroughly, so that comparisons can be made on follow-up visits. This is facilitated by adoption of a dermatological examination form (Figure 2.7). There are a few lesions or patterns of lesions that can be said to have strong diagnostic significance (Figure 2.8).

Most skin diseases, however, will present with a multitude of primary and secondary lesions and will require a systematic work-up before a therapeutic plan can be designed.

Lesion/pattern	Suggests
Petechiation or purpura	Clotting defect, vasculitis (Figure 2.9)
Telangiectasis	Connective tissue disorder, hyperadrenocorticism
Calcinosis	Hyperadrenocorticism (Figure 2.10), calcinosis circumscripta
Punched-out or V-shaped lesions at ear margins	Vasculitis (Figure 2.11), vascular defect
Acral and peri-orificial hyperkeratosis, erosion and crusting	Zinc-responsive dermatopathy, necrolytic migratory erythema (Figure 2.12), pemphigus
Erythema, excoriation and dermatitis of face, ears, feet, axilla and groin (Figure 2.13)	Allergy

2.8 Lesions and patterns with strong diagnostic significance.

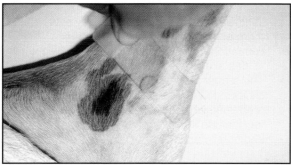

2.9 Petechiations in a young dog with vasculitis associated with hypertrophic osteodystrophy. Diascopy demonstrated failure to blanche with pressure.

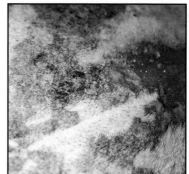

2.10 Calcinosis cutis in a Dachshund with iatrogenic hyperadrenocorticism.

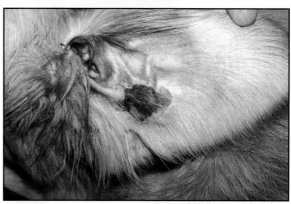

2.11 A punched-out ulcer with haemorrhagic crust on the pinna of a young dog with vasculitis associated with acute parvovirus infection.

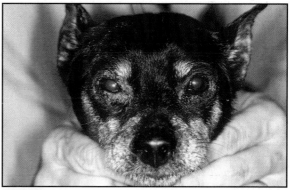

2.12 Peri-orificial facial crusting, hyperkeratosis and erosion in a Miniature Pinscher with necrolytic migratory erythema (hepatocutaneous syndrome).

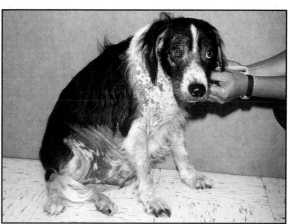

2.13 Erythema, excoriation and dermatitis of the face, ears, feet, axilla and groin in a dog with atopic dermatitis.

The problem-oriented approach to skin diseases

- Skin diseases of widely dissimilar aetiologies can be confusingly similar in their presentations
- Many common skin diseases can present with widely dissimilar appearances
- Pruritic diseases are confusing because of the self-inflicted lesions and secondary infections that often accompany them.

The practitioner should develop a systematic approach to evaluation of skin diseases which will help speed him or her towards a diagnosis. It will also allow for a more reasoned presentation to the owners of the afflicted pet if it is necessary to convince them that further diagnostic testing is required. The problem-oriented approach offers a systematic way to proceed from the basics of dermatological history taking and examination toward the goal of developing a rational therapeutic plan.

The problem-oriented approach consists of:

1. Gathering objective and subjective data by means of history, examination and further investigations to obtain a minimum database (Figure 2.14).
2. Creating the working **problem list** from the data gathered in step one. The list should include those abnormalities or complaints that require further investigation or discussion with the client or specific treatment.
3. Developing a working differential diagnosis for each problem.
4. Making a diagnostic plan to rule in or rule out the most likely items on the list of differentials.
5. Redefining the problems (into diagnoses, if possible) based on the further testing.
6. Making a therapeutic and client education plan.

Dogs
Skin scrape
Dermatophyte test medium – puppies
Malasezzia cytology
Ear swab cytology
Aspiration cytology – nodules
Trichogram; Potassium hydroxide trichogram for alopecia

Cats
Dermatophyte test medium
Potassium hydroxide trichogram
Wood's light examination
Skin scrape
Surface cytology

2.14 The minimum dermatological database.

Developing a problem list

This is the most critical and most sophisticated part of the problem-oriented approach. The key to success is defining problems that require further evaluation, while not characterizing them in more detail than is warranted by the facts. An example of listing too many problems to be useful on a list is provided by every pruritic dog, which can be found to have secondary hair loss, excoriation and, in many cases, lichenification and some scaling, all of which are attributable to the problem that will actually need to be addressed, the pruritus. If there are primary lesions, that is helpful in refining the differential diagnosis list for pruritus, while secondary lesions are rarely, if ever, helpful in this regard.

Example

- At initial evaluation the dog is noted to have the following **problems:** self-inflicted hypotrichosis; erythema; papular dermatitis; deep pustular dermatitis; pruritus; and flea infestation

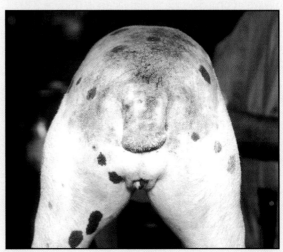

- The dog is not initially known to have the **diagnosis** of flea allergy dermatitis. The latter is not yet supported by the facts
- The **differential diagnosis list** for the problems listed includes: bacterial folliculitis, furunculosis, *Malassezia* dermatitis, demodicosis and flea allergy dermatitis
- A very experienced practitioner might have found the **problem list** papular and pustular pruritic dermatitis, tail head area, to be a sufficient working problem list. However, more experienced practitioners often commit the sin of exclusion and go straight to 'flea allergy' as the working diagnosis
- The proper problem list will allow the thorough clinician to diagnose and treat *all* of the dog's problems, which, in our illustrated case, did in fact include flea allergy, *Malassezia* dermatitis and staphylococcal furunculosis.

In defining a working problem list, it is always preferable to list all predominant primary skin lesions. Also, it is prudent to list all major client complaints.

Upon review, it may seem sensible to gather some items on the list into one problem, as they are likely all to be worked up in the same manner. Alternatively, it may be discerned that all are stages in the development of one major dermatological process, as in the papular, pruritic dermatitis and self-inflicted alopecia of the example above.

After the problem definition stage, the differential diagnosis and appropriate diagnostic tests can be pursued according to suggestions given in Part 2 of this book. For each type of problem there is a new minimum database, which is a set of tests designed specifically to rule in or rule out common causes of each presenting problem. These are given in the specific chapters in Part 2.

References and further reading

Moriello KA and Mason IS (1995) *Handbook of Small Animal Dermatology*. Pergamon, Oxford

Scott DW, Miller WH Jr and Griffin CE (2001) *Muller and Kirk's Small Animal Dermatology, 6th edition*. WB Saunders, Philadelphia

3

Investigative and laboratory techniques

Janet D. Littlewood

Whilst a complete history and thorough clinical examination are essential for dermatological cases, further diagnostic investigations are of paramount importance in reaching a definitive diagnosis. Many can be performed as part of, or at the conclusion of, the clinical examination.

Any samples sent to a laboratory are subject to national and local postal regulations.

Equipment

Hand lens

Use of a hand-held lens, in good natural light, or a combined light and magnifying lens, allows close examination of primary skin lesions. It is usually necessary to clip away surrounding hair to see the skin surface properly. This technique also enables identification of surface parasites such as fleas, lice, *Cheyletiella* mites, the larval stage of the harvest mite *Neotrombicula autumnalis* and louse egg cases.

Otoscope

Use of an otoscope is mandatory in any animal showing signs of aural irritation or inflammation, and facial or head pruritus. Sedation, or even general anaesthesia, may be necessary to allow thorough examination in fractious patients. The examination permits identification of ear mites and rules out other causes of otitis externa such as foreign bodies or tumours.

Wood's lamp

These lamps emit violet and ultraviolet light and are used to identify those dermatophyte infections that fluoresce. Lamps currently available include a magnifying lens. The lamp must be allowed to become fully warm (at least 5 minutes) and the examination should be performed in a dark room. The haircoat is examined, looking for the typical apple green fluorescence of hairs infected with *Microsporum canis*. The technique allows selection of appropriate hairs for microscopy and culture to confirm the diagnosis. Unfortunately, not all strains of *M. canis* fluoresce, the number showing positive fluorescence varying between 30 and 50%, or up to 90%, in published reports. Sometimes, the infected hairs need to warm up under the lamp before showing fluorescence and this may be a reason for false-negative examinations. Other less common dermatophytes that may

also induce fluorescence include *M. distortum*, *M. audouinii*, *M. equinum* and *Trichophyton schoenleinii*. False-positive fluorescence may be observed due to certain topical medications, dead skin scales and some bacteria.

Coat brushings

Sample collection

The coat may be brushed to collect surface debris for closer examination using a flea comb or stiff plastic hair brush into a Petri dish for examination under a microscope or hand lens.

Wet paper test

This is performed by brushing debris on to a piece of dampened white paper, for identification of flea dirt. The black flea faeces stain the damp paper reddish brown, because of the presence of soluble blood pigments.

Mackenzie toothbrush technique

This is the method of choice for screening asymptomatic cats for the presence of dermatophyte infection and for assessing whether infection has cleared in animals undergoing treatment. The whole coat is brushed with a new or sterilized toothbrush, which is then used to inoculate fungal culture medium. As an alternative, a scalp massaging brush may be used.

Samples for direct microscopy

Hair pluckings

Hair is plucked and placed on clear adhesive tape and affixed to a microscope slide or mounted under a cover slip in liquid paraffin. The tips are examined for evidence of breaking and damage, indicated by abrupt, blunt or frayed ends (Figure 3.1) instead of the tapering tips of normal hairs. This damage is evidence of either chewing and excessive grooming by the host, or diseased hairs such as in dermatophytosis (Figure 3.2). The roots are examined to assess whether hairs are in anagen (a pronounced bulb present) or telogen (club root with barbs or frayed appearance; Figure 3.3) phase. The number of hairs in anagen and telogen can be counted and an assessment made of the number of primary and secondary hairs present (see Figure 3.1), i.e. a trichogram. Abnormalities of hair structure may

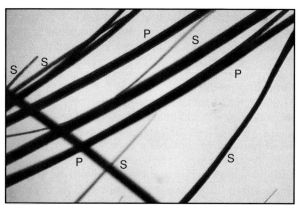

3.1 Hair pluck to show primary (P) and secondary (S) hairs. The blunt tips and frayed tips to several hairs indicate self-inflicted damage.

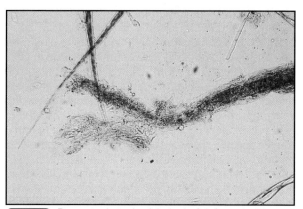

3.2 Dermatophytosis. A hair shaft infected with *Trichophyton* spp., showing disruption of the structure due to invasion of fungal elements, with ectothrix spores surrounding the damaged hair.

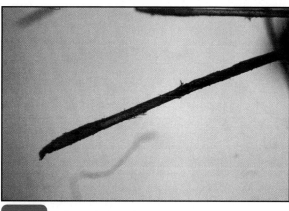

3.3 Telogen hair root.

be detected in certain deficiency diseases, dysplasias and genetic abnormalities of the hair coat. The presence of comedones or follicular plugs can also be detected, surrounding the shafts towards the root end of plucked hairs.

Examination of the roots of plucked hairs may reveal the presence of demodectic mange mites and this is a better technique than skin scraping for the confirmation of demodicosis in pododermatitis. When fungal infection is suspected, hair plucks can be taken for microscopic examination and for culture (see later).

Adhesive tape impressions

Strips of clear adhesive tape are applied to skin and then applied to glass slides for direct examination for surface parasites and eggs (Figure 3.4). This technique is particularly useful for small mammals, where skin scraping can be difficult. Tape strips of the clipped skin surface may be stained (Diff-Quick® or Gram) to look for microorganisms such as *Malassezia* (Figure 3.5).

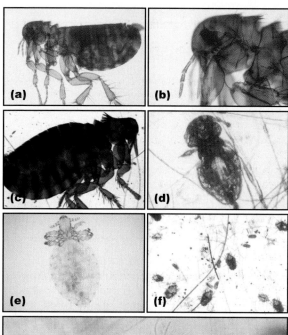

3.4 Adhesive tape detection of parasites.
(a) *Archeopsylla erinacei*, the hedgehog flea, found on a terrier dog. (b) Detail of the head and anterior thorax shows two short pronotal combs and the slanted row of short genal combs. (c) *Spilopsyllus cuniculi*, the stick-tight flea of rabbits, found on the pinna of a cat. (d) *Trichodectes canis*, the biting or chewing louse. (e) *Linognathus setosus*, the sucking louse. (f) *Cheyletiella yasguri* mites and eggs collected from the dorsum of a Boxer. (g) High-power magnification of *Cheyletiella parasitivorax* to show the globoid sense organ.

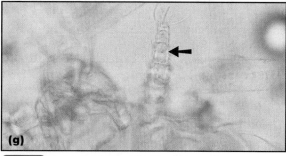

3.5 Adhesive tape strip with detail of squames with many yeast organisms in a case of *Malassezia* pedal dermatitis.

Smears of expressed follicular contents

This is a useful method for collecting *Demodex* mites from hair follicles. The skin is squeezed and a clean microscope slide is drawn across the surface to smear extruded material for subsequent examination. Alternatively material may be collected on a scalpel blade and then transferred to a slide. No staining is necessary, although a little mineral oil (liquid paraffin) may be used for coverslip mounting (Figure 3.6).

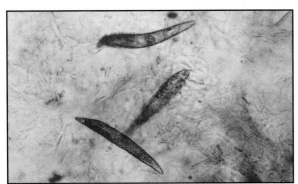

3.6 *Demodex canis* mites and cellular debris in a liquid paraffin-mounted preparation of a follicular smear.

Smears of aural wax/exudate

Debris from the external ear canal may be collected on a swab and placed on a slide. Ear mites and their eggs can be identified by microscopic examination. It may help material to adhere to the swab if it is dampened with liquid paraffin, which can also be used on the slide to disperse the sample and mount the coverslip. See Chapter 14 for further details.

Scrapings

The major secrets of success, particularly in cases of suspected sarcoptic mange, are:

* Scrape multiple sites
* Choose the sites carefully, selecting new lesions
* Scrape until capillary ooze is seen.

Papules or crusts at the edges of lesional areas are the best sites for sampling (Figure 3.7). Overlying hair is clipped away and a blunted scalpel blade is used. The sites may be moistened with saline or

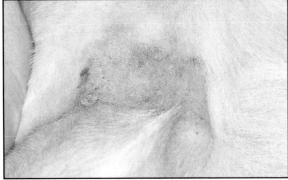

3.7 Sampling site for skin scrapes from a dog with suspected sarcoptic mange: hair clipped over lateral elbow to show early lesions of crusted papular eruptions.

mounting medium. Material can be collected directly on to microscope slides or into a test tube, if large amounts of material have been collected which require concentrating.

Mounting media

There is great debate amongst dermatologists with respect to which mounting medium is preferable for examination of skin scrapings. The choice is between liquid paraffin (mineral oil) and potassium hydroxide. Many prefer liquid paraffin since this allows immediate examination of slides and identification of live mites (Figure 3.8). It has the disadvantage of not clearing debris, in contrast to potassium hydroxide. Good separation of keratinocytes and clearing of material is obtained with 10% potassium hydroxide, but this is caustic to the skin itself and kills mites. Lower concentrations, e.g. 6% potassium hydroxide, are not lethal to mites. Material on slides is cleared in about half an hour, although this can be hastened by gentle heating. The use of a solution of 20% potassium hydroxide in 40% dimethyl sulphoxide (DMSO) will clear material on slides, without heating, in 5–10 minutes. Large amounts of material may be concentrated and cleared by mixing with the same solution in a test tube that is left to stand. The supernatant is discarded and the settled material transferred to a slide for microscopic examination. This method will also remove the bulk of liquid paraffin oil in samples, although some globules of oil tend to remain adherent to hairs. Use of other solvents first may aid in removal of oil prior to clearing and concentration. Coverslips should always be used, no matter what the mounting medium.

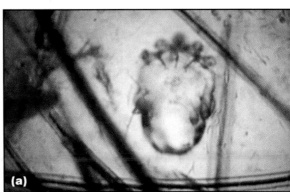

(a)

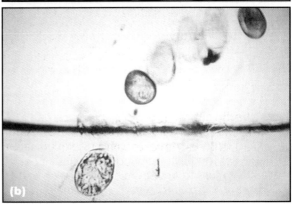

(b)

3.8 (a) *Sarcoptes scabiei* mite, adult female. (b) Group of *Sarcoptes scabiei* mite eggs from an epidermal burrow.

Dermatophytes

If dermatophyte infection is suspected, samples should be taken from the advancing edge of a new lesion, to include hair and skin scale. Fungal elements are best seen in potassium hydroxide preparations; the loss of the glassy appearance of hairs, which have become opaque through dermatophytosis, can be seen in liquid paraffin preparations. Hyphae may be seen inside hair shafts, which are often broken, or in squames. Spores may be inside (endothrix) or around hair shafts (ectothrix) (see Figure 3.2). Addition of a drop of blue–black ink or lactophenol cotton blue to the slide may permit fungal structures to be seen more easily.

Sample submission

Samples that are to be submitted to a diagnostic laboratory for fungal culture should be enclosed in paper envelopes or non-airtight containers such as Petri dishes, since bacterial contaminants tend to overgrow the sample in a moist, humid environment.

Stained smears from pustules or lesions

The microscopic examination of pustule and vesicle contents and the exfoliative cytology of the surface of lesions permits the identification of inflammatory, acantholytic and neoplastic cells and microorganisms. Ideally an intact pustule should be ruptured with a sterile hypodermic needle, its contents aspirated and smeared on to a clean slide, fixed and stained (Figure 3.9). Impression smears of ulcerated lesions or of the cut surface of excised lesions can also be made. Rapid staining techniques using Diff-Quick® or Rapistain® are ideal for practice laboratories. Other stains that may be helpful are Giemsa and methylene blue. Gram stain may be preferable for detecting microorganisms.

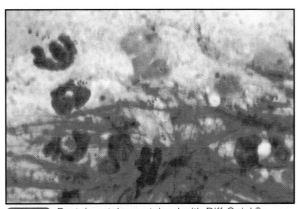

3.9 Pustule cytology, stained with Diff-Quick®, showing neutrophils with intracellular cocci in a case of staphylococcal pyoderma.

Fine needle aspirates

Examination of stained smears of aspirated cells may be helpful, particularly in cases with multiple cutaneous masses and those with lymphadenopathy.

The hair over the lesion should be clipped and its surface aseptically prepared. Samples are obtained by inserting a 21 or 22 gauge needle attached to a 10 ml syringe into the mass, retracting the plunger briskly two or three times, and withdrawing the needle

from the mass. The syringe should then be detached and a little air let in. The material in the needle and hub is then expressed on to a slide and smeared, prior to fixing and staining. Rapid air drying followed by fixing in absolute methanol is required for most of the Romanowsky (haematological) stains. However, certain pathologists have a preference for wet fixation of material, particularly with certain cytological staining methods. It is advisable to check with individual laboratories for their requirements.

The technique of fine needle aspiration allows identification of the major cell type(s) involved in a lesion and may be diagnostic for mast cell tumours, but has the serious disadvantage of giving no information about structure and cellular organization within the mass (Figure 3.10). It should not replace excision and routine histopathology, but can be a useful preoperative screening technique which, in the case of solitary mast cell tumours, might indicate the need to give a wide margin of excision.

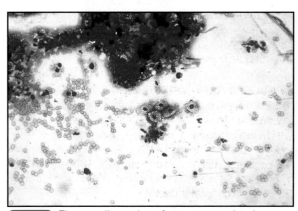

3.10 Fine needle aspirate from a mass, showing epithelial cells (large cells with central nucleus) and cellular debris. The mass was later confirmed as a sebaceous adenoma.

Culture of microorganisms

Bacterial culture

Swabs for bacterial culture should be taken from new lesions or recently ruptured pustules or vesicles, but not old, crusted, excoriated lesions. An intact pustule is ruptured with a sterile needle and the contents absorbed on to a sterile swab. Transport medium should be used for sending samples to a diagnostic laboratory. Some authorities advise sterilization of the skin surface with surgical spirit (alcohol) first, but this may lead to false-negative cultures if spirit penetrates or ruptures the fragile stratum corneum overlying the pustule, or the pustule is opened before the spirit has evaporated. Biopsy tissue may also be submitted in a sterile container for bacterial culture. For deep pyodermas, a selective culture medium for Gram-negative organisms should be inoculated in addition to routine blood agar plates, and anaerobic culture may also be indicated. For staphylococci, coagulase production is an important indicator of pathogenicity. Ideally, further biochemical tests should be employed to identify the species of *Staphylococcus* involved, although in dogs it is usually *S. intermedius*. In cases with granulomas, both fungal and mycobacterial culture may be required. Some organisms are difficult to culture, and tissue should be submitted to a mycobacterial reference laboratory.

Fungal culture

Sabouraud's dextrose agar in Petri dishes gives the best results for fungal culture, allowing the development of good colony morphology and visible pigment changes. Addition of antibiotics such as gentamicin or chloramphenicol plus actidione (cycloheximide) to the medium will prevent overgrowth of bacterial contaminants. In the UK, incubation at room temperature, rather than in incubators, is usually adequate. Plates should be examined twice weekly and discarded after 3–4 weeks.

Dermatophyte test agar contains a pH colour indicator that turns red in the presence of pathogenic dermatophytes due to the production of alkaline metabolites from utilization of protein nutrients (Figure 3.11; see also Chapter 23). The medium remains yellow–orange with the growth of contaminants, which initially metabolize carbohydrate in the medium, until the cultures become aged. Therefore, these cultures should be examined daily for the first 10 days in order to pick up the early colour change of pathogenic fungi. This medium is useful as an early indicator of the presence of pathogens, but has the disadvantages of masking typical colony morphology and the reverse pigment changes. The mycelia often fail to produce typical arthrospores on this medium. Thus subculture of positive colonies may be necessary for definitive identification of species from the reverse pigmentation and microscopic examination of macroaleurospores.

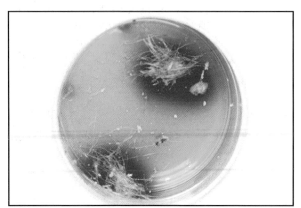

3.11 Dermatophyte test medium: colour change from yellow to red 5 days after inoculation, indicating growth of a dermatophyte.

Skin biopsy

Skin biopsy is all too often considered a last line of investigation for chronic dermatoses. This is unfortunate since dermatohistopathology can be a valuable aid to diagnosis. It is better to consider biopsy sooner rather than later in the course of investigating a case, since delay allows secondary changes to develop. Although the histological findings may not always be pathognomonic for a particular disease, the technique can be just as useful as a means of excluding some of the differential diagnoses.

Indications for skin biopsy include:

- Masses or any possible neoplastic lesions
- Persistent ulcerated lesions
- Conditions failing to respond to appropriate therapy
- Unusual or atypical dermatoses
- When a condition is suspected that requires therapy which may be expensive, of extended duration, or hazardous.

The procedure can be performed using gentle restraint and local analgesia. Local anaesthetic without adrenaline should be used to avoid the introduction of artefactual changes in the vasculature of the tissue sample. At times, sedation or general anaesthesia may be necessary, depending on the temperament of the patient, its state of health and the biopsy sites. Careful selection of lesions is important, choosing primary lesions such as pustules or vesicles and non-excoriated sites. Chronic secondary changes will often tend to obscure primary pathology. For suspected endocrine or atrophic conditions, fully developed, mature lesions give more typical histology. It is essential to take several samples and to include lesional and non-lesional skin. It is usually necessary to withdraw glucocorticoid medication and treat secondary bacterial infections for several weeks prior to taking biopsies to try and eliminate secondary or iatrogenic pathology.

Punch biopsies

Disposable 4 mm or 6 mm diameter biopsy punches that allow rapid sampling of multiple sites are available. The biopsy sample obtained with the smaller diameter punches may include only three or four hair follicle units and may be difficult to interpret histopathologically, but these are useful for sites such as the feet and the nose and for small, discrete lesions. However, the rotational force involved in obtaining the sample may disrupt vesicles or pustules. This method is inappropriate for masses or for the junctional area between lesional and normal skin. It is important, therefore, to take several biopsies of both affected and non-affected skin. Biopsy sites usually require only a single suture.

Excisional biopsies

An ellipse of tissue is excised using a surgical blade. The samples obtained are larger than those from punch biopsies. More lengthy surgical repair is required and therefore more time. This technique enables removal of whole nodules, masses or bullae, or sampling of a wedge of tissue at a junction of normal with abnormal skin. It is important that the orientation of the ellipse at such interfaces is correct, since samples are cut in half longitudinally during processing, and one half discarded. The lesion should be at one pole of the ellipse and normal tissue at the other so that examples of both are retained on the processed tissue.

The hair overlying biopsy sites should be trimmed carefully with scissors, with no surgical preparation of the site, as clipping and scrubbing destroys vital surface structure. The full thickness of skin should be taken, down to the subcutis. Excess blood should be removed and biopsies gently placed, dermis side down, on to stiff paper or cardboard before fixing to prevent curling and distortion. The usual fixative is 10% formol saline, unless immunofluorescence is required, when Michel's medium should be used. Immunohistochemical staining can be performed on formalin-fixed tissues. Tissue can also be submitted in a sterile container for bacterial or fungal culture if infection is suspected.

It is vital that adequate information regarding the patient, the history (including medication), the clinical appearance of the condition, the biopsy sites and the possible differential diagnoses are supplied to the pathologist. Only with this information can the histopathological changes be interpreted appropriately and a meaningful conclusion drawn.

Allergy testing

Restriction and provocative testing
This approach is appropriate for the diagnosis of contact allergies and food hypersensitivity.

Contact allergies
The patient is kept in a 'safe' environment, with no access to potential allergens for a period, to determine whether pruritus resolves. This is difficult to achieve in the home environment. Admission to hospital kennels and bedding on newspaper, or white cotton sheeting, while allowing exercise only on paved surfaces is the best method, allowing frequent assessment of the patient. There is usually an improvement within 7–10 days in cases of contact allergy, although it should be noted that many cases of atopic dermatitis will also improve with this regime. If improvement occurs the patient is returned home, to one room for the first week and then exposed sequentially to further rooms to identify the one that causes a return of symptoms. Attention can then be focused on individual items, such as carpets, fabrics and plants, within that environment.

Cutaneous adverse food reaction
The patient is fed a novel diet consisting, if possible, of one protein and carbohydrate source, preferably one to which the animal has never previously been exposed. All other foodstuffs should be excluded. Suitable proteins might be egg, fish, duck, chicken, rabbit or lamb, with boiled rice or potato as suitable choices of carbohydrate. The actual choice must depend on the previous dietary history of the individual case. An improvement whilst being fed this diet is suggestive of an adverse food reaction. Ideally the food should be home-prepared, although several commercial 'hypoallergenic' diets are available, including hydrolysed diets. The latter contain partially degraded proteins with peptides of approximately 10,000 daltons or less, and are presumed to have little immunogenicity.

The duration of the restriction or elimination diet ideally should be at least 3 months before the diagnosis is ruled out, although the majority of intolerant animals will improve within 6–8 weeks. Once an improvement

has been noted, dietary challenge is undertaken with reintroduction of all previously fed foodstuffs. In adverse food reaction, relapse of symptoms is often seen within a couple of days, but may take 7–10 days. To confirm the diagnosis, the symptoms should resolve again after a return to the restricted diet. Thereafter, foodstuffs may be reintroduced sequentially for a week at a time to identify the offending protein. It may be desirable from a nutritional viewpoint to change to a commercially prepared diet during the provocative phase. See Chapter 18 for more details.

Intradermal tests
Intradermal testing (IDT) is a valuable aid in the diagnosis of canine and feline atopy allowing identification of causal allergens and the formulation of appropriate vaccines for immunotherapy. Although not licensed for use in animals in the UK, allergen solutions are available from a number of sources, and are supplied either as concentrated aqueous solutions that can be diluted to testing strength on a regular basis, or ready diluted, although diluted allergens have a reduced shelf life. Testing with allergen mixes is undesirable, since the concentration of individual allergens may not be sufficient to give a positive reaction.

The selection of allergens that are relevant to the particular region is important. Figure 3.12 lists allergens selected on the basis of aeroallergens known to cause problems in humans in the UK and includes many of the allergens used by veterinary dermatologists in the UK. There are substantial regional differences to consider within the USA and Australia. A multicentre study suggested that it is an appropriate panel, although there are significant regional variations in reaction patterns, with more pollen and mould spore reactions reported in animals in South West England (Ferguson, 1992). The study also demonstrated that environmental allergens such as *Dermatophagoides* spp. and house dust predominated in cases of canine atopy in the UK. Of other groups of aeroallergens, weed pollens were found to be the most important overall. See Chapter 18 for more details.

The presence of a positive test reaction (Figure 3.13) indicates that the patient has a skin-sensitizing antibody, but does not necessarily mean that the allergen is clinically significant for that patient. Positive reactions must be interpreted in conjunction with a full knowledge of the patient's history. Other factors that may lead to false-positive reactions include irritant test solutions, contaminated allergen solutions, non-immunological histamine release, poor operator technique (traumatic needle placement, blunt needle, injection of too large a volume, injection of air) and dermatographism (pressure-induced mast cell degranulation). Many factors may give rise to false-negative reactions, the most common being the recent administration of drugs such as glucocorticoids or antihistamines. Stress at the time of induction of sedation may also give rise to false-negative skin test results. Although it is difficult to establish reliable withdrawal periods for such drugs, 1 month off alternate-day steroids and 2 weeks off antihistamines should be sufficient. Animals that have received depot steroids may need several months before reliable

Environmental
Ctenocephalides spp.
Tyrophagus putrescentiae
Acarus siro
Lepidoglyphus destructor
Dermatophagoides pteronyssinus
Dermatophagoides farinae
House dust
Human dander
Cat dander
Sheep epithelia
Kapok
Mixed feathers

Trees
Birch mix (*Betula* spp.)
Alder (*Alnus glutinosa*)
Hazel (*Corylus avellana*)
Beech (*Fagus sylvatica*)
Ash (*Fraxinus excelsior*)
Sycamore (*Platanus occidentalis*)
Poplar (*Populus alba*)
Oak mix (*Quercus* spp.)
Willow (*Salix discolor*)

Grasses
Meadow grass (*Poa pratensis*)
Fescue (*Festuca elatior*)
Cocksfoot (*Dactylis glomerata*)
Bent-grass (*Agrostis alba*)
Italian rye grass (*Lolium multiflorum*)
Timothy (*Phleum pratense*)

Weeds
Mugwort (*Artemisia vulgaris*)
Goosefoot (*Chenopodium album*)
Daisy (*Chrysanthemum* spp.)
Plantain (*Plantago lanceolata*)
Sheep's sorrel (*Rumex acetosella*)
Yellow dock (*Rumex crispus*)
Dandelion (*Taraxacum officinale*)
Red clover (*Trifolium pratense*)
Nettle (*Urtica* spp.)

Moulds
Alternaria alternata
Aspergillus fumigatus
Botrytis cinerea
Cladosporium herbarum
Epicoccum purpurascens
Fusarium moniliforme
Helminthosporium sativum
Penicillium notatum
Phoma betae
Pullularia pullulans
Rhodotorula rubra

Smuts
Barley smut
Oat smut
Wheat smut

3.12 Allergens suitable for use in the UK.

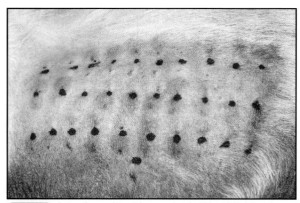

3.13 Intradermal test in an atopic West Highland White Terrier, with immediate positive reactions to housedust mites, various pollens and moulds.

skin test results can be expected. It should be noted that a negative skin test does not necessarily mean that an animal is not atopic. Many workers have observed that a number of dogs (approximately 10%) with classical signs of atopy have negative skin tests; this may indicate a failure to challenge with the appropriate allergen(s) and/or the interference of factors known to produce false-negative reactions.

The technique of intradermal testing and the interpretation of skin test reactions becomes easier with increased experience of the operator, and it is not a test that can be considered suitable for occasional use. It is preferable to refer cases to an experienced veterinary dermatologist, after other appropriate investigations have been completed.

Patch tests

Suspect materials in cases of contact allergy may be applied to the skin for 48 hours. The skin is then examined for erythema and induration, which occurs with the causal allergen. It is necessary to distinguish irritant from allergic reactions, and biopsy of the positive sites may be undertaken to document the typical histopathology of contact allergy. Specialized chambers (Finn chambers) containing potential allergens are used in human medicine and can also be used for veterinary patients. The haircoat must be clipped away the day before commencing the test and samples must be immobilized against the skin surface with bandages. This may not be tolerated by the patient and the owner may be unhappy about the removal of large areas of hair from their pet. Because contact allergy is relatively uncommon and due to the limitations of the procedure, patch testing is undertaken infrequently in veterinary dermatology.

Serological tests

Enzyme-linked immunosorbent assays (ELISAs) and radio-allergosorbent tests (RASTs) are available for the identification of allergen-specific antibodies circulating in the patient's blood. The principle of the tests is similar: patient serum is added to wells containing antigens and species-specific enzyme-linked or radiolabelled antisera to canine IgE are added. Historically there have been problems with the specificity of reagents, with polyclonal antisera recognizing and binding other classes of immunoglobulin in addition to IgE. Monoclonal antibodies to IgE are more specific, but may bind with poor affinity and are less useful in ELISA tests than in other techniques such as Western blotting and immunohistochemical staining of tissues. The most specific reagent available is a recombinant human peptide fragment of the high-affinity mast cell receptor for IgE (Allercept™ detection system, Heska Corporation), that binds to the binding site on the Fc fragment exclusive to IgE antibodies.

Wassom and Grieve (1998) reported good agreement between the results of intradermal testing using the Allercept™ detection system and an *in vitro* test in dogs in the USA. A similar study has been undertaken for dogs with suspected atopic dermatitis in the UK (Foster *et al.*, 2000). This study showed a higher prevalence of positive results by ELISA than for intradermal testing for pollens; for housedust mite allergens, the intradermal test was more sensitive than the ELISA test. Since housedust mites are known to be the most important allergens in canine atopy in the UK, most veterinary dermatologists still prefer intradermal testing to demonstrate the presence of allergen-specific antibodies in atopic patients. However, in situations where skin testing is not appropriate, or has given negative results, serum allergy testing can be helpful in demonstrating the presence of circulating IgE antibodies.

Little has been published about the usefulness of serological tests for food intolerance. In a study of diagnostic testing for food allergy, low sensitivity and high specificity were found for both skin testing and ELISA, indicating a lack of true-positive and occurrence of false-positive reactions; neither the positive nor negative predictive values adequately predicted positive and negative reactions for either test and the authors concluded that these tests cannot replace an elimination diet for food hypersensitivity testing in dogs (Jeffers *et al.*, 1991). Data validating the tests currently marketed in the UK for *in vitro* diagnosis of food allergy are lacking: dogs anecdotally reported to have improved on diets that were selected on the basis of blood test results have not been subjected to provocation testing. Restriction to a hypoallergenic diet and provocative challenge remains the only definitive test for food intolerance in animals (Hill, 1999).

Blood samples

Routine haematological and biochemical investigations are not indicated in the majority of dermatological cases, but may give useful supportive information in certain situations:

- Eosinophilia in allergic conditions, especially in cats
- White cell responses in infections
- Haematological changes in certain endocrinopathies
- Changes in serum biochemistry in endocrinopathies and hepatic disorders
- Monitoring animals treated with immunosuppressive or chemotherapeutic agents

- Investigation of malabsorption
- Measurement of antibody titres against FeLV and FIV in cats with recurrent infections
- An ELISA is available for detection of IgG antibodies to *Sarcoptes* mite antigens (Bornstein and Zakrisson, 1993) and has been shown to be helpful in the diagnosis of canine sarcoptic mange (Bornstein *et al.*, 1996; Curtis, 2001) with high positive and negative predictive values. It is of considerable assistance in those cases where sarcoptic mange is suspected but skin scrapings are negative for mites.

Hormonal assays
Hormonal assays can be performed on serum or heparinized plasma samples, usually by radioimmunoassay. Single baseline measurements of hormone concentrations are non-diagnostic, and dynamic response or suppression tests should be performed to confirm the diagnosis of an endocrinopathy (see Chapter 12).

Hypothyroidism
The routine haematological and biochemical abnormalities that may be found in cases of canine hypothyroidism are shown in Figure 3.14.

- Mild normocytic, normochromic anaemia (25–32% of cases; 35% low normal)
- Hypercholesterolaemia (33–75% of cases)
- Increased plasma lipids
- Mild to marked elevation of liver enzymes (alanine aminotransferase in 25%, alkaline phosphatase in 20–30% of cases)
- Elevation of creatine phosphokinase (10–18% of cases)

3.14 Laboratory findings in canine hypothyroidism.

Although single baseline measurements of total tri-iodothyronine (T3) or thyroxine (T4) are usually non-diagnostic, a total T4 concentration of <8.5 nmol/l is suggestive of hypothyroidism. Results in the upper normal range (30–52 nmol/l) rule out hypothyroidism. Free T4, measured by equilibrium dialysis, is less frequently reduced in non-thyroidal illnesses and should offer a more sensitive test for hypothyroidism. However, most veterinary laboratories offer an analogue assay, which is less reliable than total T4 assays; measurement of free T4 has been found to be no more useful than total T4 assay (Feldman and Nelson, 1996). A rapid semi-quantitative assay kit for measurement of serum T4 in veterinary practices was shown to be as accurate as a radioimmunoassay, but subject to the same limitations of the large overlap of T4 values in euthyroid and hypothyroid dogs (Eckersall *et al.*, 1991). If basal T3 or T4 concentrations are unusually elevated when clinical signs are consistent with hypothyroidism, the presence of anti-T3/T4 antibodies should be considered.

The best diagnostic test for confirmation of hypothyroidism is considered to be the thyroid stimulating hormone (TSH) response test. However, the bovine TSH that is commercially available is of laboratory grade and not for *in vivo* use. Human recombinant TSH can be used but is very expensive. An alternative to the above test is the thyrotropin releasing hormone (TRH) response test. Several protocols are described in the literature, but the work of Henfrey and Thoday (1991) shows the following method to be optimal:

1. Collect a blood sample for measurement of baseline total T4.
2. Inject 0.02 mg/kg TRH *slowly* intravenously.
3. Collect a second blood sample 4 hours later.

Most normal (euthyroid) dogs show a 1.2-fold increase in total T4 concentration over basal value with the results of the second sample within the normal range. It is the general opinion that this is less reliable than TSH response for the detection of hypothyroid animals.

Assays are now available to measure endogenous canine TSH (Williams *et al.*, 1996). Dogs with primary hypothyroidism would be expected to have high TSH concentrations but some confirmed cases may show values in the normal range, and some dogs with sick euthyroid disease may show elevated concentrations of TSH (Ramsey *et al.*, 1997; Scott-Moncrieff *et al.*, 1998; Dixon and Mooney, 1999a). However, for many cases the combination of a total T4 assay and endogenous TSH assay is diagnostic (Peterson *et al.*, 1997). For those cases where results are equivocal, dynamic testing or therapeutic trial (Ramsey, 1997) can be pursued. Changes in TSH concentration after administration of TRH can also be used to differentiate euthyroid from hypothyroid dogs, but the test has little advantage over measurement of baseline TSH and total or free T4 concentration (Scott-Moncrieff and Nelson, 1998).

Measurement of circulating antibodies to thyroglobulin (thyroglobulin auto-antibodies, TGAA) can also give useful adjunctive information, with positive results in 36% of hypothyroid dogs and in 43% of hypothyroid dogs that had normal TSH concentrations (Dixon and Mooney, 1999b).

Hyperadrenocorticism

The typical routine haematological and biochemical changes found in cases of canine hyperadrenocorticism are shown in Figure 3.15.

- Eosinopenia <0.2 x 10^9/l (84% of cases)
- Lymphopenia <1.5 x 10^9/l
- Neutrophilia, monocytosis
- Elevated alkaline phosphotase, often marked, fairly consistent finding
- Mild to moderate increased alanine aminotransferase
- Increased bile salts
- Hypercholesterolaemia, lipaemia
- Fasting glucose high normal or elevated (overt diabetic)
- Urea often low normal

3.15 Laboratory findings in canine hyperadrenocorticism.

Assessment of the urinary cortisol:creatinine ratio has been shown to be a reliable screening test for ruling out hyperadrenocorticism if the ratio is within the normal range, but a test of higher specificity is needed to confirm the diagnosis if the ratio is elevated (Jensen *et al.*, 1997).

Measurement of single resting cortisol concentration is non-diagnostic and dynamic testing is essential.

Adrenocorticotropic hormone (ACTH) stimulation test: The test should be performed in the morning to coincide with peak physiological cortisol concentrations. Several protocols have been published. The author's preferred method is as follows:

1. Collect blood sample for baseline cortisol estimation.
2. Inject tetracosactrin intravenously: 250 mg for dogs >10 kg, 125 mg if <10 kg bodyweight. Doses of 5 μg/kg give equally good adrenal stimulation (Kerl *et al.*,1999).
3. Collect second blood sample 1 hour (0.5–2 hours) later:
- Normal ranges: baseline cortisol 50–250 nmol/l, post ACTH cortisol <500 nmol/l;
- Abnormal results: normal to elevated baseline with post ACTH value above 600 nmol/l.

The ACTH stimulation test detects 85–90% of cases of pituitary-dependent hyperadrenocorticism and about 50% of cases of adrenal-dependent hyperadrenocorticism, but does not reliably distinguish between the two. It is the only test appropriate for the diagnosis of iatrogenic hyperadrenocorticism, indicated by low to zero baseline cortisol and absent or minimal response to ACTH. Although documented as somewhat less sensitive as a screening test, it has a higher specificity and positive predictive value than the low dose dexamethasone suppression test (Van Liew *et al.*, 1997).

Low dose dexamethasone suppression test: This is a more sensitive screening test for hyperadrenocorticism, detecting the majority of, but not all, adrenal tumours (Norman *et al.*, 1999) and 90–95% of pituitary-dependent hyperadrenocorticism. It is performed as follows:

1. Collect blood sample for baseline cortisol estimation.
2. Inject 0.01 mg/kg dexamethasone i.v.
3. Collect second blood sample 8 hours later:
- Normal dogs show suppression of cortisol concentration to less than 40 nmol/l;
- Dogs with hyperadrenocorticism fail to suppress to this degree;
- An extra blood sample at 3 hours may give an indication of aetiology, since pituitary-dependent hyperadrenocorticism may suppress to 50% of baseline at this time.

If an individual dog with HAC is not detected by one of the screening tests, it should be tested with the other (Feldman, 1983a). In the occasional animal which gives borderline results the dynamic test(s) should be repeated after 1 month.

High dose dexamethasone suppression test: This may be helpful in the differentiation of pituitary-dependent hyperadrenocorticism and adrenal tumours, but is only appropriate after a positive screening test result. The method is as follows:

1. Collect blood sample for baseline cortisol estimation.
2. Inject 0.1 mg/kg dexamethasone i.v.
3. Collect further blood samples 3 and 8 hours later:
- Cases with pituitary-dependent hyperadrenocorticism suppress to <50% of baseline at 3 hours, although some may be >50% at 8 hours;
- Cases with adrenal tumour show cortisol concentrations >50% of baseline at 3 and 8 hours.

However, the test is not a completely reliable method of differentiation. The measurement of plasma ACTH concentration offers a better method for differentiation (Feldman, 1983b), if this assay is available. However, even this test is not totally reliable, non-diagnostic results occurring in 5% of cases. Where abdominal radiography, ultrasonography and the measurement of endogenous ACTH have been compared, no one method was completely reliable in discriminating adrenal tumours from pituitary-dependent hyperadrenocorticism (Reusch and Feldman, 1991). If possible, all three investigations should be undertaken to confirm the presence of an adrenal tumour. During ultrasonography, it is important to image both adrenal glands, since adrenal tumours may be bilateral; also, functional atrophy of the contralateral gland in dogs with a functional adrenal tumour may not be apparent ultrasonographically (Hoerauf and Reusch, 1999). Further techniques to aid in the differentiation between pituitary-dependent and adrenal-dependent hyperadrenocorticism include magnetic resonance imaging of the brain, which will detect the presence of pituitary macroadenomas, but microadenomas may not be detected.

Feline hyperadrenocorticism is much less common and can be more challenging to diagnose. Hyperglycaemia is the commonest laboratory abnormality and hypercholesterolaemia is also commonly present. Elevation of alkaline phosphatase is seen in only a third of cats. ACTH stimulation tests are less reliable than in dogs, since cats may show exaggerated responses due to stress and non-adrenal illnesses and false-negative results are reported in 15–30% of confirmed cases. The urinary cortisol:creatine ratio can be helpful if owners are able to collect urine. Dexamethasone suppression testing is a more sensitive test for feline hyperadrenocorticism, using 0.2–0.15mg/kg dexamethasone and sampling protocols as for the dog (Bruyette, 2000).

Other hormone assays
Sex hormone assays are available, but the normal ranges which have been established are wide, and single baseline estimations are often unhelpful in the investigation of cases with suspected sex hormone imbalance. Elevation of hormones such as 17-hydroxyprogesterone and epiandrosterone in response to ACTH administration may be seen in dogs with adrenal sex hormone imbalance.

An assay for canine growth hormone is available in some countries and growth hormone reserve can be assessed by use of either the xylazine or clonidine response test. Concentrations of insulin-like growth factor 1 (IGF-1) correlate well with growth hormone concentrations and this assay can be used when abnormalities of growth hormone concentration are suspected. It should be noted that there is considerable overlap between growth hormone-responsive and castration-responsive dermatoses, and alopecia X of plush-coated breeds, and the distinction between the conditions is far from clear.

Faecal examination

Examination of faeces is indicated where allergy to endoparasites is suspected, or cutaneous larval migrans in cases of hookworm infestation. It may also be useful if diarrhoea is a concurrent feature, to identify forage mites (hypersensitivity reactions to these free living mites may result in cutaneous and/or enteric symptoms) or the presence of undigested food in malabsorption syndromes.

References and further reading

Bornstein S and Zakrisson G (1993) Humoral antibody response to experimental *Sarcoptes scabiei* var *vulpis* infection in the dog. *Veterinary Dermatology* **4**, 107–110

Bornstein S, Thebo P and Zakrisson G (1996) Evaluation of an enzyme-linked immunosorbent assay (ELISA) for the serological diagnosis of canine sarcoptic mange. *Veterinary Dermatology* **7**, 21–28

Bowman DD (1995) *Georgis' Parasitology for Veterinarians, 6th edn.* WB Saunders, Philadelphia

Bruyette DS (2000) An approach to diagnosing and treating feline hyperadrenocorticism. *Veterinary Medicine* **95**, 142–148

Colville J (1991) *Diagnostic Parasitology for Veterinary Technicians.* American Veterinary Publications, California

Curtis CF (2001) Evaluation of a commercially available enzyme-linked immunosorbent assay for the diagnosis of canine sarcoptic mange. *Veterinary Record* **148**, 238–239

Dixon RM and Mooney CT (1999a) Evaluation of serum free thyroxine and thyrotropin concentrations in the diagnosis of canine hypothyroidism. *Journal of Small Animal Practice* **40**, 72–78

Dixon RM and Mooney CT (1999b) Canine serum thyroglobulin autoantibodies in health, hypothyroidism and non-thyroidal illness. *Research in Veterinary Science* **66**, 243–246

Dunn K (1997) Complications associated with the diagnosis and management of canine hyperadrenocorticism. *In Practice* **19**, 246–253

Feldman EC (1983a) Comparison of ACTH response and dexamethasone suppression as screening tests in canine hyperadrenocorticism. *Journal of American Veterinary Medical Association* **182**, 506

Feldman EC (1983b) Distinguishing dogs with functioning adrenocortical tumors from dogs with pituitary-dependent hyperadrenocorticism. *Journal of American Veterinary Medical Association* **183**, 195

Feldman EC and Nelson RW (1996) *Canine and Feline Endocrinology and Reproduction, 2nd edn,* pp. 68–117. WB Saunders, Philadelphia

Ferguson EA (1992) A review of intradermal skin testing in the UK. *Veterinary Dermatology Newsletter* **14**, 13

Foster AP, Littlewood JD, Webb P *et al.* (2000) A comparative study of the Heska Allercept® test and intradermal skin testing in dogs with suspected atopic dermatitis in the UK. *Veterinary Dermatology* **11** (Suppl. 1), 17 FC-10

Frey D, Oldfield RJ and Bridger RC (1985) *A Colour Atlas of Pathogenic Fungi.* Wolfe Medical Publications Ltd, London

Henfrey JI and Thoday KL (1991) Optimising of the TSH and TRH stimulation tests for the diagnosis of canine hypothyroidism. *Proceedings of the BSAVA Congress,* 121

Herrtage ME (1990) The adrenal glands. In: *Manual of Small Animal Endocrinology,* ed. M Hutchison, pp. 73–104. BSAVA Publications, Cheltenham

Hill P (1999) Diagnosing cutaneous food allergies in dogs and cats – some practical considerations. *In Practice* **21**, 287

Hoerauf A and Reusch C (1999) Ultrasonographic characteristics of both adrenal glands in 15 dogs with functional adrenocortical tumours. *Journal of the American Animal Hospitals Association* **35**, 193–199

Jeffers JG, Shanley KJ and Meyer EK (1991) Diagnostic testing of dogs for food hypersensitivity. *Journal of the American Veterinary Medical Association* **198**, 245

Jensen AL, Iversen L, Koch J, Hoier R and Petersen TK (1997) Evaluation of the urinary cortisol:creatinine ratio in the diagnosis of hyperadrenocorticism in dogs. *Journal of Small Animal Practice* **38**, 99–102

Kerl ME, Peterson ME, Wallace MS, Melian C and Kemppainen RJ (1999) Evaluation of a low-dose synthetic adrenocorticotropic hormone stimulation test in clinically normal dogs and dogs with naturally developing hyperadrenocorticism. *Journal of the American Veterinary Medical Association* **214**, 1497–1501

Ministry of Agriculture, Fisheries and Food (1984) Bacteriology and Mycology. In: *Manual of Veterinary Investigation Laboratory Techniques Vol 1, Reference Book 389, 3rd edn.* p. 46. Her Majesty's Stationery Office, London

Ministry of Agriculture, Fisheries and Food (1986) Entomology. In: *Manual of Veterinary Parasitological Laboratory Techniques, Reference Book 418,* p. 103. Her Majesty's Stationery Office, London

Norman EJ, Mooney CT and Thompson H (1999) Dynamic adrenal function testing in eight dogs hyperadrenocorticism associated with adrenocortical neoplasia. *Veterinary Record* **144**, 551–554

Peterson ME, Melian C and Nichols R (1997) Measurement of serum total thyroxine, triiodothyronine, free thyroxine and thyrotropin concentrations for diagnosis of hypothyroidism in dogs. *Journal of the American Veterinary Medical Association* **211**, 1396–1402

Ramsey IK (1997) Diagnosing canine hypothyroidism. *In Practice* **19**, 378–383

Ramsey IK, Evans H and Herrtage ME (1997) Thyroid-stimulating hormone and total thyroxine concentrations in euthyroid, sick euthyroid and hypothyroid dogs. *Journal of Small Animal Practice* **38**, 540–545

Reedy LM, Miller WH and Willemse A (1997) *Allergic skin diseases of dogs and cats, 2nd edn.* WB Saunders, Philadelphia

Reusch CE and Feldman EC (1991) Canine hyperadrenocorticism due to adrenocortical neoplasia. *Journal of Veterinary Internal Medicine* **5**, 3

Scott-Moncrieff JCR and Nelson RW (1998) Change in serum thyroid-stimulating hormone concentration in response to administration of thyrotropin-releasing hormone to healthy dogs, hypothyroid dogs and euthyroid dogs with concurrent disease. *Journal of the American Veterinary Medical Association* **213**, 1435–1438

Scott-Moncrieff JCR, Nelson RW, Bruner JM and Williams DA (1998) Comparison of serum concentrations of thyroid-stimulating hormone in healthy dogs, hypothyroid dogs and euthyroid dogs with concurrent disease. *Journal of the American Veterinary Medical Association* **212**, 387–391

Thoday KL (1990) The thyroid gland. In: *Manual of Small Animal Endocrinology,* ed. M Hutchison, pp. 25–57. BSAVA Publications, Cheltenham

Van Liew CH, Greco DS and Salman MD (1997) Comparison of results of adrenocorticotropic hormone stimulation and low-dose dexamethasone suppression tests with necropsy findings in dogs: 81 cases (1985–1995). *Journal of the American Veterinary Medical Association* **211**, 322–325

Wade WF and Gaafar SM (1991) Diagnosis of parasitism of miscellaneous body systems In: *Diagnostic Parasitology for Veterinary Technicians,* ed. J Colville, p. 49. American Veterinary Publications Inc

Wassom DL and Grieve RB (1998) *In vitro* measurement of canine and feline IgE: a review of FcϵRIα-based assays for detection of allergen-reactive IgE. *Veterinary Dermatology* **9**, 173–177

Williams DA, Scott-Moncrieff JCR, Bruner J *et al.* (1996) Validation of an immunoassay for canine thyroid-stimulating hormone and changes in serum concentration following induction of hypothyroidism in dogs. *Journal of the American Veterinary Medical Association* **209**, 1730–1732

Yager JA and Mason K (1998) Skin and external ear. In: *Manual of Small Animal Clinical Pathology,* ed. M. Davidson *et al.*, pp. 247–260. BSAVA, Cheltenham

4

Dermatopathology

David Shearer

Dogs and cats brought to the clinic for investigation and treatment of skin disease can present with a variety of signs. The investigation into the cause of the skin disease can be planned using a problem-solving approach based on the main signs present on examination (see Chapter 2). These signs include pruritus, erythema, papules, pustules, alopecia, crusts, scales, erosions, ulcerations, nodules and pigment changes. One or more of these signs may be present and the balance of clinical features along with the signalment and history lead to a list of differential diagnoses and a plan for investigation and or treatment. Particular combinations of signs may lead to a specific test or tests in the first instance. If this is not the case, then investigation is usually based on the main presenting sign.

Gross lesions

Gross lesions are divided into primary and secondary lesions with some overlap between the types (Figure 4.1 and Chapter 2). It is important to identify lesions accurately, describe the lesions in clinical notes and to put the description on to any pathology submission form. The interpretation of the histological features in skin biopsies can be dependent upon the presenting signs and the appearance and site of the lesions.

Primary	Primary or Secondary	Secondary
Macule/patch	Alopecia	Epidermal collarettes
Papule/plaque	Scale	Excoriation
Pustule	Crust	Erosion/ulcer
Vesicle/bulla	Follicular casts	Lichenification
Wheal	Comedones	Fissure
Nodule	Pigment changes	Callus
Tumour		Scar

4.1 Gross lesions.

Histological changes

Skin biopsy may be indicated as part of the investigation of the skin disease. If biopsy and histopathology are required, a few simple rules should be applied, including:

- Apart from careful removal of hair, do not clear the biopsy site(s) or disturb surface material
- In generalized skin disease take multiple punch biopsies (minimum of three)
- Try to get the opinion of a pathologist with a specific expertise in skin pathology e.g. a member of The International Society of Veterinary Dermatopathology (ISVD).

The gross appearance of the cutaneous lesions should correlate with the histological features and in most cases the microscopic features present can be predicted from the macroscopic lesions (Figure 4.2).

If the histological features described by a dermatopathologist do not correlate with the gross appearance of the lesions then consider the following:

- The biopsy specimen(s) is/are not representative of the lesion. This may relate to the age of the lesion; most lesions have a normal progression from formation to resolution or repair. Multiple biopsies increase the likelihood of diagnosis since they increase the chance of revealing the lesion progression and one of them may contain the 'diagnostic' features required. The diagnostic material in some biopsies may be lost; an example is the superficial crust or pustule in cases of pemphigus foliaceus which can be removed during preparation of the skin for biopsy or are lost in histological processing (if they come away from the skin). For this reason the skin surface should never be prepared/cleaned before superficial biopsy (see Chapter 3)
- The appearance of the gross lesions and their clinical interpretation has been incorrect. The most common assumption made by general practitioners is 'it looks bad therefore it must be autoimmune'. Although some autoimmune dermatoses are severe, infectious agents are the most common cause of severe skin disease. Although neoplastic diseases can produce severe skin lesions, early cases of epitheliotropic lymphoma can present as a rather benign scaling, alopecic disease. In this case the clinician often asks the pathologist, 'Are you sure that this is neoplastic?'

Presenting sign	Patterns which can be seen
Pruritus	Perivascular dermatitis Nodular/diffuse dermatitis Intraepidermal vesicular/pustular dermatitis Folliculitis
Alopecia	Atrophic dermatopathy Perivascular dermatitis Intraepidermal vesicular/pustular dermatitis Folliculitis Interface dermatitis
Scaling and crusting	Atrophic dermatopathy Folliculitis Interface dermatitis Nodular/diffuse dermatitis Perivascular dermatitis Intraepidermal vesicular/pustular dermatitis Folliculitis
Pustules	Perivascular dermatitis Intraepidermal vesicular/pustular dermatitis Folliculitis
Ulcers	Perivascular dermatitis Interface dermatitis Vasculitis Intraepidermal vesicular/pustular dermatitis Subepidermal vesicular/pustular dermatitis Folliculitis/furunculosis Panniculitis
Pigment changes: hyperpigmentation	Perivascular dermatitis Nodular/diffuse dermatitis Folliculitis Atrophic dermatopathy
Pigment changes: hypopigmentation	Interface dermatitis Nodular/diffuse dermatitis
Nodules	Nodular/diffuse dermatitis Folliculitis/furunculosis Panniculitis Vasculitis

4.2 Histological patterns associated with major clinical signs.

In general, if the clinical features cannot be correlated with the dermatohistopathologist's report, the pathologist should be contacted and the case discussed. It is important to describe the clinical features accurately on the submission form and to give a brief history. The sites of the biopsies should also be recorded since the pathologist's interpretation of the histology may be affected by the sites of origin.

Generally speaking, skin sections are examined by the pathologist under low power initially and before reading the clinician's notes on the submission form. This allows an unbiased assessment and interpretation of the histology. After examination under low power the changes seen are categorized into a 'pattern' based on the pattern analysis (Figure 4.3) (Yager and Wilcock, 1995).

The biopsy sections are then examined in detail to identify dermatopathological changes in each part of the skin, usually beginning with the epidermis followed by the adnexae and dermis. The pathologist then makes an interpretation of the histological features in light of the clinical information. The pathologist's report usually includes a morphological diagnosis, aetiological diagnosis (if possible), description of changes and a discussion of the findings (Figure 4.4).

- Perivascular dermatitis (the 'dermatitis reaction')
- Interface dermatitis
- Vasculitis
- Nodular and/or diffuse dermatitis
- Intraepidermal vesicular/pustular dermatitis
- Subepidermal vesicular/pustular dermatitis
- Folliculitis/perifolliculitis/furunculosis
- Panniculitis
- Atrophic

4.3 Classification of the patterns seen in skin biopsy samples.

The pathology report should include a summary of the histological features present, a statement of the patterns seen (see Figure 4.2), an aetiological diagnosis (if possible) and a commentary outlining the conclusions that can be made. A typical report might be set out as:

Description: This is a summary of the histological features seen and usually starts with the epidermis followed by the dermis and adnexae.

Morphological diagnosis: This states the major and minor histological patterns present.

Aetiological diagnosis: This is stated if a causative agent is seen in the sections examined.

Comments: The pathologist states what can be concluded from the histological features and relates them to the clinical features. The pathologist should give a comment as to the clinicopathological correlation in this section and for this reason an accurate history and description of the gross changes is important.

4.4 The dermatohistopathology report.

Basic dermatohistopathological changes

- *Epidermal atrophy:* This is a reduction in the thickness of the epidermis. As a general rule the epidermis thickness is inversely proportional to the hair density. This change is seen in cases with alopecia and skin thinning.
- *Acanthosis (epidermal hyperplasia):* This represents keratinocyte hyperplasia and occurs in various types.
  - Regular acanthosis is a uniform increase in stratum spinosum with no rete ridges
  - Irregular acanthosis has rete ridge formation and is the commonest form in the dog and cat
  - Psoriasiform acanthosis has regular rete ridge formation with or without club-shaped tips. This is rare in the cat and dog
  - Papillated acanthosis has folding and projection above the surface. This is acanthosis with upward proliferation of dermis. It is a non-specific term
  - Pseudoepitheliomatous/carcinomatous acanthosis has an invasive appearance resembling squamous cell carcinoma. It occurs at the edge of ulcers

Acanthosis is seen in lesions with lichenification and inflammatory alopecia; typically dogs with chronic dermatitis, pyoderma and *Malassezia* dermatitis.

- *Crusts:* These are surface accumulations of squames, serum proteins, red blood cells, and white blood cells. They are classified as serous, keratinous, cellular or haemorrhagic. Crusts often contain microorganisms such as bacteria, yeasts (*Malassezia*) and occasionally dermatophytes. Crusts are most often seen in cases of pyoderma, dermatophytosis and parasitic disease but can be seen in the autoimmune disease pemphigus foliaceus.
- *Hyperkeratosis:* This is an increase in the stratum corneum. It can be orthokeratotic or parakeratotic, basket-weave or compact. Compact hyperkeratosis is associated with chronic trauma. This is seen grossly as scale and forms part of crusts.
- *Parakeratosis:* This is where there is retention of a pyknotic nucleus in the squames in the stratum corneum. It reflects increased cell turnover and a rapid response to injury. It occurs as a focal change either vertically (in episodic injury) and/or horizontally (in focal injury). Generalized parakeratosis is associated with zinc responsive dermatosis and metabolic dermatosis. This is seen grossly as scale and parakeratosis forms part of crusts.
- *Hypergranulosis:* This is an increase in the thickness of stratum granulosum and is usually associated with compact hyperkeratosis due to chronic trauma. Areas of lichenification can have hypergranulosis.
- *Hypogranulosis:* This is a decrease or loss of the stratum granulosum and is usually associated with parakeratosis.
- *Papillomatosis:* This is epidermal growth due to papilloma virus infection. This is a specific term. These are usually exophytic lesions described as 'warts' but can be endophytic in verruca-like lesions.
- *Dyskeratosis:* This is premature, faulty keratinization, which can occur in the surface or adnexal epithelium. It can be a benign change seen in various dermatoses associated with abnormal keratinization. It can also be a change in malignant lesions such as squamous cell carcinoma.
- *Spongiosis:* This is epidermal intercellular oedema which gives the epidermis a spongy appearance. This change is usually associated with exocytosis of inflammatory cells and if severe it can lead to intraepidermal vesicle formation.
- *Exocytosis:* This refers to the migration of inflammatory cells from the dermis into epidermis and adnexae. It is usually associated with spongiosis.
- *Intracellular oedema:* This appears as intracytoplasmic vacuolation and occurs in hydropic degeneration of basal keratinocytes and in ballooning degeneration.

- *Hydropic degeneration (vacuolar alteration/liquifactive degeneration):* This refers to the presence of vacuoles within the stratum basale cells. This may lead to intrabasal or subepidermal clefts. This change is seen in some ulcerative skin lesions such as dermatomyositis.
- *Ballooning degeneration:* This type of degeneration is specifically seen in herpes virus infection.
- *Reticular degeneration:* This is multilocular/intraepidermal vesicle formation due to severe epidermal oedema. Severe keratinocyte swelling can also occur in metabolic dermatosis (superficial necrolytic dermatitis/hepatocutaneous syndrome) or acute contact dermatitis.
- *Acantholysis:* This is separation of keratinocytes. Primary acantholysis is separation of normal keratinocytes as seen in pemphigus foliaceus. Secondary acantholysis occurs as the result of damage to the keratinocytes and occurs in dyskeratosis, viral infections and in association with inflammatory cells in staphylococcal pyoderma.
- *Pigment incontinence:* This refers to melanin which drops from the epidermis/adnexae into dermis where it is phagocytosed by dermal monocytes/macrophages. This is usually associated with stratum basale cell oedema. This is a feature of an interface dermatitis as is seen in cutaneous lupus.
- *Epidermal necrosis:* This can be caseous or coagulative. Caseous necrosis appears as an eosinophilic and basophilic mush. This is the most common and least specific form of necrosis and usually reflects trauma (especially scratching). Coagulation necrosis appears as eosinophilic with pyknotic nuclei and the superficial dermis is often involved. Coagulation necrosis usually occurs as the result of physical damage (burns/freezing/chemical), ischaemia or immunological mechanisms. Clinically lesions with epidermal necrosis present with ulceration.
- *Necrolysis:* This is used to describe epidermal coagulation necrosis with no dermal involvement and minimal inflammation (e.g. toxic epidermal necrolysis).
- *Apoptosis:* This is individual cell death and involves intracellular processes which require energy (compare to necrosis by oncosis which is not energy-dependent and occurs as the result of catastrophic cell damage). This can be a physiological or pathological process. These processes can be triggered in a variety of ways, one of which is cytotoxic attack by lymphocytes (satellitosis). Histologically, apoptosis appears as eosinophilic bodies which are phagocytosed by adjacent cells.
- *Satellitosis:* This refers to the appearance of cytotoxic lymphocytes surrounding an apoptotic cell; this indicates a cell-mediated immune response.
- *Civatte bodies:* These are apoptotic cells in the stratum basale of the epidermis.

33

Patterns used in dermatopathological interpretation

Perivascular dermatitis

There are prominent blood vessels (high endothelial venules), oedema of dermis and exocytosis of leucocytes into the dermis around the high endothelial venules (Figures 4.5 and 4.6). In addition to these dermal changes there are epidermal changes which may reflect the aetiology or age of the lesions. The epidermal changes (see above) include acanthosis (hyperplasia), spongiosis, intracellular oedema (basal layer in an interface dermatitis), hyperkeratosis (basket weave or compact), parakeratosis (focal or diffuse), epidermal necrosis (erosions/ulcerations) and crusts.

The perivascular dermatitis is further classified according to the vascular plexuses involved: zone 1 (superficial dermal), zone 2 (mid-dermal and perifollicular) and zone 3 (deep dermal). The type of cellular infiltrate may also reflect aetiology or pathogenesis (neutrophil, lymphocyte or eosinophil). An eosinophilic infiltrate tends to indicate a type I hypersensitivity and a parasitic or allergic aetiology.

This is a common reaction pattern, which is diagnostically weak.

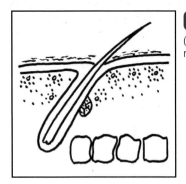

4.5 Perivascular dermatitis (the 'dermatitis reaction').

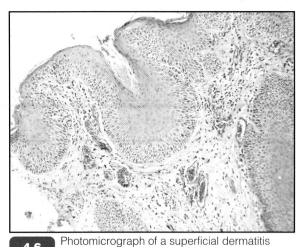

4.6 Photomicrograph of a superficial dermatitis pattern. (H&E; original magnification ×100.)

Interface dermatitis

There is hydropic degeneration of basal keratinocytes (Figure 4.7) with or without individual cell necrosis (apoptosis). There is a cell-rich or cell-poor mononuclear infiltrate at, and crossing, the dermoepidermal junction. There is pigment incontinence.

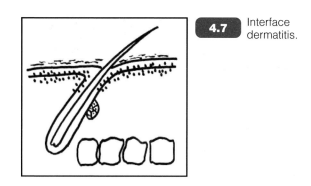

4.7 Interface dermatitis.

A cell-rich interface dermatitis is seen in cutaneous lupus and erythema multiforme (lymphocytic). A cell poor interface occurs in dermatomyositis.

Although, in some circumstances this pattern can be indicative of pathogenesis, it can be seen in many different diseases and its significance needs careful interpretation; it is a common pattern at mucocutaneous junctions/nasal planum where it is diagnostically weak compared to elsewhere.

Vasculitis

This is specific inflammation of blood vessels. Histologically there are tight perivascular cuffs of inflammatory cells (Figure 4.8) with evidence of degeneration of the vessel wall. In some circumstances there is necrosis of the inflammatory cells represented by the presence of 'nuclear dust'. A variety of cell types can be seen in cutaneous vasculitis. Microhaemorrhage should alert the pathologist to the possible presence of a vasculitis. Other changes seen in vasculitis include panniculitis, dermal necrosis and atrophy of hair follicles.

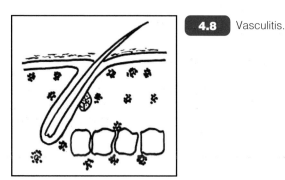

4.8 Vasculitis.

Nodular/diffuse dermatitis

Nodular and diffuse dermatitis (Figure 4.9) are considered to be one pattern but it is important to differentiate a hair follicle disease from non-follicular nodular dermatitis. The diffuse pattern reflects convergence of nodules. The cellular infiltrate gives some indication of the likely cause. A neutrophilic infiltrate occurs in response to pyogenic agents. Histiocytes/macrophages occur in response to foreign bodies and mycobacteria.

The presence of neutrophils and macrophages should alert the pathologist to the possibility of a furunculosis. An eosinophilic nodular and diffuse dermatitis raises the possibility of a parasitic aetiology. A lymphocytic infiltrate can be seen in vaccine reactions and insect bites.

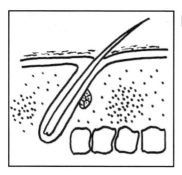

4.9 Nodular and/or diffuse dermatitis.

Intraepidermal vesicular/pustular dermatitis

Clefting leading to vesicles or pustules within the epidermis (Figure 4.10) can occur as the result of spongiosis/epidermal inflammation (parasites or infection), acantholysis (due to infection or autoimmune disease), intracellular oedema and mechanical forces (friction). The clefting may be subcorneal (pemphigus foliaceus/pyoderma), suprabasilar (pemphigus vulgaris) or with the follicular external root sheath (pemphigus foliaceus). A variety of cells can be present: neutrophils (pemphigus foliaceus / pyoderma), eosinophils (pemphigus foliaceus / parasitic disease) or mononuclear cells (macrophages in bacterial pyoderma).

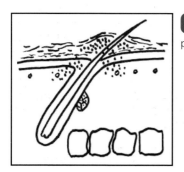

4.10 Intraepidermal vesicular/ pustular dermatitis.

Subepidermal vesicular/pustular dermatitis

(Figure 4.11) This is an uncommon pattern. It occurs in autoimmune disease such as bullous pemphigoid, thermal trauma (burns), severe dermal oedema, and severe interface dermatitis (cutaneous lupus). It can also be a histological artifact.

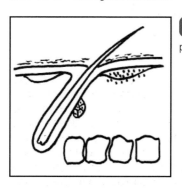

4.11 Subepidermal vesicular/ pustular dermatitis.

Folliculitis/perifolliculitis/furunculosis

Inflammation associated with the hair follicles (Figure 4.12) can affect the perifollicular vascular plexus (perifolliculitis), the outer root sheath (mural folliculitis), the entire hair follicle (luminal folliculitis), the bulb (bulbitis), the sebaceous glands (sebaceous adenitis)

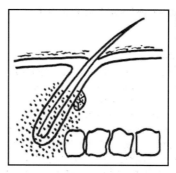

4.12 Folliculitis/ perifolliculitis/ furunculosis.

or apocrine glands (hidradenitis). Furunculosis is rupture of the hair follicle. Causes of follicular inflammatory diseases include bacteria (polymorphonuclear neutrophils and plasma cells predominate), dermatophytes (lymphocytic folliculitis), demodicosis (typically a lymphoid mural folliculitis), parasites e.g. mosquitoes/insect stings (eosinophilic folliculitis/ furunculosis), immune mediated e.g. alopecia areata (lymphocytic bulbitis).

Panniculitis

Inflammation of the subcutaneous adipose tissue (Figure 4.13) can be septal or lobular. It can also be an extension of follicular disease. Histology may indicate the cause and pathogenesis e.g. infectious agents, a vasculitis or a foreign body may be apparent.

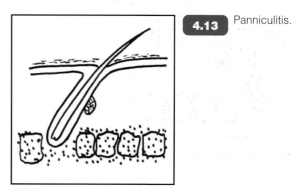

4.13 Panniculitis.

Atrophic dermatopathy

There is atrophy of the epidermis, hair follicles and sebaceous glands (Figures 4.14 and 4.15). Orthokeratotic hyperkeratosis and follicular keratosis may be present. In cases of hyperadrenocorticism there may be calcinosis cutis. The mineralized collagen is eliminated by transepidermal extrusion. This pattern is seen in a variety of endocrine dermatoses, which require a variety of hormonal assays to confirm their exact aetiology (see Chapter 3).

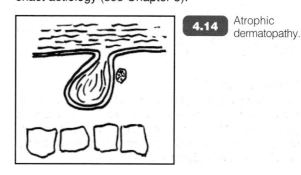

4.14 Atrophic dermatopathy.

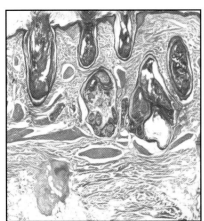

4.15

Photomicrograph of an atrophic dermatopathy. (H&E; original magnification x32.)

Conclusions

The histological diagnosis depends upon identification of the reaction patterns present and their order of importance combined with the detailed features of each component of the skin. This information is then compared to the clinical features and appearance of the gross lesions to arrive at a diagnosis, which encompasses the aetiology and pathogenesis of the skin disease. The gross and histological features should correlate. Using a problem-solving approach to the individual case based on the main clinical signs present it should be possible to predict the most likely histological patterns present (see Figure 4.2). If there is poor correlation the case should be discussed with the dermatopathologist.

References and further reading

Goldschmidt MH and Shofer FS (1992) *Skin Tumors of the Dog and Cat.* Pergamon Press, Oxford

Gross TL, Ihrke PJ and Walder EJ (1992) *Veterinary dermatopathology. A macroscopic and microscopic evaluation of canine and feline skin disease.* Mosby-Year Book Inc, St. Louis

Scott DW, Miller WH and Griffin CE (2001) *Muller & Kirk's Small Animal Dermatology, 6th edn.* WB Saunders Co, Philadelphia

Yager JA and Wilcock BP (1994) *Colour Atlas and Text of Surgical Pathology of the Dog and Cat.* Mosby-Year Book Europe, London

5

An approach to pruritus

Dawn Logas

Pruritus is defined simply as an uneasy sensation that provokes scratching and is synonymous with itch. It can be subdivided into different types of itch based on sensation, such as epicritic itch, which is a sharp, well demarcated pruritus and protopathic itch, which is a poorly localized burning sensation. It can also be subdivided by pathogenesis e.g. a physiological (short-lived) *versus* pathological, an intense severe response. Finally, itch can be divided by distribution, such as scattered or referred itch.

Although pruritus is an extremely common and uncomfortable sign of many dermatological diseases there is still a significant paucity of information on the molecular and physiological mechanisms of itching. The proposed sequence of events for pruritus starts with a stimulus in the upper layers of the skin, which leads to the release of mediators and the stimulation of neuroreceptors.

There are various mediators that can induce pruritus:

- Histamine, the first recognized pruritogen, produces pruritus via H_1 receptors
- Endopeptidases (e.g. trypsin and papain)
- Biogenic amines and kinins (e.g. serotonin, bradykinin)
- Certain neurotransmitters, such as substance P and vasoactive intestinal peptides
- Opiate peptides: can provoke pruritus or potentiate the pruritus evoked by other mediators
- Prostaglandins: more important in exaggerating ongoing itch than producing it themselves.

According to current knowledge, itch does not have its own neuroreceptors or fibres but shares with pain a group of peripheral C fibres, dorsal horn interneurons and a projection pathway in the antero-lateral spinal cord. Pruritus is initiated by intermittent discrete input volleys of C fibre origin. These activate small numbers of interneurons but do not trigger the normal concurrent central inhibition seen with more intense stimuli. After the arrival of an input volley the C fibres then exaggerate and amplify their effect on the central neurons via peptides and synaptic changes that prolong the central cells' response to an input. Therefore, if a limited number of C fibres are stimulated, a limited group of dorsal horn cells fire in an exaggerated fashion and produce itch. If rubbing or scratching occurs, the low intensity A fibres are activated and widespread inhibition results. This helps to suppress the exaggerated response of dorsal horn interneurons to the limited C fibre input thereby reducing the pruritus.

Differential diagnosis

Dogs
Pruritus is the most common presenting sign for a large number of canine dermatological diseases. The severity varies from mild to extremely severe, where the patient scratches almost continuously to the exclusion of eating and sleeping. The underlying causes range from infectious to neoplastic (Figure 5.1).

Cats
Pruritus is also a common presenting sign for feline dermatological diseases although owners are often unaware that their cat is pruritic since cats can be very secretive about their scratching. The underlying causes, like those in the dog, range from infectious to neoplastic (Figure 5.2).

Clinical approach

The clinical approach to feline and canine pruritus depends greatly on the dermatological history and physical examination of the patient.

History
The owner of a pruritic pet should be questioned about:

- Family history of the patient
- Age of onset
- Dietary history
- Pet's normal environment
- Any recent environmental changes
- Drug/insecticide history
- Areas of the body historically affected
- Type of lesions that originally occurred
- Response to previous therapies
- Current seasonality and whether this has changed over time
- Intensity of pruritus and whether this has changed over time
- Exposure to other animals
- Pruritic status of other family members and pets.

Disease	Intensity of pruritus*	
Infectious		
Superficial bacterial folliculitis	–	to +++
Deep pyoderma	–	to +++
Dermatophytosis	–	to +
Malassezia dermatitis	++	to +++
Pythiosis	++	to +++
Parasitic		
Hookworm dermatitis	++	to +++
Pelodera dermatitis	+	to +++
Schistosomiasis	++	to +++
Dracunculiasis	++	
Dirofilariasis	++	
Dermanyssus gallineae	+++	
Trombiculiasis	–	to +++
Otodectes cynotis	–	to +++
Pneumonyssoides caninum	+	
Cheyletiellosis	+	to ++
Demodicosis	–	to +
Scabies	+++	
Pediculosis	–	to +++
Hypersensitivity disorders		
Atopy	+	to +++
Contact allergy	++	to +++
Adverse food reaction	–	to +++
Flea allergy	++	to +++
Mosquito/*Culicoides* allergy	++	to +++
Hormonal hypersensitivity	++	
Immune-mediated disorders		
Pemphigus foliaceus	–	to +
Systemic lupus erythematosus	–	to +
Cutaneous drug eruptions	–	to +++
Keratinization defects		
Seborrhoea	+	to +++
Vitamin A-responsive dermatosis	+	to +++
Environmental diseases		
Irritant contact dermatitis	++	to +++
Calcinosis cutis	++	to +++
Miscellaneous skin diseases		
Subcorneal pustular dermatosis	+	to +++
Sterile eosinophilic pustulosis	++	
Waterline disease of black Labrador Retrievers	+++	
Neoplasia		
Mast cell tumour	–	to ++
Mycosis fungoides	–	to ++

5.1 Differential diagnoses for canine pruritus.

* –: no pruritus; +: mild pruritus; ++: moderate pruritus; +++: severe pruritus

Disease	Intensity of pruritus*	
Infectious		
Superficial bacterial folliculitis	–	to ++
Dermatophytosis	–	to ++
Malassezia dermatitis	+	to +++
Parasitic		
Otobius megnini	++	
Dermanyssus gallineae	++	
Lynxacarus radovsky	+	to +++
Trombiculosis	+	to +++
Otodectes cynotis	+	to +++
Cheyletiellosis	+	to +++
Demodex gatoi	+	to +++
Notoedres cati	+	to +++
Pediculosis	–	to ++
Hypersensitivity disorders		
Atopy	+	to +++
Contact allergy	++	to +++
Adverse food reaction	–	to +++
Flea allergy	++	to +++
Mosquito/*Culicoides* hypersensitivity	++	to +++
Immune-mediated disorders		
Pemphigus foliaceus	–	to ++
Systemic lupus erythematosus	–	to +
Discoid lupus erythematosus	–	to +
Cutaneous drug eruption	–	to +++
Keratinization defects		
Primary seborrhoea	–	to ++
Idiopathic facial dermatitis	+	to +++
Feline acne	–	to ++
Endocrinology		
Hyperthyroidism	–	to ++
Psychogenic diseases		
Psychogenic alopecia	++	
Environmental skin diseases		
Feline solar dermatitis	–	to ++
Miscellaneous skin disease		
Feline hypereosinophilic syndrome	++ to +++	
Idiopathic sterile granulomatous/ pyogranulomatous dermatitis	++	
Neoplasia		
Mast cell tumour	–	to ++
Cutaneous T cell lymphoma	–	to ++

5.2 Differential diagnoses for feline pruritus.

* –: no pruritus; +: mild pruritus; ++: moderate pruritus; +++: severe pruritus

If the pruritus is particularly intense the clinician should rule out adverse food reaction, contact allergy (Box 5.1), scabies, yeast dermatitis and insect hypersensitivities.

If other family members are affected the clinician must rule out dermatophytosis and parasitic infestations.

Physical examination

On the physical examination special attention should be paid to the distribution of lesions, the presence of primary/secondary lesions and the presence of secondary infections. If insect infestations or second-ary infections such as bacterial pyodermas or yeast dermatitis are present, these must be controlled before the patient can be examined accurately for allergic diseases.

Ancillary tests

Once the history and physical examination are complete, the clinician can decide which ancillary tests are necessary and will give the most valuable information. Figures 5.3 to 5.6 give a general overview of how to approach the pruritic patient, which ancillary tests to run, and the likely diagnoses.

Box 5.1: Contact dermatitis

Contact dermatitis is an inflammatory response of the skin that occurs when an irritant or allergenic substance comes in contact with the surface of the skin itself. This is due to type IV, delayed type hypersensitivity, or to an antigen-independent irritant reaction. It is an uncommon condition in both dogs and cats since the majority of their skin is covered with a dense hair coat that acts as a natural barrier to contact allergens/irritants.

Clinical signs

The clinical signs associated with contact dermatitis in the dog and the cat include erythematous papular to vesicular or erosive eruptions that can progress with chronic exposure to lichenification and excoriations.

The lesions are usually confined to the glabrous skin or lightly haired areas of the body. Therefore the lesions in the dog are usually confined to the ventrum, feet, face, perineal area and the concave surface of the pinnae. In the cat the lesions are usually confined more to the face, footpads, preauricular area, hocks and pinnae.

Diagnosis

The preliminary diagnosis of contact dermatitis is mainly based on history and clinical signs. In some incidences a patch test can be performed although these are difficult in veterinary patients. Confining the patient, using protective clothing and investigating the environment in detail are the best ways to diagnose contact allergy in the dog and cat.

Treatment

The most successful therapy for contact allergy is avoidance. When avoidance is impossible, protective clothing, pentoxifylline and glucocorticoids (systemic and/or topical) can be used.

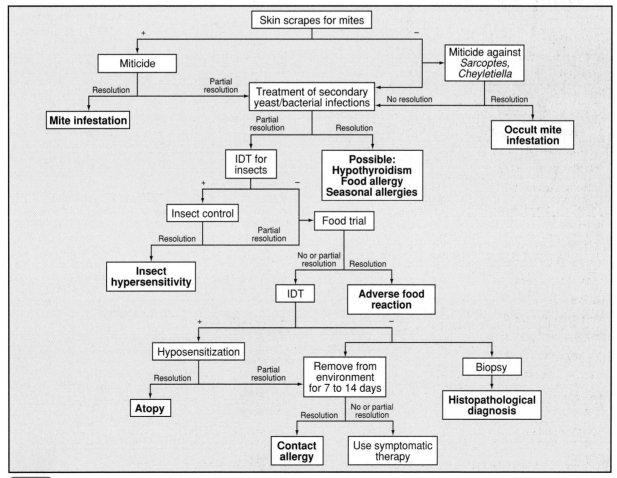

5.3 Diagnostic approach to non-seasonal canine pruritus. IDT = intradermal testing.

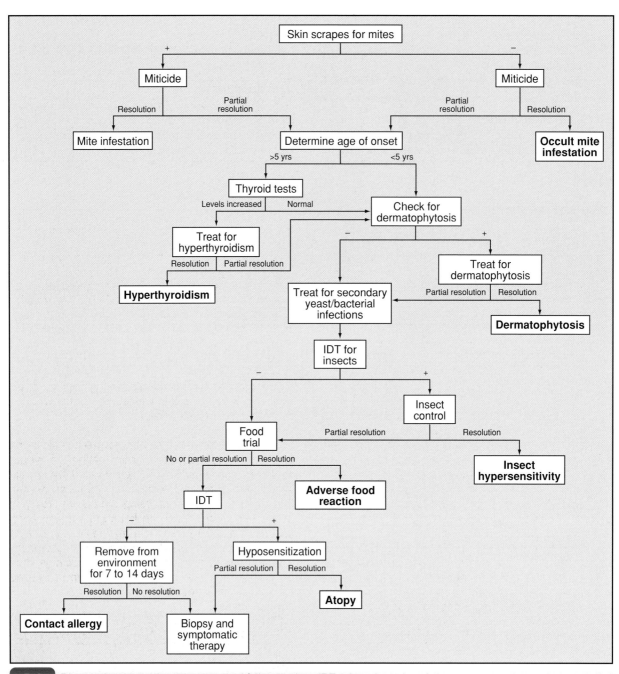

5.4   Diagnostic approach to non-seasonal feline pruritus. IDT = intradermal testing.

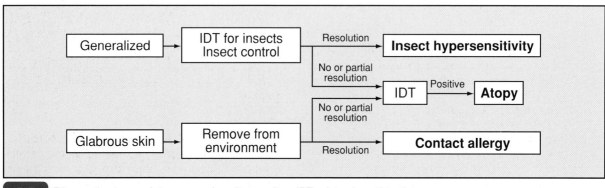

5.5   Diagnostic approach to seasonal canine pruritus. IDT = intradermal testing.

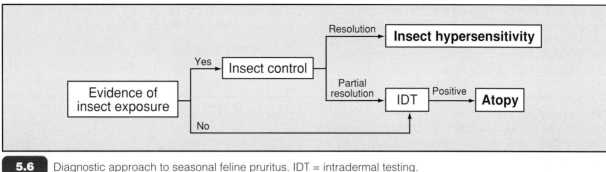

5.6 Diagnostic approach to seasonal feline pruritus. IDT = intradermal testing.

Box 5.2: Idiopathic feline facial pruritus

This syndrome is diagnosed based on the exclusion of all other known causes of feline facial pruritus.

When confronted with a case of facial pruritus, a minimum database, which includes drug history, thyroid hormone levels in cats older than 5 years, skin scrapings, ear swabs, skin cytologies, and dermatophyte cultures should be performed. If these tests are all negative, the patient should be put on a food trial for 6—8 weeks, treated with lime sulphur for occult parasitic infections, treated with intraconazole for occult yeast infection and antibiotics for possible bacterial infections. If the cat still has facial pruritus, a biopsy should be taken, the cat should be removed from the environment for 10—14 days and an Elizabethan collar applied.

At this point, if the patient is still pruritic, a diagnosis of idiopathic feline facial pruritus should be made. This occurs in approximately 10% of the cases. Unfortunately, these cases rarely respond to therapy and many are euthanased.

Therapeutic principles

The first principle a clinician should remember when dealing with a pruritic patient is that pruritus is a symptom and not a disease entity *per se*. Therefore every effort must be made to diagnose the underlying causes of the pruritus. This will enable a therapeutic plan to be formulated that can treat the underlying problems specifically. If possible, any infectious agents present should be treated completely before long-term symptomatic therapy is initiated.

If the pruritus is severe it must be controlled symptomatically for the comfort of the client and the patient. Symptomatic therapy is also needed in cases where the underlying cause cannot be determined or the pruritus does not respond to conventional therapy for the underlying disease. Symptomatic therapy is also needed to help control pruritus while other therapies have an opportunity to work.

Glucocorticoids

The most effective symptomatic therapy is provided by glucocorticoids. No matter what the underlying cause glucocorticoids will give some relief, although for a few conditions this relief may be very short-lived. Because of their potency and potential for side effects, glucocorticoids should not be used as first line drugs unless the pruritus is severe. If at all possible the glucocorticoid should be given orally instead of parenterally. This allows for better titration of the drug.

- For dogs, a good anti-inflammatory dosage of prednisolone for the first 3–5 days is 1–2 mg/kg every 24 hours or divided into two equal doses in a 24-hour period. Over the course of 2–4 weeks the dosage is decreased to 0.5 mg/kg every other day, then stopped

- For cats the dose is doubled to 2–4 mg/kg initially then tapered over 2–4 weeks to 1 mg/kg every other day, then stopped.

There are, however, several problems with using glucocorticoids without restraint. Although glucocorticoids can diminish the itch caused by certain infectious and parasitic diseases it can also worsen these conditions by decreasing the body's ability to keep these organisms in check. Long-term glucocorticoid use potentially causes a myriad of side effects (Figure 5.7) which are detrimental and occasionally fatal to the patient. Therefore, glucocorticoids should be reserved for cases of severe pruritus and only used for a short time if possible.

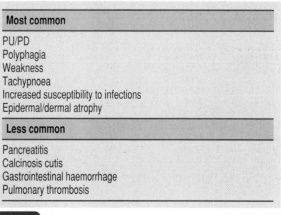

Most common		
PU/PD		
Polyphagia		
Weakness		
Tachypnoea		
Increased susceptibility to infections		
Epidermal/dermal atrophy		
Less common		
Pancreatitis		
Calcinosis cutis		
Gastrointestinal haemorrhage		
Pulmonary thrombosis		

5.7 Possible side effects of glucocorticoids.

Antihistamines and omega-3 fatty acids

Other common symptomatic therapies for pruritus include antihistamines and omega-3 fatty acids. Although not as effective as glucocorticoids, these therapies can keep the pruritus under control for many patients with mild to moderate pruritus, and are safer in the long run than glucocorticoids. These modalities will be further discussed in Chapter 18. [Editor's note: In the UK many dermatologists recommend combination products of essential fatty acids.]

Topical therapy

Topicals are another common symptomatic therapy modality that can be very helpful in some pruritic cases. Preparations may contain glucocorticoids (hydro-cortisone, betamethasone), antihistamines (diphen-hydramine), counterirritants (alcohol, camphor, menthol) and local anaesthetics (pramoxine), all of which help decrease pruritus less effectively but with much lower incidence of side effects than their systemic partners.

Cool water hydrotherapy alone or with colloidal oatmeal can also control pruritus for up to 48 hours.

Novel therapies

There are new drugs that are being used to treat refractory pruritus. These include ciclosporin and pentoxifylline. These are further discussed in Chapters 18, 31 and 32.

References and further reading

Greaves MW and Wall PD (1998) Pathology and clinical aspects of pruritus. In: *Fitzpatrick's Dermatology in General Medicine, 5th edn*, ed. IM Freedberg *et al.*, pp. 487–494. McGraw Hill, New York

Scott DW, Miller WH and Griffin CE (2001) *Muller and Kirk's Small Animal Dermatology, 6th edn*. WB Saunders, Philadelphia

6

An approach to keratinization (cutaneous scaling) disorders

Kevin Shanley and Kenneth W. Kwochka

Scaly skin in dogs is one of the most common clinical presentations seen by the small animal veterinary surgeon and can be one of the most challenging clinical situations to diagnose and treat successfully. Scaling disorders in cats are less common, although they are equally challenging diseases to diagnose and treat. Cats are inherently less likely to present with scaling disorders due in part to their physiological make-up and in part to removal of some scales via their grooming habits.

The initial question to answer in approaching scaling disorders is whether the scaling is a primary keratinization defect or if it is secondary to another primary underlying dermatosis or internal disease. Primary keratinization disorders should not be diagnosed until all secondary causes of scaling have been ruled out. Secondary causes account for at least 80% of all cases of cutaneous scaling seen in clinical practice settings.

As with most complicated medical conditions, the clinical approach to scaling disorders requires a thorough methodical diagnostic plan, a cooperative client with adequate finances, and good communication between the veterinary surgeon and the client. This approach usually results in a definitive diagnosis, which allows the best chance for specific therapy to cure the condition, or at least maximizes the possibility for adequate control with minimal long-term maintenance therapy. Most cases of secondary scaling disorders can be expected to have a successful outcome. Most cases of primary keratinization disorders are much more difficult to control adequately and often require extensive life-long topical and systemic therapy.

Cutaneous scaling disorders have typically been referred to and categorized as various types of *seborrhoea*. This nomenclature has resulted in a confusing array of clinical approaches and diagnoses, leading to inadequate treatment and a poor outcome for the patient. In this chapter, the term seborrhoea will be used to refer only to primary keratinization disorders, not in the general sense of scaling or oily coat regardless of the underlying cause. The terms 'seborrhoea sicca', 'seborrhoea oleosa' and 'seborrhoeic dermatitis' will be avoided in this chapter.

Primary disorders of keratinization produce excessive amounts of scale as a direct result of a pathophysiological defect in the process of keratinization or cornification, or in the function of cutaneous sebaceous glands. Most of these primary keratinization disorders are hereditary and have major implications for breeding, so these patients should not remain in the breeding pool.

The scope of this chapter is to describe a practical clinical approach to cutaneous scaling disorders in the dog and cat, and to help differentiate secondary scaling from primary disorders of keratinization.

Differential diagnosis

Primary keratinization disorders in the dog and cat are uncommon, are usually inherited and include specific disease entities, often limited to one or several breeds (Figure 6.1). The veterinary surgeon must be familiar with these primary disorders, their respective breed predispositions, and the type and distribution of lesions, in order to suspect them on initial examination. Some of the salient features of the most common primary disorders of keratinization are highlighted in Boxes 6.1 and 6.2. However, most patients with scaly skin disorders will not have primary keratinization diseases. Secondary scaling disorders are more common and should be considered upon initial examination in most cases.

Disorder	Breeds predisposed
Canine primary idiopathic seborrhoea	Cocker Spaniel, English Springer Spaniel, Basset Hound, West Highland White Terrier, Dobermann Pinscher, Labrador Retriever, Irish Setter, Chinese Shar Pei, German Shepherd Dog, Dachshund
Feline primary idiopathic seborrhoea	Persian, Himalayan
Feline idiopathic facial dermatitis	Persian, Himalayan
Follicular dysplasia/follicle hyperkeratosis	Dobermann, Rottweiler, Yorkshire Terrier, Irish Setter, Dachshund, Chow Chow, Standard Poodle, Great Dane, Italian Greyhound, Whippet

6.1 Breeds predisposed to primary disorders of keratinization. (continues)

Disorder	Breeds predisposed
Epidermal dysplasia?	West Highland White Terrier
Ichthyosis	American Bulldog, Golden Retriever, Jack Russell Terrier, Norfolk Terrier, Rhodesian Ridgeback, West Highland White Terrier, Yorkshire Terrier
Vitamin A-responsive dermatosis	Cocker Spaniel, Miniature Schnauzer, Labrador Retriever
Zinc-responsive dermatosis	Siberian Husky, Alaskan Malamute
Sebaceous adenitis	Standard Poodle, Akita, Vizla, Samoyed, Lhasa Apso
Nasodigital hyperkeratosis	Spaniels, Irish Terrier, Labrador Retriever
Lichenoid psoriasiform dermatosis	English Springer Spaniel
Schnauzer comedo syndrome	Miniature Schnauzer
Ear margin dermatosis	Dachshund
Acne	English Bulldog, Boxer

6.1 (continued) Breeds predisposed to primary disorders of keratinization.

Box 6.1: Spaniel seborrhoea

Predisposition
This condition is common in American Cocker and English Springer Spaniels.

Pathogenesis
Affected dogs have a two to three-fold decrease in transit time from basal cells to stratum corneum (8 days *versus* 21–23 days in normal dogs). This dramatic increase in skin cell production results in a marked increase in scale formation, which is seen clinically. A significant drive in epidermal hyperproliferation comes from inflammation associated with concurrent diseases, primarily atopy or food allergy, and also secondary bacterial and yeast infections.

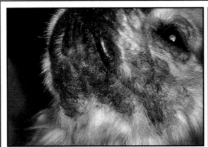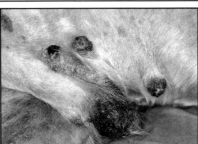

In this American Cocker Spaniel the disorder is exacerbated by facial bacterial overgrowth on the skin surface, mucocutaneous pyoderma and superficial spreading pyoderma. Note the marked hyperkeratosis on the teats. (Courtesy of C Foil)

Treatment
Controlling pyoderma, *Malassezia* dermatitis and allergic diseases allows reduced hyperproliferation and decreased scale formation. Ceruminous otitis externa is often refractory to treatment *unless* any underlying diseases are also controlled.

This hyperproliferative defect lends itself to therapeutic response. Various types of topical (sulphur, salicylic acid and tar shampoos) and oral (retinoids, linoleic acid) medications can be used for their keratoplastic effects to help normalize the hyperproliferative state and reduce scale formation.

Box 6.2: Ichthyosis

Predisposition
Ichthyosis is a rare congenital disease seen in American Bulldogs, Golden Retrievers, Jack Russell Terriers, Norfolk Terriers, Rhodesian Ridgebacks, West Highland White Terriers and Yorkshire Terriers. It is an autosomal recessive trait. One or more pups from a litter may be affected.

Clinical signs
Lesions include generalized large, thick, tightly adherent grey to yellow–brown scales over most of the body, beginning at birth or within 2 weeks after birth. There is often marked footpad and planum nasale hyperkeratosis, odour, pyoderma and *Malassezia* infection.

Diagnosis
Histopathological changes include moderate to marked compact orthokeratotic hyperkeratosis in almost all cases. In severe cases, numerous mitotic figures in basal layers, marked hypergranulosis and microvesicle formation in stratum corneum are observed.

Treatment
Treatment options include frequent bathing and emollient rinses, oil treatments, isotretinoin or acetretin.

Large flakes of scale without inflammatory skin disease on a 10-month-old Golden Retriever with ichthyosis. (Courtesy of C Foil)

Prognosis
The prognosis is variable. It is good in mildly affected dogs, some of which may improve with age but is poor in dogs affected severely from a young age.

Dogs

In dogs, the majority of common causes of secondary scaling can be categorized as:

- Allergic (Figure 6.2)
- Parasitic
- Metabolic
- Endocrine
- Infectious
- Autoimmune.

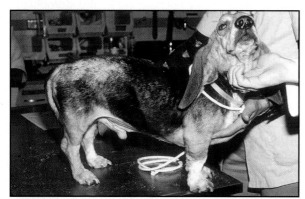

6.2   Significant secondary keratinization disorder in a Basset X Beagle with atopy and flea allergy. (Courtesy of C Foil)

One disease initially classified as a primary keratinization defect, epidermal dysplasia of West Highland White Terriers, is now thought to be a severe manifestation of hypersensitivity in this breed, illustrating the difficulty in making distinctions (Box 6.3). Figure 6.3 highlights keratinization disorders in allergic diseases.

- Pro-inflammatory changes from allergies increase epidermal cell proliferation and scale formation
- Pruritus induces scratching, chewing, etc., which damages epidermal surface and epidermal barrier function, exacerbates epidermal hyperproliferation, and increases susceptibility to secondary bacterial and yeast infections
- Management of the primary allergic disease dramatically improves response to therapies directed at seborrhoea

6.3   Keratinization disorders secondary to allergy.

Cats

Primary idiopathic seborrhoea has been recognized in Persians, Himalayans and several other exotic pure-bred cats. An idiopathic facial dermatitis of Persian (Figure 6.4) and Himalayan cats has also been reported.

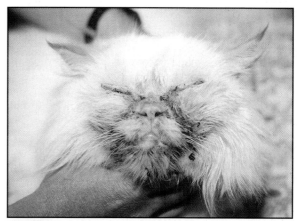

6.4   Idiopathic facial dermatitis in a Persian cat; this disorder is classified by some as a primary keratinization disorder. (Courtesy of C Foil)

Secondary scaling disorders in cats may be due to:

- Parasitic diseases (cheyletiellosis, notoedric mange, demodicosis, pediculosis)
- Allergic diseases (flea allergy, food allergy, atopic dermatitis)
- Infectious diseases (pyoderma, dermatophytosis, *Malassezia* dermatitis)
- Metabolic/endocrine diseases (diabetes mellitus, hyperadrenocorticism, liver disease)
- Neoplasia (paraneoplastic alopecia, thymoma-associated dermatosis).

Clinical approach

Signalment
Signalment can provide useful information for distinguishing between primary disorders of keratinization and secondary scaling disorders.

Box 6.3: Epidermal dysplasia of West Highland White Terriers

Pathogenesis

Since first reported and recognized as a clinical entity, this condition has been considered an inherited disease specific to West Highland White Terriers and commonly referred to as 'Armadillo Westie Syndrome' or 'Westie Seborrhoea' due to the marked hyperpigmentation, lichenification, skin fold prominence and scaling. There is not total agreement on the aetiology. Rather than an inherited keratinization disorder, this condition is probably a severe inflammatory or hypersensitivity reaction of these dogs to *Malassezia* or may be due to marked self-trauma secondary to an underlying allergy (atopic dermatitis or food allergy).

Diagnosis

An important histological feature of skin biopsies is marked epidermal dysplasia, wherein the epidermis is markedly hyperplastic and the epidermal basal keratinocytes are not orderly and columnar but are altered in shape and lack perpendicular orientation (polarity) to the basement membrane zone.

Treatment

Treatment is to address any secondary bacterial, yeast, fungal or parasitic infections, bathe frequently with keratoplastic, keratolytic shampoos, and identify and control any underlying allergic skin diseases.

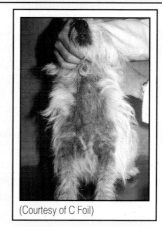

(Courtesy of C Foil)

Age of onset

Young animals: Most primary disorders of keratinization are inherited and will typically present within the first 2 years of life, often within the first 6 months. This is particularly true of:

- Primary idiopathic seborrhoea
- Ichthyosis
- Epidermal dysplasia
- Schnauzer comedo syndrome
- Canine and feline acne.

The common causes of secondary scaling in this age group are:

- Infectious (superficial pyoderma, dermatophytosis, *Malassezia* dermatosis)
- Parasitic (cheyletiellosis, demodicosis, scabies, endoparasitism)
- Allergic (flea allergy dermatitis, adverse food reaction dermatitis, atopic dermatitis).

Middle age: Primary keratinization defects are uncommon in middle-aged animals. Secondary scaling disorders are commonly present due to endocrinopathies such as hypothyroidism (canine; Figure 6.5) or hyperadrenocorticism, allergic diseases (as listed above) and autoimmune diseases (pemphigus foliaceus).

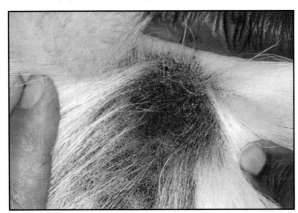

6.5 Close-up of a lesion on a profoundly hypothyroid Akita, illustrating the keratinization disorder that may accompany hypothyroidism. (Courtesy of C Foil)

Older animals: These are more likely to have secondary disorders of scaling due to:

- Endocrinopathies (as with middle-aged patients)
- Neoplastic diseases such as cutaneous lymphosarcoma (canine) or paraneoplastic alopecia (feline)
- Metabolic disorders such as hepatocutaneous syndrome (necrolytic migratory erythema, diabetic dermatopathy, metabolic epidermal necrosis, superficial necrolytic dermatitis) or diabetes mellitus (canine mean age of onset is 8 years, range of 4–14 years; feline age range is 8–13 years).

Breed

The breed of the patient can be tremendously helpful in suggesting a particular primary keratinization disorder (see Figure 6.1). It is also quite helpful in identifying predispositions for underlying diseases that lead to secondary scaling disorders. The West Highland White Terrier, Golden Retriever, Labrador Retriever, Dalmatian, Wire-Haired Fox Terrier, Chinese Shar Pei and numerous other breeds are genetically predisposed to developing atopy. Hypothyroidism, hyperadrenocorticism, cutaneous lymphosarcoma and pemphigus foliaceus also have breed predispositions.

Sex

The sex of the patient is usually of little value in offering diagnostic clues to the underlying disease. The sexual status (intact *versus* neutered) can lead towards particular types of sex hormone imbalances as primary causes of secondary scaling.

History

The history can be helpful, particularly when the scaling disorder is seasonal. All primary and most secondary scaling skin diseases are non-seasonal (year round), although in warm humid climates, clinical manifestations can be exacerbated in a seasonal manner. If a seasonal history is present, it is most indicative of an underlying flea allergy or atopic dermatitis.

Other historical clues and their associated diseases include heat-seeking, decreased appetite, weight gain, altered bark (hypothyroidism); polyuria, polydipsia, polyphagia, muscle weakness (hyperadrenocorticism); or abnormal urination posture, ie. not lifting a leg in males or lifting a leg in females (sex hormone imbalance).

The degree of pruritus (Figure 6.6) is often a tremendously helpful clue in dermatology in general, but is less

Invariably pruritic
Flea allergy
Atopic dermatitis
Adverse food reaction
Pyoderma
Scabies
Malassezia dermatitis
Variably pruritic
Cheyletiellosis
Pediculosis
Pemphigus foliaceus
Cutaneous lymphosarcoma
Dermatophytosis
Non-pruritic
Uninfected demodicosis
Hypothyroidism
Hyperadrenocorticism
Sex hormone abnormality
Metabolic disease
Low ambient humidity
Endoparasitism
Leishmaniasis
Inappropriate shampoo usage

6.6 Pruritus in secondary scaling in dogs and cats.

helpful in scaling disorders as they are often complicated by secondary bacterial or yeast infections, which typically induce pruritus in addition to excessive scaling. What is more helpful is the degree of pruritus remaining *after* the secondary pyoderma or yeast dermatitis has been treated and removed. Once secondary infections are resolved, a more accurate assessment of pruritus is possible. Pruritus usually indicates allergic (atopy, food allergy, flea allergy or contact allergy) or parasitic (cheyletiellosis, notoedriasis or scabies) primary underlying diseases. The degree of pruritus caused by particular diseases can vary tremendously from one patient to another, or even in the same patient as the disease progresses. An example of a scaling disease with highly variable levels of pruritus is pemphigus foliaceus.

Distribution of lesions

The distribution of lesions provides additional diagnostic clues.

Primary disorders

Primary disorders of keratinization are often multifocal and can become generalized (primary idiopathic seborrhoea, follicular dystrophy, vitamin A-responsive dermatosis, ichthyosis), but may also be site-specific (ear margin dermatosis (Figure 6.7), chin acne, nasodigital hyperkeratosis):

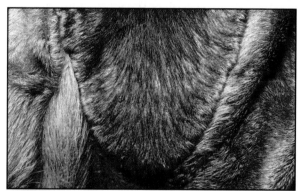

6.7 Ear margin dermatosis, as seen on this Bloodhound, is characterized as a localized primary keratinization disorder. (Courtesy of C Foil)

- Primary idiopathic seborrhoea often begins in intertriginous areas (Figure 6.8) and around nipples
- Sebaceous adenitis tends to affect the dorsum of the head, neck and chest initially and progresses to involve the majority of the trunk and proximal extremities
- Zinc-responsive dermatosis involves the periocular and perioral areas, dorsal bridge of the nose, pinnae, footpads, scrotum, vulva, elbows and pressure points
- Vitamin A-responsive dermatosis usually begins on the ventral neck (Figure 6.9), ventral and lateral chest and ventral abdomen, and frequently presents along with marked ceruminous otitis externa
- Lichenoid psoriasiform dermatosis of Springer Spaniels presents with erythematous papules and plaques on the inner pinnae, external ear canal and inguinal region.

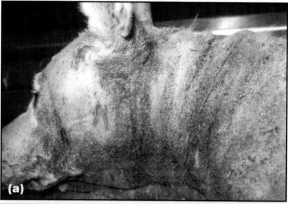

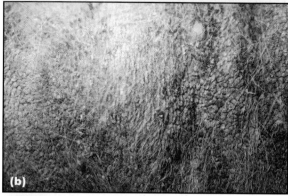

6.8 Severe primary keratinization disorder in a white German Shepherd Dog, illustrating distribution on neck folds. The close-up shows marked greasy hyperkeratosis. (Courtesy of C Foil)

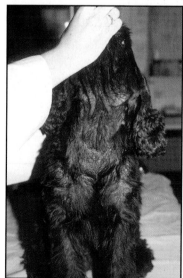

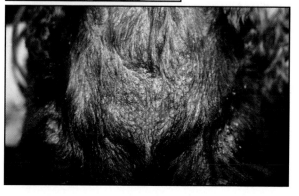

6.9 Marked ventral neck hyperkeratosis in an American Cocker Spaniel with vitamin A-responsive dermatosis. The close-up shows the severe keratinization disorder in this dermatosis. (Courtesy of C Foil)

Secondary scaling diseases

Lesion distribution in secondary scaling diseases is often based on the underlying predisposing cause:

- Scabies causes marked pruritus, with alopecia, erythema, papules, crusts and scaling involving the ventrum, pinnal margins, face, elbows, hocks and legs
- Atopy involves the feet, face, ear canals and ventrum
- Food allergy has multiple presentations from multifocal (involving the ears, feet, face, eyelids, ventrum and perineal area) to generalized
- Flea allergy presents with pruritus, scaling, alopecia, crusts and erythema involving the dorsal lumbosacrum, ventrum, hind legs and front legs.

Therapeutic principles

Topical treatment

Topical therapy plays an important role in resolving scaling disorders and there is a wide array of shampoos, conditioners, dips, lotions, creams, sprays, gels, ointments and powders (Figure 6.10). Topical medications may be anti-pruritic, antibacterial, antifungal, antiparasitic, keratoplastic, keratolytic, degreasing, astringent, moisturizing and anti-inflammatory. Product selection depends on the desired effects.

Keratolytic
Sulphur
Salicylic acid
Tar
Selenium sulphide
Benzoyl peroxide
Propylene glycol
Fatty acids
20% Urea

Keratoplastic
Sulphur
Salicylic acid
Tar
Selenium sulphide
Alpha-hydroxy acids

Barrier restoration
Linoleic acid
Free fatty acids
Lanolin
Mineral oil
Vegetable oils
Vitamin E

6.10 Topical agents useful in keratinization disorders.

The severity of the condition will determine the frequency of application. For most moderate to severe cases of multifocal or generalized seborrhoea and secondary scaling disorders, twice weekly bathing is a reasonable starting frequency. Shampoo contact time of 10–15 minutes is tremendously important in achieving desired results. Thorough rinsing will minimize shampoo residue and lessen the potential for irritation.

Epidermal cell health and renewal

Topical medications may be effective on one or more processes involved with epidermal cell health and renewal. Proliferation, differentiation and desquamation are the three main processes involved.

Proliferation: Proliferation occurs in the basal cell layer. The rate of proliferation is increased in most keratinization disorders and can be reduced by using topical keratoplastic agents in shampoo therapy. A key principle in understanding scaling disorders is to appreciate the fact that any inflammatory condition often leads to epidermal hyperproliferation, which leads to excessive scale formation.

Histologically, the epidermis is hyperplastic and often spongiotic. Therefore, controlling the inflammation helps to return epidermal proliferation to normal and reduce scale formation. Keratoplastic agents help normalize basal keratinocyte proliferation by methods such as decreasing DNA synthesis and slowing mitosis.

Differentiation: Keratin formation and protein cross-linkage occur during differentiation as the epidermal cells mature and migrate superficially into the spinous layer of the epidermis. Abnormalities in either of these processes can lead to excessive scaling. No current therapy, with the possible exception of retinoids, is known to affect these processes.

Desquamation: This is the release of keratinocytes from the surface of the epidermis. This process is highly orchestrated and normally involves many factors. The lack of any of these factors can alter normal desquamation and result in increased scaling. Increased visible scale is due to increased numbers of desquamating keratinocytes and larger numbers of keratinocytes sloughed en mass, attached to each other. This is due in part to persistent intercellular bridging between adjacent keratinocytes, resulting in larger, more visible scales.

Water loss

Normal skin is constantly losing water via transpiration. The epidermal barrier is responsible for maintaining adequate hydration of the epidermis and a balance of microbes on the surface of the stratum corneum. It is highly dependent on the presence of three intercellular lipids: sphingolipids, free fatty acids and free sterols. Disruption of the epidermal barrier integrity leads to increased transepidermal water loss (TEWL) and an altered microbial milieu. In addition to proinflammatory conditions, disruption of the epidermal barrier also results in an increased epidermal drive to hyperproliferate, leading to epidermal hyperkeratosis and increased scale formation. This emphasizes the need to control underlying allergic diseases, superficial pyoderma, *Malassezia* dermatitis infections and other proinflammatory diseases in order to help minimize excessive scaling. Increased TEWL also results in reduced epidermal barrier function and the skin becomes drier.

Keratolytic agents help remove excessive scales by decreasing keratinocyte cohesion and increasing epidermal cell desquamation, resulting in scale removal. Dry scaling diseases will respond to treatment with emollient or moisturizing therapy (such as water, oils, lanolin, colloidal oatmeal, propylene glycol, urea, sodium lactate), which help by rehydrating the epidermis or reducing TEWL, and keratolytic agents (such as sulphur and salicylic acid). Dogs with scaling dermatoses have a higher TEWL than control dogs. Conversely, improved barrier function results in decreased TEWL and improved hair coat and skin condition. Oral zinc and linoleic acid have been shown to reduce TEWL significantly.

Vitamin A and synthetic retinoids

Vitamin A (retinol) functions to maintain normal keratinization of skin and epithelial cells. Vitamin A deficiency and toxicosis have similar signs, which underscores the importance of diagnosing accurately vitamin A-responsive dermatosis (i.e. 'vitamin A deficiency localized to the skin'). The maximum recommended dose of vitamin A is 800–1000 IU/kg/day orally. A frequently recommended dose for vitamin A-responsive dermatosis is 10,000 IU once daily.

Retinoids are synthetic vitamin A derivative drugs that have higher potency and lower toxic potential than natural vitamin A (Figure 6.11). Their main physiological effect is on epithelial cell keratinization, via regulating growth, proliferation and differentiation. Retinoids are highly teratogenic and so the implications for women and intact female dogs and cats with regards to reproduction are tremendous. Isotretinoin was the first clinically available retinoid and has been studied the most in veterinary medicine. Etretinate has also been extensively studied in veterinary medicine but is no longer manufactured. It has been replaced by acetretin, which is the active metabolite of etretinate. The elimination half-life of acetretin is only 2 days, thus it is less likely to cause birth defects than etretinate. Retinoids should be administered with food as their absorption is highly variable if administered on an empty stomach. Side effects in dogs include keratoconjunctivitis, decreased tear production, vomiting, diarrhoea, stiffness, pruritus and mucocutaneous junction erythema in dogs. In addition, hypertriglyceridaemia, hypercholesterolaemia and increases in alanine aminotransferase, aspartate aminotransferase and serum alkaline phosphatase

Drug	Isotretinoin	Acetretin
Formulation	10, 20, 40 mg capsules	10, 25 mg capsules
Dose	1–3 mg/kg once daily	0.5–1.0 mg/kg once daily
Diseases that may respond	Schnauzer comedo syndrome; sebaceous adenitis (especially Poodles, Vizsla and other shorthaired breeds); ichthyosis; feline acne; epitheliotropic lymphoma; keratoacanthoma; sebaceous gland hyperplasia/adenoma	Primary idiopathic seborrhoea of spaniels (probably); sebaceous adenitis?; solar dermatosis; squamous cell carcinoma

6.11   Synthetic retinoids.

can be seen in a small percentage of dogs. In cats, vomiting, diarrhoea, inappetence and conjunctivitis are the most common side effects. Skeletal abnormalities may occur with long-term usage, particularly with isotretinoin. These side effects are uncommon and are usually mild. Switching to a low-fat diet can minimize hypercholesterolaemia and hypertriglyceridaemia. Artificial tears and ocular lubricants can minimize problems associated with keratoconjunctivitis and decreased tear production. The primary deterrent in using retinoids in most clinical situations is the expense, particularly with acetretin.

References and further reading

Kwochka KW (1993a) Overview of normal keratinization and cutaneous scaling disorders of dogs. In: *Current Veterinary Dermatology: The Science and Art of Therapy*, ed. CE Griffin *et al.*, pp.167–175. Mosby Year Book, St Louis

Kwochka KW (1993b) Primary keratinization disorders of dogs. In: *Current Veterinary Dermatology: The Science and Art of Therapy*, ed. CE Griffin *et al.*, pp. 176–190. Mosby Year Book, St Louis

Kwochka KW (1993c) Symptomatic topical therapy of scaling disorders. In: *Current Veterinary Dermatology: The Science and Art of Therapy*, ed. CE Griffin *et al.*, pp. 191–202. Mosby Year Book, St Louis

Nett CS, Reichler I, Grest P *et al.* (2001) Epidermal dysplasia and *Malassezia* infection in two West Highland White Terrier siblings: an inherited skin disorder or reaction to severe *Malassezia* infection. *Veterinary Dermatology* **12**, 285–290

Scott DW and Miller WH (1996) Primary seborrhoea in English Springer Spaniels: a retrospective study of 14 cases. *Journal of Small Animal Practice* **37**, 173–178

Scott DW, Miller WH and Griffin CE (2001) Keratinization defects. In: *Muller and Kirk's Small Animal Dermatology, 6th edn*, pp.1025–1054. WB Saunders, Philadelphia

7

An approach to pustules and crusting papules

Karen A. Moriello

This chapter will review the diagnostic and clinical approach to patients presenting with pustular and/or papular lesions. Unless otherwise specified, comments will apply to both cats and dogs.

The lesions and their development

Papules

A papule is a small solid elevation of the skin <1 cm across. Because these lesions are small and can be hidden by the hair coat, they are often first found by palpation of the skin during the physical examination. Papules tend to be erythematous and are the result of an accumulation of inflammatory cells in the dermis, intraepidermal oedema, superficial dermal oedema or epidermal hypertrophy. Papules may or may not be associated with hair follicles. Papules may or may not develop crusts consisting of serum, pus or blood. The development of a crust on a papule may be part the result of self-trauma from pruritus or be part of the 'natural life' of the papule.

Individual papules may enlarge to form *nodules* (>1 cm across). A group of papules may coalesce into a raised lesion called a *plaque*.

Pustules

A pustule is a small (<1 cm across) elevation of the skin that is filled with pus (Figure 7.1). Pustules are small abscesses. These lesions often start as small papules and develop into pustules as the result of the breakdown of epidermal cells and the accumulation of inflammatory cells at the peak of pustule. Pustules may be intraepidermal, subepidermal or follicular in location. Pustules vary in colour and may be white, yellow, green or red. Because of the fragile nature of pustules, rupture and crusting is common. Ruptured pustules commonly appear as 'epidermal collarettes' (a circular spreading ring of crusts) (Figure 7.2) or honey-coloured crusts adhered to the skin. Pustules may or may not contain microorganisms. *Impetigo* is a term used to describe a pustular eruption in sparsely haired areas of the skin.

Folliculitis

Folliculitis refers to inflammation of the hair follicle. Hair follicles have a 'goose bump' appearance and close examination of the skin may reveal an intact pustule, papule, or crusted papular lesion at the base of the hair.

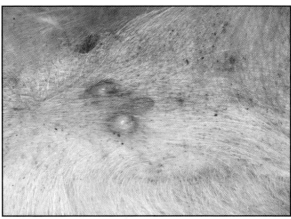

7.1 Intact pustules on the ventral abdomen of a puppy with impetigo.

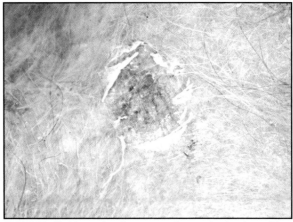

7.2 Epidermal collarette on the trunk of a dog with staphylococcal folliculitis.

Primary and secondary lesions

Papules and pustules are commonly referred to as primary lesions. A primary lesion is simply the initial eruption that develops spontaneously as a direct result of the underlying disease. In everyday practice it is rare to see a patient present with just primary lesions.

Secondary lesions evolve either as a result of self-trauma or as a progression in the 'life of a lesion'. They include, but are not limited to: crusting and scaling, epidermal collarettes, alopecia, hyperpigmentation, lichenification, erosions or ulcers, excoriations, oiliness to the hair coat and erythema. Owners may complain of 'odour'.

Differential diagnosis

Figures 7.3 and 7.4 summarize common and uncommon causes of pustules and papules in dogs and cats. The most common cause of a pustular and/or papular eruption in dogs is a bacterial pyoderma. Crusted papules are more common in cats with skin disease and are referred to as 'miliary dermatitis' (Figure 7.5). As with all skin diseases, the history and physical examination findings are the most helpful sources of information in early case diagnosis. Many skin diseases present similarly, especially in cats, and it is the history, physical examination findings and the results of diagnostic tests which lead to a definitive diagnosis.

Pemphigus

Pemphigus presents as a pustular crusting dermatosis and is an important differential diagnosis in dogs and cats. It should be suspected if the patient has pustules and/or crusting on the face, inner pinnae, nail beds and footpads. Bacterial pyodermas in dogs can produce extensive pustular eruptions and crusting on the trunk; there are, however, a few clinical clues that should raise suspicion that this may not be a bacterial pyoderma:

- It is rather odd for a case of bacterial pyoderma to present with a lot of primary lesions all in the same stage (pustules). The clinician should consider pemphigus as a possible differential diagnosis if there are large numbers of easily found pustules that span several hair follicles
- Cytological examination of pustular contents may reveal rafts of acantholytic cells, which it is uncommon to see in bacterial pyodermas
- Early stages of pemphigus may masquerade as a bacterial pyoderma and failure to respond to appropriate antibiotic therapy should make the clinician at least consider the possibility that another disease may be present.

Pemphigus is discussed in detail in Chapter 26.

Skin disease	Clinical presentation	Comments
Superficial bacterial pyoderma	Impetigo	Intact pustules common on ventrum, lesions will crust and spread to form epidermal collarettes
	Folliculitis	'Goose bump' appearance to hair coat, may look like or be described as 'hives' by owners
	Acne	Intact pustules or papules on chin
Ectoparasites	Flea bites	Flea bites commonly present as crusted papules that do not spread
	Sarcoptes	Presents as diffuse papular eruption that does not spread
	Demodex	Early lesions may be papular
Insect bite reactions	Insect bite hypersensitivity	Mosquito bites are most common cause, enquire about history of exposure; usually acute
Fungal infections	Dermatophytosis	May present as a papular eruption, especially on the face
	Malassezia	May present as oily papular eruption
Allergic disorders	Flea bite hypersensitivity	Most common in a caudal distribution
	Atopic dermatitis	Bacterial pyoderma is common, look for face/ears, feet and ventral distribution
	Food intolerance/hypersensitivity	
	Contact reaction	Can be generalized from a shampoo reaction, but usually ventral
Autoimmune disorders	Pemphigus complex	Large, green pustules that span several hair follicles are common
	Bullous pemphigoid	Usually vesicular in presentation
Uncommon disorders	Subcorneal pustular dermatitis	Rare disorder
	Sterile eosinophilic pustular dermatitis	Rare disorder
	Drug eruptions	Pemphigus-like lesions can develop acutely, there is usually a history of drug administration
	Irritant reactions	Usually acute and located in contact areas, exposure to fibreglass insulation is one source
	Juvenile cellulitis	Early lesions may present as intact pustules/papules on the muzzle or inner pinnae, may occur periocularly in older dogs

7.3 Differential diagnosis of pustular or papular lesions in dogs.

Skin disease	Clinical presentation	Comments
Superficial bacterial pyoderma	Chin acne	May start as comedones and can progress to furunculosis
	Folliculitis	Intact pustules are rare, most common presentation is dorsal scaling with hair shafts piercing scales
	Impetigo	Intact pustules may be seen in cats with abnormal hair coats, e.g. Devon Rex
Dermatophytosis	Folliculitis Miliary dermatitis-like lesions	
Parasitic	Insect bite hypersensitivity	Variable presentations; may present as papules on ears; cat has history of exposure outdoors
	Flea bites	Common on neck
	Cheyletiella	Dorsal to generalized papular eruption
Allergic	Atopic dermatitis Food allergy	Papular crusted lesions on face and body are common
	Flea allergy dermatitis	Neck and caudal aspect of cats
Autoimmune	Pemphigus complex	Intact pustules may be seen on inner ear pinnae or around mammae
Neoplasia	Mast cell tumour	Skin tumours may present as crusted lesions
	Cutaneous lymphoma	
Miliary dermatitis	Focal or diffuse small erythematous crusted lesions	See Figure 7.5

7.4 Differential diagnosis of pustular or papular lesions in cats.

Common causes of miliary dermatitis in cats	
Microbial	Bacterial folliculitis Dermatophytosis *Malassezia* Pox virus
Parasitic	Fleas Lice (*Felicola subrostratus*) *Cheyletiella* *Otodectes cynotis* Chiggers (*Trombicula* spp.) Fur mite (*Lynxacarus radovsky*) *Demodex* spp. *Notoedres* and *Sarcoptes* (rare)
Allergic	Flea allergy dermatitis Atopic dermatitis Food allergy Systemic drug reaction Localized drug reaction (e.g. ear medications) Contact reaction (e.g. grooming shampoo)
Miscellaneous	Nutritional deficiencies (essential fatty acids, biotin, generic diet) Epitheliotropic lymphoma Immune mediated skin disease (e.g. pemphigus) Endoparasites (rare) Idiopathic miliary dermatitis
Cutaneous sign of systemic disease	Feline leukemia virus infection Feline immunodeficiency virus infection Hyperthyroidism Hypereosinophilia syndrome

7.5 Differential diagnosis of miliary dermatitis in cats.

Clinical approach

The clinical approach described below assumes that the clinician has obtained a thorough general and dermatological history and physical examination. In a work-up of patients with pustular and papular eruptions, it helps to keep two points in mind: common things occur commonly; and more things are missed through not looking than by not knowing.

History

Pruritus

In patients with the problem of 'pustules/papules' it is very important to clarify the issue of whether or not the patient is pruritic, and if so, how pruritic. Scabies causes a papular eruption and is associated with severe pruritus that is poorly responsive to glucocorticoids. Other parasitic infestations are less pruritic when compared to scabies. Parasitic infestations tend to be contagious so it is helpful to know if other in-contact animals are affected; lice are host-specific. If owners report lesions associated with touching the pet, cheyletiellosis, fleas and scabies should be suspected. Allergic skin diseases are not contagious and usually respond well to glucocorticoids.

Microbial infections may or may not be pruritic depending upon the agent and the host. Some dogs with superficial pyodermas are pruritic while others are not. Bacterial pyodermas are not considered contagious diseases. In cats, pruritus from dermatophytosis can vary from none to severe and the disease is contagious. Autoimmune skin diseases are considered 'non-pruritic' disorders, however many patients with these diseases exhibit pruritus. This may be due to the inflammatory mediators or due to pruritic secondary infections.

Previous treatment

Response to prior treatment often provides key information. Appropriate treatment for fleas can rule out flea, louse, *Cheyletiella* and fur mite infestations. Treatment with ivermectin at an appropriate dose and interval can rule out scabies, lice, fur mites, *Notoedres* and *Otodectes* infestations. Response or lack of response to appropriate systemic antibiotic and/or antifungal therapy may help rule in or rule out yeast and staphylococcal infections in dogs.

Onset of lesions

Whether or not the eruption is acute or chronic can help narrow the list of differential diagnoses. Acute eruptions of papular lesions on thinly haired areas, especially the face may suggest an insect hypersensitivity in either dogs or cats. It is also important to ask owners about travel histories, home remodelling or their hobbies.

Waxing and waning of lesions

It is very helpful to clarify if the there is any waxing and waning of lesions, waves of lesions, or if the patient seems to become depressed or febrile. Autoimmune skin diseases have a tendency to wax and wane and patients may become febrile and depressed shortly before or during an active wave of lesions.

Previous diagnostic tests

Finally, the results of previous diagnostics may contain very useful information, even if it is necessary to repeat a diagnostic test. For example, no growth on a bacterial culture may be key information in a patient with a pustular eruption that is not responding to appropriate antibiotic therapy. This might be a clinical clue that the patient has an autoimmune skin disease. In general, serum chemistries and complete blood counts are not very helpful in the diagnosis of skin diseases but the information may be helpful in older animals with no prior history of skin disease that suddenly develop a bacterial pyoderma, for example.

Physical examination

It is very important when examining patients with papular and pustular lesions to note the distribution of lesions, the variety of lesions, and the numbers of early and late lesions. For example, in dogs with bacterial pyodermas it is common to find papules, pustules, crusted pustules, epidermal collarettes, target lesions, scales pierced by hairs and scales adhered to the skin. In other words, dogs with bacterial pyodermas tend to show the whole 'life cycle of a pustule'. What should catch the clinician's attention are deviations from this. If, for example, you easily find a large number of pustules widely scattered throughout the hair coat, you may have a patient with pemphigus or a pemphigus drug eruption. This is especially true if the pustules are large, span several hair follicles and are greenish in colour. In the average case of canine pyoderma, you usually need to hunt to find intact pustules and they are still not too numerous nor too large. On the other hand, if you are examining a patient with a papular eruption and you note the absence of any other stages of the life cycle of a pustule, it may a case of scabies. The primary lesion in scabies is a papule and many dogs present with only a papular eruption and a key clinical clue is the absence of epidermal collarettes, target lesions and pustules.

In dogs, bacterial pyoderma rarely affects the face, except in long standing cases. The suspicion of a possible autoimmune skin disease increases in dogs presented with recently developed pustular and/or crusting lesions on the face.

In cats, intact pustules are rare, and when they do occur they are mostly found around the nipples. Their presence strongly suggests a possible immune-mediated skin disease. In cats, palpation of the skin often reveals more than a visual examination. Lesions of miliary dermatitis (small red crusted papules) are often felt before they are seen.

Diagnostic tests

Core tests

Skin scraping: The author considers skin scraping to be a core diagnostic test. The primary reason is to rule out demodicosis. This is a costly and difficult disease to treat. It is helpful to know that it is not the primary cause of the skin disease seen that day, or is not present concurrently. Numerous deep skin scrapings should be performed from lesional areas. *Demodex* mites are part of the normal skin flora, but they are not easily found. If they are easily found, then demodicosis is present.

Flea combings: Flea combings are easy and inexpensive and can reveal evidence of a flea, louse, *Cheyletiella* or fur mite infestation. In addition, hairs can be examined for the presence of louse and *Cheyletiella* eggs adhered to hair shafts.

Impression smears of the skin: Cytological examination of skin impression smears from the surface of the skin, cracks and crevices of lichenification, intact pustules or nail bed exudates can reveal valuable information. Numerous slides should be made and several should be heat fixed with a match and examined for *Malassezia* organisms.

Dermatophyte culture: The author always performs a fungal culture (or repeats one) for all cats presented with skin disease, and for puppies, elderly dogs and dogs with facial lesions.

Response to therapeutic trials

Dogs: In dogs, if the initial skin scrapings and flea combing are negative and there is no strong suspicion of an autoimmune skin disease (pemphigus), the author will treat aggressively for a suspected bacterial infection. If *Malassezia* organisms are found on cytological examination of the skin or ear swabs, the author will treat concurrently with a systemic antifungal drug. In these patients, cefalexin 30 mg/kg orally bid for at least 30 days with appropriate topical therapy is instituted. Obviously, glucocorticoids are not used! At the end of the antibiotic treatment trial, the results of the fungal culture should be finalized and the patient re-evaluated.

Cats: Miliary dermatitis is the most common presentation of pustular/papular lesions in cats. There are two possible initial responses to treatment trials at this stage. The first, and most traditional, is to treat the cat with flea control under the assumption that the miliary dermatitis is due to fleas. In suspect cases, multiple cat households, indoor/outdoor cat situations, or in flea-endemic areas, this is probably the best approach. The second approach is to consider miliary dermatitis to be a manifestation of a bacterial and/or yeast infection in cat. If the owner is practising flea control and/or the miliary dermatitis has not responded to flea control this is a viable second option. Also, if cytological examination of skin impression smears shows predominantly neutrophils (with or without cocci), the cat should be treated with oral antibiotics for 30 days. A careful search for *Malassezia* is also warranted. It is important to remember that concurrent yeast infections occur in cats and that *Malassezia* organisms are smaller in cats than in dogs, and newly budded organisms appear as 'large cocci'.

Secondary diagnostic testing

The choice of secondary diagnostic tests depends upon the results of the initial diagnostic testing and any response to therapy trials. There are several possible outcomes at this stage:

- Lesions resolved, but the patient is still pruritic
- No change in the lesions or the patient has worsened
- Patient initially responds to treatment, but relapses shortly after therapy has concluded.

Lesions resolved, but still pruritic: If the patient is still pruritic, a diagnostic work-up for pruritus should be pursued (see Chapter 5). This may include the following:

- Repeat skin scraping to rule out *Demodex* mites
- Treatment trial for scabies and fleas; this is recommended prior to doing a food trial or expensive allergy testing

- Treat for *Malassezia* infection, if this has not been done
- Skin biopsy procedure
- Food trial and/or *in vitro* allergy test or intradermal skin test

No change or worsened: If there is no change in lesions or the patient has worsened, the following diagnostic tests may be helpful:

- Repeat skin scrapings to rule out *Demodex* mites
- Repeat impression smears to look for microbial organisms or acanthocytes
- Culture of an intact pustule to determine if bacterial resistance is present and/or if the pustule is sterile. Antibiotic therapy should be discontinued for at least 72 hours prior to culture of the pustule
- Biopsy of representative lesions particularly intact pustules and papules or miliary dermatitis lesions
- If systemic signs of illness are present a complete blood count, urinalysis and serum chemistry panel may be helpful.

Relapse after conclusion of therapy: If the patient initially responded to therapy but relapsed shortly after therapy concluded, the following should be considered:

- Initial therapy was correct but too short in duration. Also consider owner compliance issues, dosage and dose errors
- If the patient is non-pruritic during these relapses, consider an underlying endocrine or metabolic disease and test appropriately
- Possible case of primary bacterial pyoderma (skin immune system defect manifesting in recurrent bacterial infections).

Further reading

Paterson S (2000) *Skin Diseases of the Cat.* Blackwell Science, Oxford
Paterson S (2000) *Skin Diseases of the Dog.* Blackwell Science, Oxford
Mason I (1993) Pustules and crusting papules. In: *Manual of Small Animal Dermatology,* ed. PH Locke *et al.,* pp. 60–64. BSAVA Publications, Cheltenham
Scott DW, Miller WH and Griffin CE (2001) *Muller and Kirk's Small Animal Dermatology, 6th edn.* WB Saunders, Philadelphia

8

An approach to nodules and draining sinuses

David Shearer and Jane Dobson

Nodules, tumours and sinus tracts are common signs in small animal dermatology. Some of these lesions may be common, as in a cat bite abscess, or rare, as in the case of some mycoses. Nodules and tumours are solid, cystic or oedematous elevations of the skin that may extend into subcutis, panniculus and/or muscle. Microscopically, they are made up of accumulations of cells and fluid within the epidermis, dermis and hypodermis. These cells may be neoplastic, inflammatory/reactive or both. Disruption of the epidermis over nodules occurs frequently as a result of inflammation or ischaemia. The clinical features associated with the necrosis and inflammation are sinus tracts and/or ulceration.

A sinus tract represents an attempt at rejection and removal of various types of material from the dermis and subcutis. The material can enter the skin by penetration, via the hair follicles, by systemic routes or may be formed within the skin and subcutis.

Differential diagnosis

Nodules and tumours may be classified as:

- Inflammatory
  - Infectious inflammatory
  - Non-infectious inflammatory
- Neoplastic.

Inflammatory nodular lesions

Infectious and parasitic causes
Nodules comprised of inflammatory cells, with sinus tract formation (e.g. abscesses, Box 8.1) or without may be the sequel of a folliculitis, furunculosis or panniculitis (Box 8.2), depending on the focus of the inflammatory response. A variety of organisms can cause nodules, including mycobacteria, *Actinomyces/ Nocardia*, *Staphylococcus*, *Leishmania* and various fungi (Figure 8.1).

Non-infectious causes
Nodules are also seen with accumulations of inflammatory cells without the involvement of microorganisms (Figure 8.2). These nodules may occur with or without sinus tract formation. Debris may be released into the dermis from ruptured hair follicles, producing a 'foreign body' response. Other

Box 8.1: Abscesses

Clinical presentation
Abscesses are common in cats and seen occasionally in dogs. The lesions are usually single, occasionally multiple, subcutaneous, painful nodules, with or without ulceration and discharging sinus formation. Abscesses are usually caused by penetrating injury and infection (bite, claw injury, foreign body).

Diagnosis
Diagnosis is usually based on clinical examination and surgical exploration.

Prognosis
The prognosis following appropriate treatment is usually good. In immunosuppressed individuals, however, the causative organism may spread to involve internal organs.

Treatment
Drainage and systemic antibiotics for 5 days is usually effective. In poorly responsive cases, samples should be collected for microbiology and sensitivity testing.

Bacterial
- Furunculosis secondary to staphylococcal folliculitis and/or *Demodex*
- *Actinomyces/Nocardia* infections
- Cutaneous mycobacterial infections
- Post-traumatic and foreign body abscesses (Box 8.1)
- Feline mycoplasmal abscesses
- Cutaneous bacterial granuloma
- Focal adnexal dysplasia (usually the result of chronic focal folliculitis/furunculosis)

Fungal
- Subcutaneous dermatophytic granuloma
- Sporotrichosis
- Opportunistic subcutaneous fungal infections: eumycetoma; phaeohyphomycosis; zygomycosis; hyalohyphomycosis
- Cutaneous involvement with systemic mycoses: cryptococcosis; coccidioidomycosis; blastomycosis; histoplasmosis

Parasitic
- Leishmaniasis
- Rhabditic dermatitis
- Disseminated infections with Protista

Other
- Protothecosis
- Pythiosis
- Lagenidiosis

8.1 Infectious and parasitic causes of inflammatory nodular lesions.

Box 8.2: Panniculitis

Clinical presentation

Panniculitis is inflammation of the subcutaneous adipose tissue and is not a specific disease. Focal panniculitis can occur as a bystander effect in follicular disease (especially furunculosis) or it can be a process specifically involving the adipose tissue. The lesions present as single or multiple, discrete or diffuse, subcutaneous nodules, with or without ulceration and discharging sinus formation. The lesions may be painful.

Diagnosis

A variety of causes have been reported in dogs and cats and include:
* Infectious (bacteria, mycobacteria, fungi)
* Parasitic (arthropod bites)
* Immune-mediated (lupus erythematosus, drug reaction, vasculitis)
* Physicochemical (mechanical trauma, foreign materials)
* Pancreatitis/pancreatic neoplasia
* Nutritional (Vitamin E deficiency)
* Idiopathic.

The diagnosis is based on ruling out these potential causes through appropriate diagnostic techniques. Biopsy and histopathology/microbiology are essential in confirming the panniculitis and attempting to rule out an infectious cause. A sterile idiopathic nodular panniculitis is diagnosed on the basis of histological and microbiological results. In the future, further specific causes, especially unidentified infectious agents, are likely to be identified in cases that are currently diagnosed as sterile idiopathic nodular panniculitis.

Prognosis

The prognosis depends upon the aetiology.

Treatment

The treatment depends upon the aetiology. Single lesions due to trauma or injection sites can be surgically excised. Animals with multiple sterile lesions usually respond to glucocorticoids, e.g. prednisolone at 2 mg/kg orally sid (dogs) and 4 mg/kg orally sid (cats).

Mast cell degranulation
Urticaria
Angiogenic oedema
Degenerated collagen
Arthropod-bite granuloma
Eosinophilic granuloma
Fatty acids/lipids
Sterile nodular panniculitis
Traumatic panniculitis
Post-injection panniculitis
Xanthoma
Calcium
Calcinosis cutis
Calcinosis circumscripta
Extravasated blood (haematoma/seroma)
Vascular disease, vasculitis, thrombosis
Clotting disorders
Amyloid
Nodular cutaneous amyloidosis
Idiopathic
Sterile nodular granuloma and pyogranuloma
Canine juvenile cellulitis syndrome
Canine histiocytosis
Nodular dermatofibrosis in German Shepherd Dogs

8.2   Non-infectious causes of inflammatory nodules.

endogenous substances recognized as 'foreign' and targeted by the immune/inflammatory response are fatty acids/lipids released on adipocyte breakdown (sterile panniculitis) and the products of dermal mineralization (calcinosis circumscripta, calcinosis cutis).

Neoplastic and non-inflammatory nodular lesions

Nodule/tumour formation is classically associated with the accumulation of neoplastic cells (Figure 8.3), and again may be seen with or without sinus tract formation. Neoplasms of the skin are the most frequently diagnosed tumours of domesticated animals. The prevalence varies depending on the study, but in dogs and cats they represent between 25% and 58% of all neoplasms seen. More than 25 morphologically distinct cutaneous neoplasms have been described. Skin tumours may arise from epithelial elements (epidermis, hair follicles, sweat and sebaceous glands), mesenchymal tissue (including round and spindle cells of the skin) and melanin-producing cells. Skin tumours may also arise from cells of the haemopoietic system, including cells of macrophage/histiocytic lineage, plasma cells and lymphoid cells, which normally pass through the dermis. In addition, neoplasms of non-cutaneous origin may metastasize to the skin.

Other non-neoplastic non-inflammatory conditions may cause nodule formation (Figures 8.4 and 8.5). These may include: hyperplastic, dysplastic or developmental accumulations of cells; excesses of non-cellular tissue components, such as collagen; and benign cystic structures.

Tumours of epithelial origin

Epidermal cells
   Squamous papilloma/papillomatosis
   Squamous cell carcinoma
   Multicentric squamous cell carcinoma in situ (Bowen's syndrome)
   Basal cell tumour (including the rarer basal cell carcinoma)
   Keratoacanthoma/intracutaneous cornifying epithelioma

Follicular hair matrix/follicular epithelial components
   Trichoepithelioma
   Pilomatrixoma

Sebaceous/hepatoid gland cells/apocrine/ceruminous
   Adenoma/adenocarcinoma

Tumours of melanocyte origin

Melanoma
   Benign dermal
   Malignant

Tumours of round cell origin

Mast cell tumour

Plasmacytoma

Lymphoma
   Epitheliotropic
   Non-epitheliotropic
   Angiotropic lymphoma (lymphomatoid granulomatosus)

Histiocytoma
Histiocytic tumours
   Histiocytic sarcoma – localized
   Histiocytic sarcoma – disseminated (malignant histiocytosis)
Transmissible venereal tumour

Tumours of mesenchymal origin

Spindle cell sarcomas
   Haemangiopericytoma (dogs)
   Schwannoma (nerve sheath origin)
   Fibrosarcoma (fibroblast origin)
   Myxosarcoma

Blood and lymphatic vessels
   Haemangioma/haemangiosarcoma
   Lymphangioma/lymphangiosarcoma

Adipose tissue
   Lipoma/liposarcoma
   Fibrolipoma
   Infiltrative lipoma

Fibrous tissue
   Fibroma

Miscellaneous/other
   Fibropapilloma (feline sarcoid)
   Benign fibrous histiocytoma
   Leiomyosarcoma
   Dermatofibroma

Metastatic neoplasms

Many, e.g. carcinomas

8.3 Neoplastic causes of nodular lesions.

Benign nodular sebaceous hyperplasia (Figure 8.5)
Skin tag (skin polyp, acrochondron)
Naevi/Hamartomas:
Collagenous
Vascular
Follicular
Sebaceous
Fibroadnexal dysplasia
Dermoid cyst/dermoid sinus
Follicular cyst/epidermoid cyst/epidermal inclusion cyst
Lipomatosis
Nodular dermatofibrosis
Apocrine cystomatosis

8.4 Other causes of non-inflammatory nodular lesions.

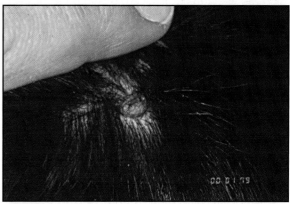

8.5 Nodular sebaceous hyperplasia: one of several similar lesions in the skin of this elderly dog.

Clinical approach

Skin scraping and hair pluck examination
It is important not to forget to perform the basic tests such as scrapings/hair pluckings for the identification of *Demodex* spp. or dermatophytes, which can present clinically as discharging sinuses and nodules.

Cytology
Cytology is a useful screening tool for obtaining rapid diagnostic information but the technique requires some practice (see Chapter 3). It is most useful when performed in practice before carrying out more invasive techniques.
   Material for cytology may be collected by:

- Fine needle aspiration
- Impression from the lesion (especially a freshly cut surface or exudates) or a scraping
- Smears or touch impressions of sinus tract contents.

Gloves should always be worn and it should be assumed that the lesions are infectious in origin until proven otherwise.

If the specimen is acellular, the lesion should be reaspirated or skin biopsy undertaken to gain samples for culture and histopathology. An easy mistake to make is to miss the lesion on aspiration and obtain adipocytes that wash off in fixation and staining, leaving a blank slide.

Microbial culture and identification

The cytology result may indicate whether the lesion is likely to be inflammatory rather than neoplastic. If inflammatory, then collection of material for microbiology may be indicated. In general, a representative tissue sample such as from a wedge incision biopsy or punch biopsy is the most rewarding type of material. However, if tissue grains or granules are present within a tumour or a sinus tract then they may be packed with organisms and some material should be collected for culture. Cytology may already have given the clue if this is the case.

Cultures from swabs rarely identify the causative agent and superficial samples commonly collect secondary invaders, particularly where the lesions are ulcerated. It is important to consider which organisms are likely to be involved, based on the clinical features and cytological results, so that the correct choice of culture media can be used and potential safety hazards assessed.

The differential diagnoses should be clearly stated on the microbiology submission form so that the laboratory will perform the appropriate type(s) of culture from the submitted specimen(s). Subsampling and transport to a reference laboratory for particular organisms may be required (e.g. for the culture and identification of mycobacteria). Apart from swabs in transport media, solid tissue samples can be submitted in sterile universal containers with a drop of sterile saline to prevent them drying out (it is not necessary to submerge the sample in sterile saline).

If an infectious agent is not immediately suspected or cannot be identified, multiple representative skin biopsy samples should be submitted for histopathology. Before placing all samples in formalin, several biopsies should be frozen for future microbiological diagnosis. Histopathology samples should be accompanied by a differential diagnosis and requests for special staining to rule out difficult microbial infections; most pathologists will perform these if the histological pattern raises the possibility of an infectious cause. Some organisms, such as some forms of mycobacteria, are not easy to culture or may take some months to grow *in vitro*.

Skin biopsy and histopathology

General considerations

There are no general contraindications for skin biopsy. Sedation and local anaesthesia are sufficient for most techniques other than total surgical excision of large nodules. Potential bleeding disorders should be evaluated prior to biopsy, including punch biopsy. The theory that biopsies hasten the growth or dissemination of malignant neoplasms is unfounded, but the soft tissue tract through which the biopsy is collected should be removed in its entirety at subsequent excision of the tumour, as tumour cells may be spread locally on instruments or through haemorrhage. The growth of neoplasia is determined by the innate ability of the malignant cells to avoid self-death and thus support their own replication, and the inability of the host defence mechanisms to prevent establishment of tumour foci in tissues distant from their original site.

Biopsy technique

For inflammatory lesions, multiple deep punch biopsy samples may be taken. However, the best sample for histopathology is from an elliptical incision biopsy that includes the margin of the nodule. If this is excisional, the whole nodule should be positioned in the centre of the ellipse. Using this technique the sample will be cut in half along the long axis, thus providing an excellent margin in which to evaluate the invasiveness of the lesion. It is important to be sure that the biopsy sample is removed *en bloc* to ensure that there is representative deeper tissue available for evaluation. It is impossible to confirm surgical excision from routine histological examination, though it may be possible to confirm that there is no surgical margin of excision.

Biopsy of the local lymph node

Correctly staging a tumour for oncological management requires evaluation of the draining lymph node. Enlarged soft nodes may be seen with inflammatory nodules due to antigenic stimulation, lymphatic spread of infectious foci or inflammatory reaction to neoplasia. All enlarged lymph nodes should be aspirated for cytology. If a firm lymph node is negative for neoplasia on fine needle aspiration, a biopsy should be performed under general anaesthesia. Infiltration with local anaesthetic can destroy lymph node architecture. Although the sample provided by a Tru-cut needle might be sufficient, excisional biopsy of the affected lymph node provides the best information, particularly in cats.

Immunohistochemistry

The cell types in lesions can, in some cases, be identified on the basis of cell surface molecules (markers) using immunocytochemistry. This technique employs immunoglobulins directed at the cell surface molecules. These immunoglobulins may not bind to all types of sample and, although some may work with formalin-fixed tissues, most work best on fresh-frozen specimens. These technical aspects of immunohistochemistry may limit the use of this technology in practice but many reagents are being developed that appear to work on formalin-fixed specimens.

Immunohistochemistry can be used to identify the phenotype of the cells within neoplasms. However, this depends upon the expression of phenotype-specific molecules by the tumour cells. Since tumours may share surface molecules it is usual to employ a panel of reagents against a variety of markers; the 'profile' of positive markers obtained leads to the identification of the phenotype.

It is important to note, however, that anaplastic tumours, whose histogenesis and phenotype cannot be identified by microscopy, can also lose their expression of characteristic markers. Hence, anaplastic tumours, in which one might hope to use immunocytochemistry for phenotyping, can have equivocal staining. In this circumstance the results of immunohistochemistry add nothing to the microscopic examination and interpretation by a pathologist.

Neoplastic lesions in the dog and cat

Clinical presentation

Most cutaneous neoplasms (see Figure 8.3) present as a solitary lesion of the skin with or without involvement of the subcutis. The majority of neoplasms are slow growing and not painful.

The clinical appearance may vary:

- Exophytic/pedunculated mass, e.g. squamous papilloma, sebaceous adenoma
- Superficial, ulcerated lesion, e.g. squamous cell carcinoma (basal cell carcinoma, Figure 8.6)
- Dermal nodule (± ulceration), e.g. histiocytoma, plasmacytoma, mast cell tumour, basal cell tumours (trichoepithelioma, pilomatrixoma) dermal melanoma, etc.
- Subcutaneous mass, e.g. lipoma, fibroma, any of the soft tissue sarcomas.

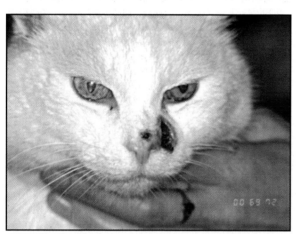

8.6 Basal cell carcinoma on the face of a cat. This is much less common than the feline benign basal cell tumour. (Courtesy of D Bostock.)

Cutaneous neoplasia tends to be seen in the older animal with a mean age in the dog of 8.3 ± 3.7 years, and 8.6 ± 4.7 years in the cat (Goldschmidt and Shofer, 1992). A notable exception is the canine cutaneous histiocytoma, which is most common in dogs under the age of 2 years.

Neoplastic lesions may present as multiple skin nodules. Examples of these are:

- Cutaneous lymphoma
- Epitheliotropic lymphoma (mycosis fungoides)
- Non-epitheliotropic lymphoma (primary cutaneous lymphoma)
- Angiotropic (lymphomatoid) granulomatosis
- Papillomatosis (Box 8.3)
- Malignant tumours which metastasize to the skin, carcinomas, mast cell tumours (see Chapter 30)
- Multicentric squamous cell carcinoma in situ (Bowen's disease) especially cats (see Chapter 29)
- Basal cell carcinoma in cats may be multicentric
- FeSV-associated fibrosarcoma in cats.

Box 8.3: Papillomatosis

Clinical presentation

Canine papillomatosis occurs in various syndromes in the dog, including oral and cutaneous forms. Lesions can be single or multiple and can occur in a variety of cutaneous sites. They can be exophytic, pedunculated or cauliflower-like, inverted or pigmented plaque-like lesions. In the dog, exophytic/pedunculated lesions usually occur on the head and feet. Inverted papillomas occur on the ventral abdomen and multiple papillomas may occur on the pads. Cutaneous horns may develop over papillomas. In the cat, multiple papillomas may develop anywhere on the body and papilloma virus is involved in the development of multicentric squamous cell carcinoma.

Diagnosis

Biopsy, incisional or excisional, and histopathology are required for confirmation of the diagnosis. Immunohistochemistry and PCR are used to confirm a viral aetiology.

Prognosis

Assuming that the individual does not have an abnormal cutaneous cell-mediated immunity, the prognosis is good. Spontaneous regression occurs in most cases.

Treatment

Although spontaneous regression occurs in most cases various forms of treatment can be considered. These include surgical excision, autogenous vaccines, cryosurgery. Other reported treatments include interferon and retinoids.

In the dog there are notable breed predispositions to certain cutaneous tumours. Specific tumours are described in Figures 8.7, 8.9, 8.11 and 8.13. Reactive histiocytoses are discussed in Box 8.4. See Box 8.6 for a description of feline injection-associated sarcoma.

Establishing a diagnosis

An indication of the histogenesis of a skin mass may be gained by assessing the location of the tumour within the skin; epithelial tumours tend to be superficial and exophytic whilst adnexal, round cell and mesenchymal tumours present as endophytic, intradermal or deeper/subcutaneous masses. Ulceration occurs with cutaneous tumours of different types and is not indicative of histogenesis.

Where the lesion is nodular, cytological examination of fine needle aspirates may differentiate between neoplastic and non-neoplastic conditions and differentiate between round cell, epithelial and mesenchymal neoplasms. In some cases, such as mast cell tumours, cytology can be diagnostic.

Histological examination of skin punch or incisional (or excisional) biopsy samples is usually required to provide a definitive diagnosis of histological type and to grade the tumour.

Prognosis

The majority of solitary neoplasms of the skin and subcutis in the dog are benign and many of those classified as malignant, e.g. squamous cell carcinoma (SCC), are locally invasive rather than highly metastatic tumours.

Malignant neoplasms form a greater proportion of skin tumours in the cat, especially SCC.

Squamous cell carcinoma (see also Chapter 29)	
Incidence/epidemiology	Relatively common in both cat and dog. Affects older animals: mean age 9 years; dogs >6 years; cats >5 years. Strong aetiological association with exposure of non-pigmented, lightly haired skin, especially in cats
Site predilection	Cats: pinnae, nasal planum and eyelids
Clinical features/prognosis	Epidermal and dermal lesions. Usually solitary, proliferative or erosive lesion, often ulcerated. Locally invasive growth. Local recurrence if incompletely excised. Metastasis is uncommon but usually via lymphatic route
Treatment	Wide surgical excision/radiotherapy
Basal cell tumour (see also Trichoepithelioma, Pilomatrixoma, Tricholemmoma, Sebaceous epithelioma)	
Incidence/epidemiology	Common in both dogs and cats; 4–11% of canine skin tumours; 14–34% of feline skin tumours but accurate figures quite hard to find for many of these tumours Affects middle-aged to older animals. Dog, mean age 6–7 years; Cat, 9 years. No sex predisposition reported. Reported predisposition in Cocker Spaniel, Poodle and Kerry Blue Terrier
Site predilection	Head, neck and shoulders
Clinical features/prognosis	Usually a solitary, discrete, firm, well circumscribed mass 0.5–2.0 cm, although may be larger. May be pigmented or cystic. Recurrence and metastasis both rare. Occasionally basal cell carcinomas occur that are more locally aggressive
Treatment	Wide surgical excision
Trichoepithelioma, Pilomatrixoma, Tricholemmoma	
Classification	Tumours of hair follicles/with differentiation to hair follicle structures; classified as basal cell tumours with various types of hair follicle differentiation
Incidence/epidemiology	Occur in cats and dogs >5 years of age. No sex predisposition. Kerry Blue Terrier and Poodle predisposed to pilomatrixoma, Cocker Spaniel and Basset Hound predisposed to trichoepithelioma
Site predilection	Lesions are dermal. Cat: head; Dog: back, rump, shoulder
Clinical features/prognosis	Solitary, well circumscribed, slow-growing, non-invasive lesions. May attain large size. Local recurrence and metastasis are rare
Treatment	Wide surgical excision
Intracutaneous cornifying epithelioma/keratocanthoma	
Incidence/epidemiology	Accounts for 5% of canine epithelial tumours. Rare in cats. Older dogs >5 years. Possible male predisposition. Recognized in Keeshund, German Shepherd Dog, collies, Old English Sheepdog and Norwegian Elkhound
Site predilection	Dermal or subcutaneous mass, usually on back or tail
Clinical features/prognosis	Usually solitary but some dogs have multiple tumours, non-invasive benign lesions characterized by pore opening to surface through which grey-brown keratin can be expressed. Multiple lesions reported in Norwegian Elkhound
Treatment	Wide surgical excision. Retinoids have been reported for multiple lesions
Sebaceous gland tumours	
Tumour types	Nodular sebaceous hyperplasia, Sebaceous gland adenoma, Sebaceous epithelioma (basal cell tumour with sebaceous differentiation)
Incidence/epidemiology	Common tumours in the dog (6–21% skin tumours; nodular hyperplasia 50%; sebaceous epithelioma 30–40%; sebaceous adenoma 8%; sebaceous carcinoma 1–2%). Tend to occur in older dogs, mean age 9–10 years. No sex predisposition. Cocker Spaniel is predisposed. Also common in Poodle, Kerry Blue Terrier, Boston Terrier, Beagle, Dachshund and Basset Hound. Rare in the cat
Site predilection	Trunk, head, eyelids and lips
Clinical features/prognosis	Nodular sebaceous hyperplasia and sebaceous adenoma are superficial lesions that may arise at any site. Sebaceous epithelioma (basal cell tumour with sebaceous differentiation) are dermal. Lesions may be solitary or multiple in predisposed animals. Slow-growing, well circumscribed benign lesions
Treatment	Wide surgical excision
Hepatoid (perianal) gland adenoma/hyperplasia	
Incidence/epidemiology	Not reported in cats. Tumour of old male dogs >8 years; but up to 25% occur in females. Also occurs in neutered animals. This is benign growth and is usually androgen-dependent. No breed predisposition reported but common in Cocker Spaniel, English Bulldog, Samoyed and Beagle
Site predilection	Usually arise in the perianal skin (Figure 8.8) but may also occur around the base of the tail, prepuce, caudal ventral abdomen or occasionally elsewhere
Clinical features/prognosis	Present as nodule with or without ulceration. The prognosis is good
Treatment	Wide surgical excision

8.7   Epithelial tumours. (continues)   ▶

Apocrine (epitrichial) gland tumours (adenoma/adenocarcinoma)	
Incidence/epidemiology	Uncommon in dog and cat. Usually dogs and cats >10 years, no sex predisposition in dog or cat. Golden Retriever, Cocker Spaniel and German Shepherd Dog may be predisposed
Site predilection	In the dog, head, neck, dorsal trunk and limbs. In the cat, head, pinna, neck, axilla, limb and tail
Clinical features/prognosis	Usually solitary tumours. Respond to wide surgical excision. Adencarcinomas occasionally metastasize to lymph nodes, lungs and bones
Treatment	Wide surgical excision
Eccrine (atrichial) gland tumours (adenoma/adenocarcinoma)	
Incidence/epidemiology	Rare in dog and cat
Site predilection	Footpad/digit
Clinical features/prognosis	Often malignant and metastasize rapidly to the local lymph nodes
Treatment	Wide surgical excision, castration, oestrogen therapy (transient effect with recurrence after withdrawal)

8.7 (continued) Epithelial tumours.

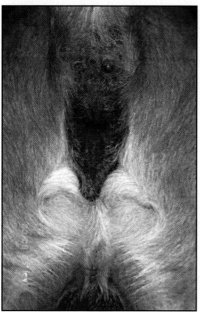

8.8 Hepatoid (perianal) gland tumours – a common benign lesion in older male dogs.

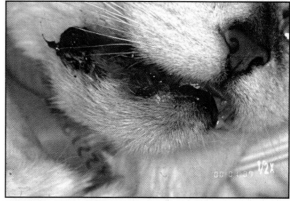

8.10 Malignant melanoma originating from the mucocutaneous junction of the lower lip in a cat.

Melanoma (Malignant melanoma/benign dermal melanocytoma)	
Incidence/ epidemiology	Relatively uncommon tumours of the skin in cats and dogs: 4–6% of all canine skin tumours and 1–2% of all feline skin tumours. Dogs: mainly affects older animals (7–14 years of age) and is most common in Scottish Terrier, Boston Terrier, Airedale Terrier and Cocker Spaniel. Cats: affects older cats, mean age 8 years, no sex or breed predisposition
Site predilection	Lesions usually dermal, and may arise on the head (Figure 8.10), eyelids, trunk, digit and scrotum
Clinical features/ prognosis	Usually solitary, slow-growing, circumscribed, pigmented lesions. Most cutaneous melanomas follow a benign course but those sited on mucocutaneous junctions (e.g. eyelid or lip) and those affecting the digit may be malignant with widespread metastasis
Treatment	Wide surgical excision

8.9 Melanocytic tumours.

Box 8.4: Reactive histiocytoses

Clinical presentation
Reactive histiocytoses in the dog present as either systemic histiocytosis or cutaneous histiocytosis. Male Bernese Mountain Dogs and Golden Retrievers are predisposed to systemic histiocytosis. The clinical signs include lethargy, anorexia, weight loss, respiratory stertor, conjunctivitis, episcleritis, lymphadenopathy, papules, plaques and nodules. Lesions occur over the entire body but the face, dorsum, flanks and scrotum are often most affected. At post mortem examination lesions are present in lungs, liver, spleen, bone marrow and lymph nodes.

Collies and Shetland Sheepdogs may be predisposed to cutaneous histiocytosis. Nodules and plaques occur any at any site.

Diagnosis
The diagnosis of systemic histiocytosis is based on the clinical signs and the histological features of biopsies from the various organs affected. Biopsy and histology are required for the diagnosis of cutaneous histiocytosis. Immunocytochemistry will support the histological diagnosis in both systemic and cutaneous histiocytosis.

Prognosis
Systemic histiocytosis disease can be rapidly fatal or follow a fluctuating course of remission and recurrence.

Treatment
High doses of glucocorticoids and other immunosuppressive drugs are effective in managing these diseases.

Canine cutaneous histiocytoma (CCH; Langerhans' cell tumour)	
Incidence/epidemiology	Common cutaneous tumour in dogs (Figure 8.12), represents up to 10% of all canine skin tumours. Does not occur in cats. Most common in young dogs, over half of CCHs occur in dogs <2 years of age. Boxer and Dachshund are reported to be predisposed to CCH and it is also common in the Flat-Coated Retriever
Clinical features/prognosis	Dermal lesion common on the head, especially the pinna, limbs, feet and trunk. Lesions are usually solitary, and present as a rapidly growing, well circumscribed nodule, often hairless and sometimes ulcerated. Despite rapid early growth, this is a benign tumour which will usually undergo spontaneous regression
Treatment	Wide surgical excision
Histiocytic sarcoma	
Incidence/epidemiology	Rare. Bernese Mountain Dog, Rottweiller, Golden Retriever, Labrador Retriever and Flat-Coated Retriever appear to be predisposed
Clinical features/prognosis	Solitary or multiple cutaneous/subcutaneous nodules
Treatment	Wide surgical excision. Early wide surgical excision may be curative
Disseminated histiocytic sarcoma (malignant histiocytosis)	
Incidence/epidemiology	Rare. Bernese Mountain Dog, Rottweiller, Golden Retriever, Labrador Retriever and Flat-Coated Retriever appear to be predisposed. Male Bernese Mountain Dogs
Clinical features/prognosis	Usually spleen, liver, lymph nodes and lungs affected. Occasionally multiple dermal and subcutaneous nodules. Other signs are lethargy, weight loss, lymphadenopathy, hepatomegaly, splenomegaly and pancytopenia. Grave prognosis
Treatment	None effective reported
Plasmacytoma	
Incidence/epidemiology	Common in dogs, rare in cats. Usually affects older dogs (mean 9 years). No breed or sex predilection reported
Site predilection	Intradermal lesion. Common on the ear, digit and lip. May also arise at mucocutaneous junctions
Clinical features/prognosis	Lesions are usually solitary and present as a raised red or ulcerated, well defined mass. The clinical course is benign with good prognosis following surgical resection. Metastasis does not occur although second tumours at different sites may occur in a small percentage of cases. Tumours containing amyloid appear to be at greater risk of local recurrence
Treatment	Wide surgical excision
Mast cell tumour	
See Chapter 30	
Lymphoma: cutaneous and epitheliotropic	
See Box 8.5	
Lymphomatoid granulomatosus/angiotropic lymphoma	
Incidence/epidemiology	Very rare, reported in dogs
Site predilection	Usually visceral lesions in dogs (especially cardiopulmonary/skeletal muscle). Skin lesion on face, mucocutaneous junctions, elbows, trunk
Clinical features/prognosis	Multiple chronic non-healing ulcerative lesions and subcutaneous plaques/nodules
Treatment	No useful therapy reported
Transmissible venereal tumour	
Incidence/epidemiology	Very rare in UK; rare to uncommon elsewhere. Occurs in young, sexually active dogs
Site predilection	Usually urogenital as opposed to cutaneous
Clinical features/prognosis	Usually vegetative, papillary or nodular lesions of the penis/vulva. Does not commonly metastasize but may be transplanted to other areas of the body, through trauma or grooming. Usually responds to treatment
Treatment	Vincristine 0.025 mg/kg i.v. weekly for 4–6 weeks; radiotherapy; wide surgical excision

8.11 Round cell tumours.

Box 8.5: Cutaneous lymphosarcoma (lymphoma)

Clinical presentation

Cutaneous lymphoid tumours present as (multi)focal or generalized skin conditions. The clinical appearance of the lesions can be very variable and cutaneous lymphosarcoma should thus be considered as a differential diagnosis for many ulcerative or nodular skin conditions.

Cutaneous epitheliotropic lymphoma covers a spectrum which includes mycosis fungoides, Sézary syndrome and pagetoid reticulosis. The first signs of epitheliotropic lymphoma may be generalized scale and pruritus. Foci of erythroderma, crusting, ulcerated lesions, multiple dermal nodules or erythematous plaques may feature in both epitheliotropic and non-epitheliotropic lymphoma in the dog. In some cases lesions may affect or be restricted to mucocutaneous junctions. Cats may present with a single plaque which may be pruritic.

Lymph nodes may become involved as the disease progresses.

Epitheliotropic lymphoma giving rise to multiple non-pigmented nodules in the muzzle/nasal tissues. This dog also had nodules on the eyelids, digits and perianal region.	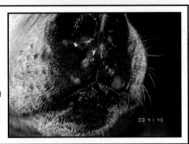

Primary cutaneous lymphoma forming multiple, coalescing dermal nodules.	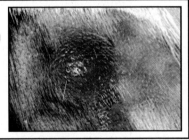

Diagnosis

Fine needle aspirate cytology may be indicative of a diagnosis of a round cell or lymphoid tumour. Histological examination of incisional or excisional biopsy material is really required to distinguish between non-epitheliotropic lymphosarcoma, where the neoplastic lymphoid cell infiltrate is in the dermis, and the epitheliotropic form.

Prognosis

Non-epitheliotropic lymphosarcoma is an aggressive disease which progresses rapidly to involve lymph nodes and other organs and is ultimately fatal.

Epitheliotropic lymphosarcoma is a much more chronic disease that may wax and wane over periods of months before the true tumour stage develops and disseminates to other organs.

Treatment

Chemotherapy is the treatment of choice for lymphosarcoma but both forms of cutaneous lymphosarcoma have proved difficult to treat with conventional chemotherapeutic protocols showing poor initial response rates and short remission times.

Surgical resection or radiotherapy may be indicated for localized lesions, but the disease is rarely solitary.

There are some reports of improvement of epitheliotropic lymphoma lesions following treatment with retinoids.

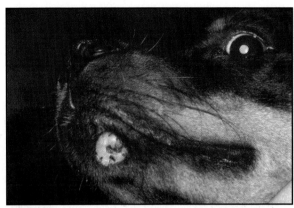

8.12 Canine cutaneous histiocytoma. This lesion, sited on the lower lip of a young cross-bred dog, is the typical appearance. (Courtesy of S Baines)

Box 8.6: Feline injection-associated/ vaccine-associated sarcoma

Clinical presentation

These present as firm white/grey subcutaneous tumours with necrotic cores at the site of previous injection (usually, but not always vaccines). They usually present as masses between the scapulae. This phenomenon is well recognized in North America, where vaccines are now given in a variety of sites amenable to complete excision if a sarcoma forms (limbs and tail). The sarcomas are usually fibrosarcoma; however, some other phenotyes are seen, including osteosarcoma, malignant fibrous histiocytoma, rhabdomyosarcoma and liposarcoma. In the United Kingdom, lesions that fit the gross and histological features of injection-associated sarcomas described in North America have been observed; however, they have not been extensively reported.

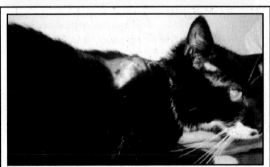

Interscapular fibrosarcoma. This locally aggressive tumour recurred following surgical removal. The site and aggressive behaviour of this tumour are typical of the so-called vaccine-induced sarcoma, although there is no evidence that this particular tumour was associated with vaccination.

Diagnosis

Although fine needle aspiration cytology may indicate a sarcoma, non-neoplastic proliferating fibroblasts in reactive lesions can be indistinguishable from neoplastic cells. The lesions have inflammatory and neoplastic components when examined histologically. Diagnosis is based on biopsy and histology. To date there is no correlation between histological grading and behaviour.

Prognosis

The prognosis is guarded with a high local recurrence potential. Metastasis to the lungs and elsewhere occurs in between 10% and 24% of cases.

Treatment

Early wide surgical excision is essential. Aggressive surgery and radiation therapy are advocated in North America. The role of chemotherapy, in addition to surgery and radiotherapy, is still to be determined.

Spindle cell tumours/Spindle cell sarcoma (fibrosarcoma/canine haemangiopericytoma, schwannoma, myxosarcoma)	
Incidence/epidemiology	Common tumours in both dogs and cats. Although these tumours may be subdivided according to their supposed tissue of origin, they are similar in their clinical appearance and behaviour. Tend to occur in older animals (mean age 8.6 years in dogs, 9.2 years in cats), but may affect young animals of either species. No sex predisposition in either species. Retriever breeds may be at increased risk in the dog
Site predilection	Suggested association of fibrosarcoma with vaccine/injections sites in cats. May be dermal, subcutaneous or arise in deep fascia. Some site variation with different types e.g. haemangiopericytoma most commonly arises on the limbs, fibrosarcoma on the limbs head and trunk
Clinical features/prognosis	Most tumours in this group present as a solitary, relatively slowly growing mass. Often give the appearance of being well circumscribed, or even encapsulated, but in fact are very infiltrating in their pattern of growth. Often incompletely excised at surgery leading to high rate of local recurrence. Rate of metastasis low
Treatment	Wide surgical excision
Haemangioma	
Incidence/epidemiology	Relatively common tumours in dogs and cats. Tend to occur in older animals (mean 8.7 years in dogs). No reported sex or breed predisposition but Boxer, German Shepherd Dog and Golden Retriever may be at increased risk. Possible association with exposure to sunlight especially in short-haired breeds
Site predilection	Dermal or subcutaneous in site. Occur on the limbs, trunk and tail
Clinical features/prognosis	Usually solitary although multiple lesions have been reported. Usually presents as a soft, fluctuant dermal or subcutaneous mass, more superficial lesions may be blue to red-black in colour. Solitary lesions are amenable to surgical resection and the prognosis is good
Treatment	Wide surgical excision
Haemangiosarcoma (primary cutaneous haemangiosarcoma)	
Incidence/epidemiology	Relatively common tumour in the dog and cat. In the dog, haemangiosarcoma (HSA) of the skin is distinct from that of internal viscera (spleen and heart); however, HSA arising in internal viscera may metastasize to the skin so it is important to ascertain that a cutaneous lesion does not represent metastatic disease from a distant primary site. Tends to occur in older animals (mean 9.6 years in the dog; 9.4 years in the cat). No sex predisposition has been reported. The German Shepherd Dog is at increased risk of visceral HSA, but cutaneous HSA appears to be more common in other breeds including Irish Wolfhound, Whippet and Golden Retriever
Clinical features/prognosis	Tumours may be cutaneous or subcutaneous. The site may be of prognostic importance in the dog. Tumours may arise at any site, the trunk and limbs are equally represented. In the dog: truly cutaneous HASs are usually quite well differentiated, well circumscribed tumours which are amenable to surgical excision and carry a favourable prognosis with low rates of metastasis. However, tumours which are sited in the subcutis tend to be more aggressive locally and carry a higher risk of metastasis. In the cat haemangiosarcoma may be locally infiltrating, leading to problems of local recurrence. Metastasis is uncommon
Treatment	Wide surgical excision
Lipoma/infiltrating lipoma	
Incidence/epidemiology	Common tumours in the dog, occur occasionally in the cat. Occur in older animals (mean age 8.8 years in dogs). Predilection in female dogs (entire and neutered) and neutered male cats. Obesity may also be a predisposing factor for development of these tumours
Site predilection	Dermal or subcutaneous in site. Most commonly arise on abdominal or thoracic wall
Clinical features/prognosis	May be solitary or multiple, usually soft mobile, well circumscribed, encapsulated tumours. Surgical resection is curative. The infiltrating variant is not encapsulated and infiltrates widely through connective tissue and muscle. Surgical resection is often not effective in eradicating this form of lipoma and local recurrence rates are high. Metastasis does not occur in either form
Treatment	Wide surgical excision
Fibroma/dermatofibroma/collagenous naevi	
Incidence/epidemiology	Relatively uncommon in dogs. Uncommon in cats; tumours which have the histological appearance of fibroma are uncommon in cats and represent well differentiated fibrosarcomas (Goldschmidt and Shofer, 1992). Occur in older dogs (mean 8.4 years), no breed or sex predisposition reported
Site predilection	Limbs and head most common sites
Clinical features/prognosis	Intradermal or subcutaneous mass. Solitary, soft to firm masses, overlying epithelium may be hyperplastic. Clinical behaviour is benign; surgery is the treatment of choice and the prognosis is good
Treatment	Wide surgical excision

8.13 Mesenchymal/spindle cell tumours

Tumour location may influence clinical behaviour. For example, melanoma of the canine digit carries a higher risk of metastasis than melanoma elsewhere in the skin.

Malignant adnexal tumours (sebaceous carcinoma, apocrine carcinoma) are rare but when they do occur they can follow a very aggressive course with local infiltration and metastasis.

Treatment

Most solitary skin tumours are adequately treated by local/wide surgical excision.

References and further reading

Goldschmidt MH and Shofer FS (1992) *Skin Tumours of the Dog and Cat.* Pergamon Press, Oxford

Gross TL, Ihrke PJ and Walder EJ (1992) *Veterinary Dermatopathology. A Macroscopic and Microscopic Evaluation of Canine and Feline Skin Disease.* Mosby-Year Book, St. Louis

McEntree MC and Page RL (2001) Feline vaccine-associated sarcomas. *Journal of Veterinary Internal Medicine* **15,** 176–182

Scott DW, Miller WH and Griffin CE (2001) *Muller & Kirk's Small Animal Dermatology, 6th edn.* WB Saunders, Philadelphia

Yager JA and Wilcock BP (1994) Dermatopathology and skin tumours. In: *Colour Atlas and Text of Surgical Pathology of the Dog and Cat.* Mosby-Year Book Europe Limited, London

9

An approach to disorders of pigmentation

Zeineb Alhaidari

In veterinary dermatology, disorders of pigmentation are disorders of melanogenic pigmentation; the role of other factors contributing to pigmentation in hairless skin, such as haemoglobin or carotenes, is anecdotal.

Melanin pigments are synthesized in specialized cells, the melanocytes, which are present in the hair follicle and in the epidermal basal layer. Melanocytes are dendritic cells sending connections to a determined number of neighbouring keratinocytes, to form a pigmentary functional unit. In the epidermis every melanocyte is associated with 36 keratinocytes while the bulbar melanocyte is associated with only four cortical keratinocytes. These follicular melanocytes have specific properties. They are taller than epidermal melanocytes and synthesize bigger melanosomes which are distributed individually to the cortical cells. They are characterized by a cyclic activity, synthesizing melanin during the anagen phase, and entering apoptosis during the catagen phase, to be replaced at the next cycle by non-differentiated cells residing in the permanent upper part of the outer root sheath.

The precursors of the melanocytes, melanoblasts, originate in the neural crest. After migration to their final locations in skin, eyes, inner ears and leptomeninges, these precursor cells proliferate and differentiate into melanin-producing melanocytes. These cells are characterized by highly organized membrane-bound organelles called melanosomes in which melanin biosynthesis takes place. Melanin synthesis is dependent on the production of competent melanogenic enzymes. Tyrosinase is the critical and rate-limiting enzyme in melanin production.

Once established, the melanocyte, a fragile cell almost devoid of proliferation potential, is unable to produce growth factors, and is dependent on the neighbouring keratinocytes and fibroblasts to survive.

Ultra-violet light is the most potent stimulus for melanogenesis. It has both direct and indirect effects on melanocytes resulting in an increased dendricity, and increased synthesis of both melanosomes and tyrosinase. The result of these effects may be seen as tanning in alopecic dogs (Figure 9.1).

Pigmentation disorders occur when any one of these distinct and specific mechanisms is disturbed. They are, therefore, common clinical problems. Pigmentation disorders not only have a cosmetic importance, but sometimes have a medical or zootechnical significance as they can reflect systemic diseases or

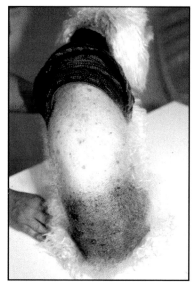

9.1 Tanning observed in an alopecic white poodle incompletely protected from the sun by a coat.

genodermatoses. Their differential diagnosis requires a methodical approach based on the three classical major steps of every dermatological examination: history, physical examination and diagnostic tests.

An approach to hypopigmentation disorders

Differential diagnoses
These are listed in Figure 9.2.

History

Breed
Certain breeds are recognized as being at risk for most non-infectious circumscribed hypomelanoses:

- *Vitiligo (Box 9.1):* This is most prevalent in the Belgian Shepherd, Rottweiler, Dobermann, Rough Collie, Newfoundland, German Shorthaired Pointer, German Shepherd Dog and Old English Sheepdog and in the Siamese cat.
- *Uveodermatological syndrome (Box 9.2):* This is reported mainly in northern breeds of dog such as the Siberian Husky, Akita Inu and Samoyed
- *Lupus:* Lupus predominantly affects the Rough Collie and German Shepherd Dog

Box 9.1: Vitiligo

Vitiligo is a circumscribed melanocytopenic amelanosis resulting from the selective destruction of melanocytes.

Pathogenesis
The pathogenesis of vitiligo is still a matter of debate, though the autoimmune hypothesis prevails.

Autoimmune theory
According to this theory, vitiligo is due to an autoimmunization process directed against a component of the melanogenic system, resulting in the progressive loss of melanocytes. It has been demonstrated in cultures of human melanocytes that melanocyte-specific antibodies are able to induce necrosis. These antibodies have also been demonstrated in humans to correlate with the extent and severity of the disease.

Neurogenic theory
The neurogenic theory is based on the hypothesis that there is an increased release of a neurochemical mediator derived from catecholamines and inhibiting melanogenesis. This theory is strengthened by the fact that vitiligo sometimes follows neural paths, but on the other hand, vitiligo has never been associated with destruction of nerves.

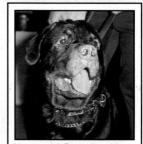

Young adult Rottweiler with acquired vitiligo and poliosis.

The melanocyte self-destruction theory
This theory postulates that a normal compound of melanogenesis is cytotoxic for the melanocyte. A mechanism which would usually protect the melanocyte from this aggression is thought to be ineffective in certain genetically predetermined cells.

In fact none of these theories is fully satisfying and, as they are not necessarily exclusive, several mechanisms could be involved.

Predisposing factors
Various breeds are predisposed (see main text). In the USA, most cases are recognized in Rottweilers.

Clinical signs
Vitiligo is characterized by the development of achromic macules on facial mucocutaneous junctions in young animals. With time, these macules spread progressively and symmetrically, and could extend to the footpads, nails and hairs, without any other accompanying skin pathology.

Diagnosis
Biopsies of depigmenting lesions demonstrate an active process with discrete superficial perivascular lymphocytic inflammatory infiltrate. Established lesions are characterized by the absence of melanocytes and the absence of inflammatory infiltrate.

Treatment
Classically, there is no treatment for vitiligo in animals and the development of the condition is unpredictable. However, in some early cases, glucocorticoids are useful and may give a satisfying repigmentation.

Extensive lesions

Inherited
  Piebaldism
  Waardenburg syndrome
  Oculocutaneous albinisms
  Chediak–Higashi syndrome
Acquired
  Nutritional imbalances
    Copper deficiency, zinc deficiency, severe protein
    deficiencies

Circumscribed lesions

Acquired
  Traumatic
    Physical trauma: X-rays, burns, cold, mechanical
    Chemical trauma, surgical scars
  Immune-mediated
    Vitiligo
    Uveodermatological syndrome
    Sutton's halo
  Post-inflammatory
    Lupus
    Bullous autoimmune dermatoses
    Contact dermatitis
    Any inflammatory dermatitis
  Infectious
    Mycobacterium leprae (humans)
    Malassezia furfur (humans)
    Leishmaniasis (humans and dogs)
  Idiopathic
    Idiopathic nasal hypopigmentation
    Periocular depigmentation of the Siamese cat

9.2 Differential diagnoses for hypopigmentation disorders.

Box 9.2: Uveodermatological syndrome

Uveodermatological syndrome has been described mainly in northern breeds of dog. It is the equivalent of the Vogt–Koyanagi–Harada syndrome in humans, in whom it combines neurological symptoms (meningitis) with ophthalmological (uveitis) and cutaneous manifestations (alopecia and depigmentation). It is secondary to an immune-mediated reaction directed against the melanocytes of these different organs.

Clinical signs
Dogs classically present with a severe uveitis, which may precede or follow depigmentation of the facial mucocutaneous junctions, extending sometimes to the hair (poliosis), other mucocutaneous junctions or the footpads. Until recently, neurological manifestations were not recognized in the dog. Necropsy of a Siberian Husky which did not present any neurological symptoms, demonstrated a subacute

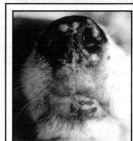

Uveodermatological syndrome in a Siberian Husky, with partial depigmentation of the nose, muzzle and lips.

meningitis, suggesting that neurological expression of the disease could have been missed in the dog so far (Denerolle *et al.*, 2000).

Diagnosis
Skin histology is diagnostic and characterized by a granulomatous lichenoid infiltrate. Histopathological findings in the eye demonstrate a granulomatous panuveitis and retinitis.

Treatment
Treatment involves a combination of oral immunosuppressive doses of corticosteroids and/or cytotoxic drugs with topical corticosteroids and cycloplegics. The ophthalmological prognosis is poor while the skin lesions generally repigment fairly easily.

- *Dermatomyositis:* This is described mainly in the Rough Collie, Shetland Sheepdog and Beauceron Shepherd Dog
- *Acquired nasal idiopathic hypopigmentation:* This condition is more frequently observed in the Labrador, Siberian Husky, Samoyed, Poodle and German Shepherd Dog

Age of onset

The age of onset of hypomelanosis is of major diagnostic importance. If the lesions are present at birth or appear early in life, they are indicators of genodermatoses, such as the Waardenburg syndrome (Figure 9.3), albinism (Box 9.3), or dermatomyositis.

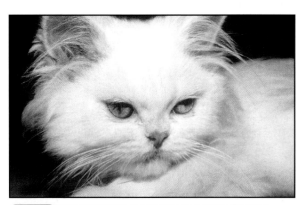

9.3 Waardenburg syndrome in a white Persian kitten, presenting with complete deafness and heterochromic irides.

Box 9.3: Albinism

The different forms of albinism result from disorders of melanocyte functions and are characterized by homogeneously reduced pigmentation usually due to deficient melanin biosynthesis. The defect can be restricted to melanocytes, as in oculocutaneous albinisms (OCAs), or can affect organelles with a similar cellular origin, such as lysosomes or platelets.

OCA type 1

Type 1 OCAs are a consequence of mutations affecting the gene for tyrosinase. The most common mutations are associated with no residual enzyme activity and are called tyrosinase-negative OCA. These mutations lead to the most obvious phenotype: white hairs and skin, translucent irides, severe photophobia and nystagmus. Other tyrosinase mutations have been associated with residual enzyme activity, and are associated with variable amounts of pigmentation.

Temperature-sensitive OCA

Temperature-sensitive OCA is associated with unusual enzyme activity, the tyrosinase being inhibited in warmer areas of the body, and activated in cooler areas such as the extremities. This form of OCA has been reported in humans, and is the result of genetic selection in Siamese cats, Himalayan cats, mice and rabbits.

Chediak–Higashi syndrome

Chediak–Higashi syndrome combines hypomelanosis of the skin, immunodeficiency and bleeding diathesis, as a consequence of a mutation affecting the *beige* gene. This gene codes for a protein involved in the genesis of cellular organelles such as platelets, lysosomes and melanosomes. The syndrome is characterized by the presence of giant cytoplasmic inclusions in leucocytes, melanocytes and other cell types, which impair cell function. Chediak–Higashi syndrome has been described in several species including humans, Persian cats, Aleutian mink, beige mice, blue and silver foxes, Hereford cattle and killer whales.

The development of achromic macules on the mucocutaneous junctions in young adults points towards vitiligo or lupus. Old animals are more prone to develop hypomelanoses associated with neoplastic diseases, such as cutaneous lymphoma.

Development of disease

The development of the hypopigmentation should be carefully documented. Circumstances of onset should be considered. Any trauma can potentially induce spongiosis, which interferes with the distribution of melanosomes to adjacent keratinocytes. It can even result in the death of melanocytes, with subsequent irreversible amelanosis. Any preceding drug administration should be reported.

The location of the initial lesion is of great importance, particularly if dealing with nasal depigmentation:

- Achromic macules appearing at the junction of the nasal planum with hairy skin are suggestive of bullous autoimmune dermatoses (BAID)
- The rostral nares are often a primary site for contact dermatitis
- If the depigmentation is unilateral, mostly located on the floor of the nares, and associated with purulent discharge, aspergillosis is a likely diagnosis.

Seasonality of depigmentation is an indicator for lupus and pemphigus erythematosus, as the lesions in these diseases are photoaggravated.

Physical examination

General examination

Sometimes, hypomelanoses are associated with multisystemic diseases:

- Joints are involved in both systemic lupus erythematosus (SLE) and leishmaniasis
- Eye involvment is reported in leishmaniasis, systemic mycoses such as cryptococcosis, or uveodermatological syndrome
- Blood is affected in SLE or canine cyclic haematopoiesis, a rare genodermatosis described in the Rough Collie

Dermatological examination

A thorough dermatological examination must be carried out to ascertain whether depigmentation is the only cutaneous lesion present. If this is the case, and if lesions are limited to the nose, the persistence of nasal markings suggests a non-inflammatory dermatosis, such as acquired idiopathic nasal hypopigmentation (Figure 9.4) or vitiligo. However, sunlight can induce an actinic dermatitis upon any unpigmented, initially uninflamed lesion with subsequent disappearance of nasal markings.

When depigmentation is associated with other skin lesions, the type of lesion may point towards a possible diagnosis:

- Scales: consider leishmaniasis
- Crusts and ulcers: consider BAID
- Nodules: consider systemic mycoses and tumours.

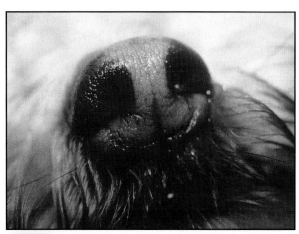

9.4   Persistence of nasal markings in a case of idiopathic acquired nasal hypopigmentation.

Diagnosis

Skin biopsy

Skin biopsy is the fundamental diagnostic test when dealing with hypopigmentation.

- Absence of both inflammatory infiltrate and melanocytes points towards a post-inflammatory depigmentation or vitiligo
- If melanocytes are present, and there is no inflammatory infiltrate, acquired idiopathic nasal hypopigmentation is suspected
- Lichenoid infiltrates are of particular interest: if lymphocytic, lupus and epitheliotropic lymphoma are possibilities; a granulomatous lichenoid infiltrate is pathognomonic for uveodermatological syndrome
- When dealing with granulomatous or pyogranulomatous nodular to diffuse infiltrates, special stains should be used to try to demonstrate infectious agents such as *Leishmania*, mycobacteria or fungal organisms.

Ancillary tests

Diagnosis should be completed with CBC, serum chemistry profile, urinalysis, cultures, serologies for leishmaniasis or systemic mycoses, antinuclear antibody (ANA) test and Coombs' test.

Figure 9.5 summarizes the approach to hypopigmentation disorders.

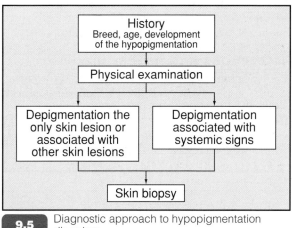

9.5   Diagnostic approach to hypopigmentation disorders.

An approach to hyperpigmentation disorders

Differential diagnoses

These are listed in Figure 9.6.

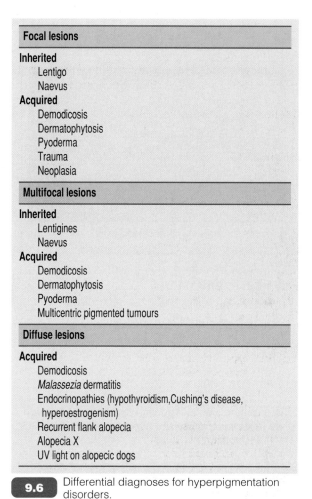

Focal lesions
Inherited
Lentigo
Naevus
Acquired
Demodicosis
Dermatophytosis
Pyoderma
Trauma
Neoplasia
Multifocal lesions
Inherited
Lentigines
Naevus
Acquired
Demodicosis
Dermatophytosis
Pyoderma
Multicentric pigmented tumours
Diffuse lesions
Acquired
Demodicosis
Malassezia dermatitis
Endocrinopathies (hypothyroidism,Cushing's disease, hyperoestrogenism)
Recurrent flank alopecia
Alopecia X
UV light on alopecic dogs

9.6   Differential diagnoses for hyperpigmentation disorders.

History

Predisposing factors

Lentigo (Box 9.4) is a hereditary hypermelanosis. Demodicosis and most endocrinopathies are highly prevalent in certain breeds (see Chapters 12 and 21).

Age of onset

Young animals are prone to infectious disorders, either parasitic or bacterial. Older animals are prone to endocrinopathies and neoplastic diseases.

Development of condition

Circumstances of onset and development of the hyperpigmentation should be detailed. Any trauma can result in residual hyperpigmentation, secondary to an increased epidermal turn-over. Itch is a frequent cause of cutaneous trauma, observed in every pruritic dermatitis, either allergic, parasitic, or bacterial, and as such, is a fundamental differential diagnostic criterion for hyperpigmentation. Usually, a contagious condition is an acariosis or a dermatophytosis.

Box 9.4: Lentigo

Clinically, lentigo is a black macule resulting from an increased number of basal melanocytes, and increased basal melanin load. Lentigo may present as either single or multiple lesions (lentigines). It is the only recognized inherited form of hypermelanosis in animals.

Ginger cats frequently present with multiple lentigines affecting the facial mucocutaneous junctions, which progressively increase in number and size with ageing , and generally end up coalescing.

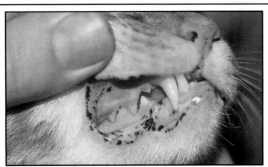

Three-year-old Domestic short-haired calico cat with lentigo simplex.

Physical examination

The distribution of the lesions is important:

• A focal lesion may be caused by trauma, demodicosis, dermatophytosis or neoplasia
• Multifocal lesions may be associated with pyoderma, demodicosis (Figure 9.7) or dermatophytosis
• Diffuse hyperpigmentation may be caused by demodicosis or endocrinopathies. Endocrinopathies are usually associated with systemic signs such as lethargy and obesity hypothyroidism, and PU/PD in Cushing's disease.

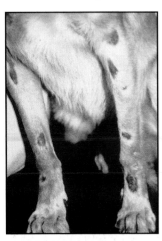

9.7 Multifocal alopecic hyperpigmented lesions in a case of demodicosis.

Diagnosis

Biopsy
Biopsies are usually not very rewarding when dealing with hypermelanoses, although some conditions may be diagnosed histologically, such as recurrent flank alopecia or neoplasia. A biopsy should be taken if these conditions are strongly suspected.

Simple tests
Basic simple tests are the main diagnosic tools:

• Skin scrapings are mandatory in all cases of hyperpigmentation
• Direct examination
• Wood's lamp examination
• Fungal culture
• Cytology should be used in every case to check for presence of *Malassezia*.

In cases of multifocal lesions in the dog, if these tests fail to reveal any aetiological agent, empirical antibacterial therapy is given for 3–4 weeks, at the end of which the dog is rechecked.

In cases of diffuse hyperpigmentation, CBC, serum chemistry profile and urinalysis may suggest a possible hormonal imbalance. A stress leucogram, elevated ALP and/or cholesterol may indicate Cushing's disease; elevated cholesterol is a pointer for hypothyroidism. In such cases, specific endocrine tests should be used.

Figure 9.8 summarizes the approach to hyperpigmentation disorders.

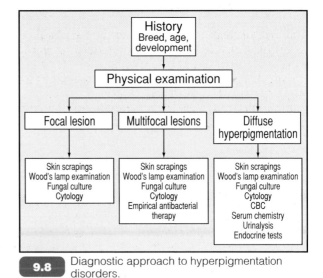

9.8 Diagnostic approach to hyperpigmentation disorders.

References and further reading

Busca R and Ballotti R (2000) Cyclic AMP a key messenger in the regulation of skin pigmentation. *Pigment Cell Research* **13**, 60–69

Denerolle P, Tessier M and Molon-Noblon S (2000) Nerve lesions in a Siberian Husky suffering from a uveodermatological syndrome. *Pratique Médicale et Chirurgicale de l' Animal de Compagnie* **35**, 273–278

10

An approach to alopecia in the cat

Petra Roosje and Julie Henfrey

Feline alopecia is defined here as a partial, diffuse or total loss of hairs. Alopecia can be congenital or acquired and various patterns occur, such as focal, multifocal, diffuse or symmetrical. Feline symmetrical alopecia is a clinical reaction pattern with a myriad of underlying causes and not a disease on its own. Successful management of alopecia hinges on an accurate diagnosis and it is the purpose of this chapter to provide an overview of alopecia in cats and indicate a suitable diagnostic approach to such cases.

Congenital or hereditary conditions causing feline alopecia are described in Box 10.1.

Acquired focal alopecia

The division between diseases that cause focal or extended alopecia is somewhat arbitrary, as many causes of focal alopecia can also cause extended or symmetrical alopecia. In addition, a focal alopecia may develop into a multifocal or extended alopecia. Some of the causes of focal alopecia will therefore be discussed under causes of extended or symmetrical alopecia.

Differential diagnosis

Differential diagnoses are listed in Figure 10.1.

Dermatophytosis
Demodicosis
Injection site reaction
Local glucocorticoid reaction
Idiopathic lymphocytic mural folliculitis
Pseudopelade
Psychogenic alopecia
Alopecia areata
Alopecia mucinosa
Pinnal alopecia
Traction alopecia

10.1 Differential diagnoses for acquired focal alopecia.

Clinical approach

The clinical approach to feline acquired focal alopecia is illustrated in Figure 10.2.

Dermatophytosis

Clinical signs of dermatophytosis are variable and include focal, multifocal or 'symmetrical' alopecia.

Box 10.1: Congenital or hereditary alopecia and hair abnormalities

Clinical presentation

These conditions are uncommon except in hairless breeds (Sphinx cats and Canadian Hairless cat). The clinical presentation is variable and depends on the extent of the defect. Other ectodermal defects may occur: defects of claws, whiskers, papillae on tongue or adnexae (sebaceous glands, sweat glands, arrector pili muscles), and absence of thymus. Affected cats can be alopecic at birth or have a normal coat and develop hypotrichosis or alopecia within 2 weeks and have severe hypotrichosis at 6 months of age. Deposits of lipid material in nail folds and paronychia may occur.

Described diseases
- Alopecia universalis (Sphinx cat, Canadian Hairless cat)
- Hereditary hypotrichosis (reported in Burmese, Birman, Devon Rex, Siamese; Burmese kittens were born without a thymus)
- Follicular dysplasia (one case of a tricoloured Cornish Rex cat)
- Hairshaft disorders in Abyssinian cats
- Pili torti.

Diagnosis

Definitive diagnosis of all the congenital/hereditary alopecia syndromes is by biopsy and trichogram.

Therapy

There is no therapy. 'Naked' cats are more at risk for development of solar changes, so protection from ultraviolet light is indicated. *Malassezia* infections may occur in cats with a seborrhoea oleosa; regular bathing with shampoos is recommended.

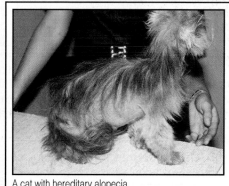

A cat with hereditary alopecia.

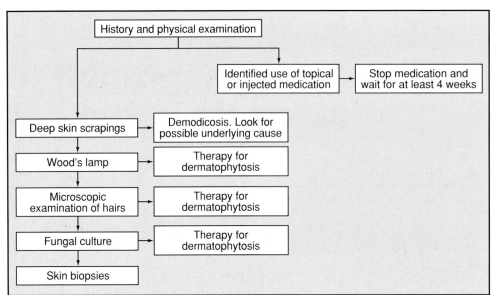

10.2 The clinical approach to a cat with acquired focal alopecia.

Classically, dermatophyte infections are considered non-pruritic but intense pruritus can occur. Detailed information on dermatophytosis can be found in Chapter 23.

Demodicosis
Demodicosis is uncommon in cats. The clinical signs vary. Pruritus is variable and skin lesions may be focal, multifocal or generalized. Lesions consist of alopecia, erythema, scaling or crusting. Detailed information on demodicosis can be found in Chapter 21.

Injection site reactions
Cats can develop adverse reactions to subcutaneous injections. Reactions have been associated with vaccines, ivermectin, praziquantel, antibiotics and glucocorticoids. Lesions are present at sites where injections are given. The inflammatory reaction can present initially as a circular or oval, alopecic, erythematous, non-pruritic plaque. A pruritic ulcerative form has also been described. The panniculus may be involved. Diagnosis is based on the lesion itself, the location and a compatible history. Biopsies are helpful to establish the diagnosis and rule out other causes of focal alopecia. Therapy is usually not required. Hair regrowth may take several months to a year. In some cases the alopecia is permanent.

Idiopathic lymphocytic mural folliculitis
An idiopathic lymphocytic mural folliculitis has been described in cats that have one or more well circumscribed annular areas of alopecia that may be total or diffuse. The lesions were seen on the head, limbs and trunk, and scaling and pruritus were variable.

Lymphocytic folliculitis in the cat is a reaction pattern and not a disease in itself (Scott *et al.*, 2001). There are many conditions that show this pattern but have different aetiologies. Examples are early stages of epitheliotropic T cell lymphoma, feline immunodeficiency virus infection, demodicosis, dermatophytosis, pseudopelade, sebaceous adenitis, drug reactions and food intolerance. The histological patterns can be differentiated to a certain extent by the different parts of the hair follicle or the sebaceous glands that are specifically targeted. To differ-

entiate between these various causes, a complete history, skin scrapings and fungal culture are indicated. In addition, multiple biopsies are important and repeated biopsies may be necessary to document the development of, for example, epitheliotropic T cell lymphoma.

Because the histopathological diagnosis may be associated with various diseases, a specific therapy cannot be recommended and the prognosis is variable depending on the aetiology. Only a few cases and their variable response to therapy such as oral glucocorticoids or systemic retinoids have been described. Spontaneous remission has been reported.

Local reaction to glucocorticoid
A thorough and complete history is important to identify iatrogenic focal alopecia caused by the application of a glucocorticoid-containing cream or a glucocorticoid injection. A local skin atrophy may also be observed. Treatment consists of stopping the glucocorticoid therapy. Hair regrowth will occur, depending on the type of steroid used and the frequency and duration of treatment.

Alopecia areata
Although alopecia areata is said to occur in cats, definitive case reports have not been published. Alopecia areata in humans and dogs is characterized by an immune-mediated attack on the follicular bulb. Anti-follicular autoantibodies and T lymphocytes have been described in the dog. In cats, focal or multifocal patches of non-inflammatory alopecia can be found. Animals are not pruritic. Typical findings for alopecia areata as described in dogs and horses are apoptotic or necrotic bulbar keratinocytes. The intensity of the lymphocytic attack in and around the hair bulb may vary. Therapy and prognosis for alopecia areata in the cat are unclear. Spontaneous recovery is said to occur but may take a long time.

Feline pinnal alopecia
Some cats develop a non-pruritic, bilateral alopecia of the pinnae that is diffuse or patchy, with underlying normal skin. This may be physiologically similar to the pre-auricular alopecia that is prominent in some cats.

Bilateral alopecia was described primarily in Siamese cats in which hair regrowth was described after several months. The aetiology is unknown and histopathology has not been described.

Traction alopecia

Focal to multifocal alopecia may occur after clipping of a matted coat in long-haired cats. The alopecia may be total or diffuse. Hair will regrow spontaneously.

Extended or symmetrical feline alopecia (FSA)

FSA is defined here as either total or partial loss of hair, often in a symmetrical pattern without any gross skin lesions, on the ventral, lateral, perineal and dorsal aspects of the trunk of the cat. The hair loss may extend to the head, neck or legs. Of importance to the clinical approach is whether the alopecia is self-induced due to pruritus or over-grooming, or spontaneous. Pruritus is the most common cause of FSA.

Differential diagnosis

Many diseases can cause extended or symmetrical acquired alopecia (Figure 10.3).

Clinical approach

The clinical approach to FSA is illustrated in Figure 10.4.

With pruritus or over-grooming
Flea bite hypersensitivity
Atopic dermatitis
Food hypersensitivity
Ectoparasite infestation: fleas; pediculosis; *Otodectes cynotis*; scabies; demodicosis; cheyletiellosis
Dermatophytosis
Psychogenic alopecia
Hyperthyroidism

Without pruritus or over-grooming
Hyperadrenocorticism
Paraneoplastic alopecia
Demodicosis
Systemic and metabolic diseases: feline leukaemia virus infection; feline immunodeficiency virus infection; end-stage renal disease; diabetes mellitus; hypothyroidism; chronic hepatic disease
Cheyletiellosis
Dermatophytosis
Telogen and anagen defluxion
Iatrogenic alopecia
Alopecia areata
Idiopathic lymphocytic mural folliculitis
Alopecia mucinosa
Pseudopelade
Trichorrhexis nodosa

10.3 Differential diagnoses for extended or symmetrical feline alopecia.

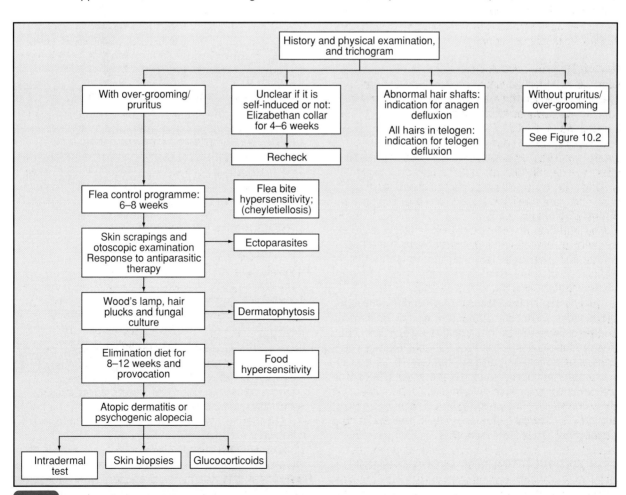

10.4 The clinical approach to a cat with extended or symmetrical feline alopecia.

FSA with pruritus or over-grooming

Hypersensitivity
Atopic dermatitis and, to a lesser extent, food intolerance are common causes of symmetrical alopecia in cats. In both diseases the presence of skin lesions is variable. Differentiation between atopic dermatitis and psychogenic alopecia (see Box 10.2) can be difficult. Most cats with atopic dermatitis will respond to glucocorticoids and have positive intradermal skin test results. In contrast, skin biopsies from cats with psychogenic alopecia will usually reveal a basically normal skin. Further information on allergic skin disease is available in Chapter 18.

Box 10.2: Psychogenic alopecia

Clinical presentation
Feline psychogenic alopecia or dermatitis is produced by chronic licking, and is thought to be due to an anxiety neurosis. Various patterns of alopecia may occur as long as the alopecia is in a place that the cat can reach with its tongue. Usually the skin is intact but sometimes excoriations due to the intensive licking may occur. Although a predilection for breeds like Siamese and Abyssinian has been described by some authors (Scott *et al.*, 2001), others have seen this problem more frequently in European short-haired cats (Willemse, 1997). Cats of all ages and both sexes can be affected. Almost any change in the environment may cause stress, particularly when it affects the perceived territory of the cat. Whilst a new baby, new home or new pet are obvious triggers, marked stress may be caused by a new cat in the area which the owners may be unaware of.

Diagnosis
Before making a diagnosis of psychogenic alopecia, it is mandatory to rule out all other causes of self-induced alopecia. Trichograms show hairs that do not epilate easily and have barbered tips. Hair regrows if an Elizabethan collar is placed on the cat but there is usually no response to prednisolone therapy. Histology of skin biopsies reveals normal skin sometimes with increased numbers of mast cells.

Prognosis
The prognosis is good if the stress trigger can be identified and removed. This is unfortunately often difficult. Anxiolytic drugs may be beneficial (see Chapter 31).

Ectoparasites
Flea infestation or flea bite hypersensitivity is a very common cause of symmetrical alopecia in the cat. In one study, flea infestation was the cause in 82% of definitively diagnosed cases (Thoday, 1990). Diagnosis and therapy are discussed in Chapter 19.

Lice and mite infestations such as cheyletiellosis, otodectic mange, sarcoptes and demodicosis may occasionally cause patchy to diffuse alopecia in cats. The presence of skin lesions is variable. Management and therapeutics are found in Chapters 14, 20 and 21. Some dermatologists advocate therapeutic trials with antiparasiticidal agents (avermectins, lime sulphur) in early work-up of this presentation. This is sensible in regions where infestations with *Cheyletiella* and *Demodex gatoi* are commmon.

FSA without pruritus or over-grooming

Paraneoplastic alopecia
This is described in Box 10.3.

Box 10.3: Paraneoplastic syndrome

Clinical presentation
The dermatological changes are variable and have been associated with various forms of neoplasia. These changes usually develop in middle-aged to older cats that often display inappetence, weight loss and lethargy. Three different manifestations have been described so far but other clinical manifestations may occur.

Paraneoplastic alopecia associated with pancreatic carcinoma and bile duct carcinoma
A rapidly developing alopecia of the ventrum and legs, characterized by smooth glistening skin in alopecic areas, with easy epilation of remaining hairs. Painful footpads that may fissure are also a feature. Some cats groom excessively. Histological changes consist of telogenization of hair follicles, follicular and adnexal atrophy and miniaturized hair follicles. Focal areas of hyperkeratosis (orthokeratotic and parakeratotic) and areas of hypokeratosis are present and a superficial perivascular lymphocytic dermatitis.

Exfoliative dermatitis and thymoma
Cats initially have a non-pruritic scaling dermatitis of the head and pinnae that progresses to the body. In more chronic cases alopecia develops together with large adherent scales. Histology will reveal a lymphocytic interface dermatitis that may involve the hair follicles.

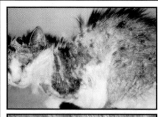
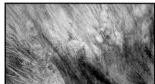

A cat with exfoliative dermatitis and thymoma. The close up of the head shows large scales.

Necrolytic migratory erythema and pancreatic carcinoma
Cats have been described with anorexia, depression and skin lesions on the legs and body consisting of thickened skin with scales and exudative lesions with alopecia and erythema. Histological changes of early lesions consisted of parakeratotic hyperkeratosis, upper-level epidermal oedema and a superficial perivascular infiltration with lymphocytes and plasma cells ('red, white and blue'). In more chronic lesions bacteria, dermatophytes or yeast may be found in the stratum corneum.

Diagnosis
Skin biopsies. Depending on the localization of the suspected neoplasm, diagnostic imaging of the thorax and abdomen and /or exploratory laparotomy are indicated. Haematological and biochemical results may be unremarkable.

Prognosis
The prognosis is often grave because many animals are diagnosed in a late stage of the disease and are in poor condition. Additionally, metastasis may have occurred (e.g. pancreatic carcinomas). Depending on the size and localization of the neoplasm, and exclusion of metastasis, surgery is the treatment of choice. If a cat with a thymoma survives the surgical procedure, it can recover fully with disappearance of the skin lesions. In one cat with paraneoplastic alopecia, pancreatectomy was performed and the cat showed complete hair regrowth. Unfortunately, alopecia recurred and metastasis was confirmed on necropsy.

Diabetes mellitus
This is reported to cause symmetrical alopecia in cats. However, in view of the high incidence of diabetes mellitus in cats with hyperadrenocorticism, all diabetic cats with symmetrical alopecia should be evaluated for hyperadrenocorticism.

Systemic, metabolic and nutritional disease

Hair formation and epidermal keratinization requires up to 30% of the recommended daily protein intake of adult cats. Chronic hepatic or renal disease and malabsorption syndromes may cause patchy to diffuse alopecia with poor hair quality in cats but these animals are ill and should have other apparent problems in their history and physical examination.

Feline leukaemia virus (FeLV) infections have been associated primarily with non-alopecic dermatoses, e.g. seborrhoea, poor wound healing, exfoliative dermatitis and a pruritic crusting dermatitis.

Feline immunodeficiency virus (FIV) infections may occasionally cause a generalized non-pruritic papulocrustous dermatitis with alopecia and scaling. On histology giant keratinocytes are found and a hydropic interface dermatitis. These cats are unresponsive to therapy. Clinical signs of FeLV and FIV infections can overlap and co-infection occurs. Therefore, suspect cats should be tested for both viruses.

Endocrine disorders that can be associated with alopecia are described in Box 10.4.

Telogen or anagen defluxion

Both these disorders are associated with stress caused by sudden illness, surgery or chemotherapy, for example, which arrests the hair cycle. If arrested in anagen, hair loss will occur in a few days of the insult. If arrested in catagen or telogen, hair loss will present several weeks after the insult. Diagnosis is on history, physical examination and results of a trichogram. Anagen defluxion hairs are irregular and have dysplastic changes. Telogen hairs are characterized by a shaft of uniform diameter and a non-pigmented root end that does not have a root sheath. Details of hair structure are discussed in Chapter 1. Depending on the stage, biopsies may show normal skin or all hairs in the same phase of the growth cycle (telogen defluxion). In anagen defluxion, apoptosis and fragmented cell nuclei in the keratinocytes of the hair matrix of anagen hair follicles, and eosinophilic dysplastic hair shafts within the pilar canal can be seen (Yager and Wilcock, 1994). If the cause is removed, the hair will regrow without therapy.

Box 10.4: Dermatological symptoms associated with endocrine disorders

Hyperadrenocorticism

Clinical presentation

Hyperadrenocorticism is a relatively uncommon disease of cats. It may be iatrogenic or occur naturally.

In naturally occurring hyperadrenocorticism, the lesion may be in the pituitary (PDH; 80% of cases) or may be due to adrenal neoplasia (ADH; 20%). Most affected cats are middle-aged or older. Most manifest with polydipsia, polyuria and polyphagia, diabetes mellitus (90% of cats are either prediabetic or overtly diabetic), and thinning of the hair coat. Lethargy, a pendulous abdomen and thin, hypotonic and extremely fragile skin may be seen. Symmetrical alopecia affecting the trunk, neck and proximal limbs is seen in approximately 50% of cases. Hypercholesterolaemia (50%), elevated alanine aminotransferase (40%) and alkaline phosphatase (20%) may be seen but there are no consistent haematological or biochemical changes. Hepatomegaly may be seen on ultrasonography, but adrenal mineralization is of no diagnostic significance.

Iatrogenic hyperadrenocorticism in cats may be associated with focal or symmetrical alopecia. Medial curling of the ear tips may be a feature of this syndrome.

Diagnosis

The diagnosis of spontaneous hyperadrenocorticism is difficult and clinicians are advised to consult their own laboratory for advice or refer to a specialist. Diagnostic tests should include a chemistry panel and urinalysis. ACTH stimulation testing usually gives hyper-responsiveness with a dose of 125 μg cosyntropin per cat i.m. or i.v. with samples for cortisol assay taken at 0, 30 and 60 minutes. There is usually no suppression of cortisol concentrations with a dexamethasone suppression test – 0.1 mg/kg i.v. with samples for cortisol assay taken at 0, 4 and 8 hours.

Another option is a modified high-dose dexamethasone screening test (HDDST). The owner has to collect urine at home under stress-free conditions on three consecutive days. Aquarium gravel can be used instead of the normal cat litter to collect the three morning urine samples. After collection of the urine on the second day the owner administers dexamethasone (0.1 mg/kg tid orally). The urinary cortisol:creatinine ratio (C:C ratio) is measured before and after administration of a high dose of dexamethasone. Reference values for the urinary C:C ratio in healthy cats are 2–36 x 10^{-6}. In cats with PDH, increased C:C ratios are expected with 50% suppression after dexamethasone.

Ultrasonography is a sensitive way to differentiate pituitary-dependent from adrenal-dependent hyperadrenocortism. Magnetic resonance imaging or computed tomography is indicated for visualization of a pituitary mass.

Therapy and prognosis

Bilateral adrenalectomy followed by lifelong medication for hypoadrenocorticism has been reported to be more effective than medical management in the treatment of feline PDH. The prognosis is still guarded because of a high rate of postoperative complications. Hypophysectomy is another option (Meij *et al.*, 2001) with a fair to good prognosis depending on the skill of the surgeon and on postoperative recovery. Medical management of hyperadrenocorticism with mitotane or ketoconazole has resulted in very little success. Therapy with metyrapone at a dosage of 250–500 mg/cat/day orally was more successful in the short term. However, cats may suffer a rebound increase in ACTH and thus increased cortisol levels in the long term (Daley *et al.*, 1993).

Hyperthyroidism

Clinical presentation

Hyperthyroidism is a common multisystemic disorder in middle-aged to older cats. Most cats show evidence of weight loss despite a normal to increased appetite. Cutaneous signs are uncommon but can include seborrhoea, dull matted hair coat and, rarely, patchy or symmetrical alopecia due to over-grooming.

Diagnosis

Beside the history and clinical findings, high basal serum total T4 concentrations are diagnostic. In some cases additional measurement of free T4 can be necessary.

continues ▶

Box 10.4: Dermatological symptoms associated with endocrine disorders (continued)

Therapy

Radioactive iodine, surgical excision and antithyroid drugs such as methimazole or carbimazole. Methimazole is given orally, initially at a dose of 5–15 mg daily in divided doses for 3 weeks, depending on the degree of hyperthyroidism. Cats are monitored every 3 weeks for efficacy and adverse effects. The dose is adjusted according to serum T4 levels.

Hypothyroidism

Clinical presentation

Spontaneous adult-onset hypothyroidism is extremely rare in cats. Iatrogenic impairment or removal of the thyroid gland can induce hypothyroidism in mature cats. If undiagnosed, these cats can have seborrhoea, a dull coat, easily epilated hairs, symmetrical alopecia and poor hair growth in clipped areas. The congenital form has been reported sporadically and affected kittens are lethargic with stunted growth. The coat may be full and consist of mainly secondary hairs or display a generalized thinning of the hair coat with only a few primary hairs.

Diagnosis

In both adult-onset and congenital hypothyroidism a low serum total T4 is expected. A definitive diagnosis, however, needs a TRH stimulation test, a TSH stimulation test, or measurement of freeT4 (determined by dialysis). Because the diagnosis of both adult-onset and congenital hypothyroidism is complex, clinicians are advised to consult their own laboratory for advice or refer to a specialist.

Therapy

Cats with hypothyroidism are treated with L-thyroxine at an initial dose of 10–20 µg/kg/day orally sid or bid. The dose is adjusted according to the clinical response of the cat and post-pill serum T4 evaluation.

Alopecia mucinosa

Two adult cats have been described with non-pruritic alopecia with fine scaling of the head, neck and ears. Histopathology revealed mucinosis of the epidermis and the outer root sheath of the hair follicle. In both cats an epitheliotropic T cell lymphoma was diagnosed after several months. Because only two cases have been described, it is not clear if feline alopecia mucinosa always develops into epitheliotropic T cell lymphoma or whether other forms exist.

Pseudopelade

Recently, a cat was described with non-pruritic and non-inflammatory alopecia of the ventrum and legs. Onychomadesis (loss of claws) was present as well. The histopathological pattern was characterized by an early stage, with lymphocytes and dendritic cells in and around the follicular isthmus, and a late stage with follicular atrophy that resembles pseudopelade (of Brocq) in humans (Olivry *et al.*, 2000). In addition, circulating anti-follicular antibodies were found. As only one cat has been described, therapy and prognosis are hard to give. This cat was unresponsive to treatment with prednisolone at an immunosuppressive dose and showed a temporary regrowth of hair during cyclosporin therapy.

Trichorrhexis nodosa

Acquired trichorrhexis nodosa has been described in two cats, associated with excessive trauma to the hair. A trichogram will reveal abnormal hair shafts with focal hair shaft swelling associated with cuticular damage and splaying of cortical cells. In one cat an association with chronic use of a flea shampoo was described. The problem resolved after discontinuation of the use of the shampoo.

References and further reading

Daley CA, Zerbe CA, Schick RO *et al.* (1993) Use of metyrapone to treat pituitary-dependent hyperadrenocorticism in a cat with large cutaneous wounds. *Journal of the American Veterinary Medicine Association* **202**, 956–960

Goossens MMC, Meyer HP, Voorhout G *et al.* (1995) Urinary excretion of glucocorticoids in the diagnosis of hyperadrenocorticism in cats. *Domestic Animal Endocrinology* **12**, 355–362

Meij BP, Voorhout G, van den Ingh TSGAM *et al.* (2001) Transsphenoidal hypophysectomy for treatment of pituitary-dependent hyperadrenocorticism in 7 cats. *Veterinary Surgery* **30**, 72–86

Olivry T, Power HT, Woo JC *et al.* (2000) Anti-isthmus autoimmunity in a novel feline acquired alopecia resembling pseudopelade of humans. *Veterinary Dermatology* **11**, 261–270

Scott DW, Miller WH and Griffin CE (2001) *Muller & Kirk's Small Animal Dermatology, 6th edn.* WB Saunders, Philadelphia

Thoday KL (1990) Aspects of feline symmetric alopecia. In: *Advances in Veterinary Dermatology*, ed. C Von Tscharner *et al.*, pp. 47–69. Baillière Tindall, London

Willemse T (1997) Psychogenic alopecia in cats and the role of the opioid and dopaminergic systems. In: *Consultations in Feline Internal Medicine, vol. 3*, ed. JR August, pp. 224–230. WB Saunders, Philadelphia

Yager JA and Wilcock BP (1994) *Color Atlas and Text of Surgical Pathology of the Dog and Cat.* Mosby-Yearbook, London

11

An approach to focal alopecia in the dog

Sue Paterson

Focal alopecia may be of two types:

- True alopecia results when the hair is lost from the hair follicle. Any disease that affects hair growth can lead to true alopecia
- Apparent alopecia occurs when the hair shaft is damaged, usually by self-inflicted trauma. In these cases the hair is not actually lost from the hair shaft but cropped short. Any cause of pruritus can cause apparent alopecia.

True alopecia can be caused by agents that damage the hair follicle unit directly, or by factors that cause inadequate or defective hair growth. Direct damage to the hair follicle unit can be mediated by infections or follicular parasites, or through immune-mediated or neoplastic mechanisms (Figure 11.1). More widespread damage to the skin, through burns, trauma or vascular injury, can produce similar signs. Where the hair follicle is destroyed rather than merely damaged, cicatricial scarring occurs and hair loss is permanent.

Hair growth follows an orderly progression: anagen (growth); catagen (intermediate); and telogen (resting) phases. Hair growth may fail through lack of stimulation of the anagen growth phase or through elongation of the telogen resting phase. Defective hair growth due to abnormal growth factors can lead to miniaturized or dysplastic hairs that are often subsequently shed.

Hypothyroidism and hyperadrenocorticism can lead to failure of hair growth and are well recognized causes of alopecia. Sex hormones may play a role in promoting hair growth which is not yet fully understood. Hair follicle dysplasia and endocrine alopecia often cause bilaterally symmetrical alopecia and are discussed in Chapter 12.

Apparent alopecia usually occurs when the animal chews, rubs or scratches an area, leading to shortening of the hair. Close inspection of the 'alopecic' site reveals short stubble rather than absolute hair loss. Non-follicular parasitic diseases and allergy are the most common causes.

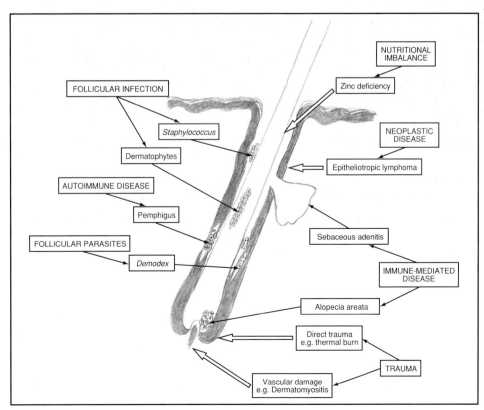

11.1 Factors causing damage to the hair follicle.

Differential diagnosis

Figure 11.2 lists the different causes of true and apparent alopecia.

True alopecia
Failure of hair growth
Endocrine disease
Follicular dysplasia
Hair cycle arrest alopecia
Damage to hair follicle
Follicular infections
Follicular parasites
Neoplasia
Immune-mediated/autoimmune disease
Trauma (direct or through vascular damage)
Nutritional deficiency

Apparent alopecia
Pruritic skin disease
Flea allergy
Scabies
Atopy
Food allergy/intolerance
Contact allergy
Malassezia infection
Cheyletiella infestation
Otodectes infestation

11.2 Conditions causing focal alopecia in the dog.

Clinical approach

Before examining the animal it is possible to formulate a short list of differential diagnoses by taking a thorough general and dermatological history. Pertinent questions for focal alopecia must include the presence or absence of pruritus as an initial presenting sign. With the possible exception of infectious causes, few of the causes of true alopecia are highly pruritic.

General history

Age
The age at onset of disease is an important diagnostic clue, especially when the condition is of long standing and there are chronic lesions. Diseases such as demodicosis and dermatophytosis are most commonly seen in young puppies. Dermatomyositis (Box 11.1) is an immune-mediated disease that causes vascular damage and subsequent hair loss; it is also seen in young dogs. Most cases of atopy occur between 6 months and 3 years. An important neoplastic cause of hair loss, epitheliotrophic lymphoma, is seen in older dogs; few cases occur in animals under 7 years.

Breed
- Dermatomyositis is commonly seen in the Rough Collie, Shetland Sheepdog and the Beauceron Shepherd
- Dysplastic hair conditions are recognized in the Dobermann
- Small terriers and Boxers are predisposed to hyperadrenocorticism

Box 11.1: Dermatomyositis

Clinical presentation

Dermatomyositis is a hereditary idiopathic inflammatory condition of the skin and muscles of young Rough Collies, Shetland Sheepdogs and Beauceron Shepherd Dogs. It is also recognized in other breeds, although a familial basis is unproven in those.

Lesions first occur in dogs under 6 months old. The severity and progression of the disease is variable but the most severe symptoms usually occur at 12 months of age. Skin signs are evident at areas of mechanical trauma, especially the face, ear tips, carpal and tarsal areas, digits and tail tip. Less commonly, nails may show signs. Primary vesicular lesions are rare; affected animals tend to present with erythema, scaling, alopecia and crusting. Ulceration can occur in severe cases.

Manifestations of myositis occur after cutaneous lesions and are varied; affected dogs may have problems eating, and a high-stepping gait. [Editor's note: In the USA, a very similar clinical presentation is found in the recently described post-vaccination ischaemic folliculopathy, in which alopecia is induced by low-grade vasculitis as a late-onset adverse reaction to vaccination. This can be seen in any breed and the condition is managed similarly to familial dermatomyositis.]

Diagnosis

Typically a history of cutaneous and muscular disease in a predisposed breed is highly suggestive of dermatomyositis. Biopsy of affected skin and muscle is important to establish a diagnosis. Histopathology of skin reveals hydropic degeneration of basal cells of skin and hair follicles, follicular atrophy ('faded follicles') and vasculitis. Muscles show signs of fibre necrosis and atrophy. EMG abnormalities include positive sharp waves and fibrillation potentials in muscles of head and extremities.

Prognosis

The prognosis is dependent on the severity of signs. Lesions in mildly affected dogs will heal spontaneously, although they may be left with areas of scarred alopecia. Moderately affected dogs can be treated and kept as pets with a good quality of life for extended periods. In severe cases, where dogs have widespread skin disease and multiple muscle involvement, the disease can be uncontrollable and euthanasia is the most humane option.

Treatment options

Sunlight and trauma aggravate the disease, so management should aim to avoid both insults. Vitamin E at 200—800 IU/day or marine oil supplementation appears to be useful for skin lesions. Prednisolone may be necessary at doses of 1 mg/kg daily. This is best used in short courses to deal with flare-ups although some dogs need continuous glucocorticoid therapy. Pentoxifylline can be used as a glucocorticoid-sparing drug. This should be given whole, with food, at a dose of 200–400 mg every 24–48 hours; 2—3 months may be needed to assess response to therapy with this drug.

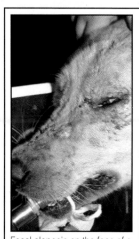

Focal alopecia on the face of a dog with long standing dermatomyositis.

- Sebaceous adenitis is frequently identified in the Standard Poodle, Akita, Samoyed and Viszla
- The Husky is prone to developing zinc-responsive dermatosis (Figure 11.3)
- Two forms of pattern baldness (Box 11.2) are recognized in Dachshunds.

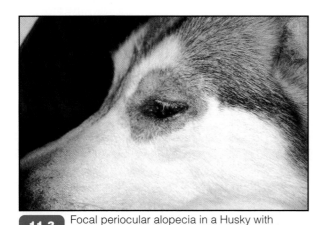

11.3   Focal periocular alopecia in a Husky with zinc-responsive dermatosis.

Box 11.2: Pattern baldness

Clinical presentation

This is a rare disease, found in four forms:
- Pinnal alopecia is seen in male and, rarely, female Dachshunds and occasionally in other breeds. Progressive hair loss occurs from the ear pinnae, starting at 6–9 months of age and being complete by 8–9 years. Chronically the skin becomes hyperpigmented. The dog's general hair coat is unaffected
- In American Water Spaniels and Portuguese Water Dogs hair is lost exclusively from the ventral neck, caudomedial thighs and tail, from 6 months of age
- In Greyhounds hair loss begins on the caudal thighs and may evolve into extensive ventral alopecia
- Most commonly in Dachshunds, but also in Boston Terriers, Chihuahuas, Whippets, Manchester Terriers, Greyhounds and Italian Greyhounds, hair loss starts at about 6 months of age. Alopecia is progressive but restricted to the post-auricular region, ventral neck, ventrum and caudomedial thighs. This usually occurs in bitches.

Diagnosis

A history of non-inflammatory hair loss in predisposed breeds with typical age of onset and distribution is helpful. Definitive diagnosis is made by biopsy. Typical signs include miniaturization of hair follicles and hair shafts, whilst adnexal structures remain unchanged.

Prognosis

Response to therapy is variable and often unsuccessful. The disease is unsightly but benign.

Treatment options

Melatonin has been used with variable success at a dose rate of 3–6 mg orally qid.

Gender

With the exception of sex hormone imbalances, the gender of an animal is not a useful diagnostic pointer.

Diet

Dietary deficiencies are now rare in domestic pets. Zinc-responsive dermatosis can still be identified in dogs fed an unbalanced diet, especially if it is cereal-based. High levels of calcium supplementation may also interfere with zinc absorption. Careful questioning regarding the quality of a pet's diet can help to establish a link with cutaneous lesions. Food intolerance can lead to pruritus and localized areas of self-inflicted trauma. Affected dogs often have a history of gastrointestinal disturbance.

Other

Where systemic disease such as hyperadrenocorticism or hypothyroidism is suspected, a more general history is useful. Polyphagia and polydipsia are commonly seen in hyperadrenocorticism. Reduced exercise tolerance, weight increase and heat-seeking activity can be associated with hypothyroidism.

The animal's lifestyle may give an important clue to the aetiology of lesions. Jack Russell Terriers and other small hunting dogs are predisposed to *Trichophyton* infection (Figure 11.4) due to their contact with rodents and hedgehogs. The presence of lesions on the owner or on in-contact animals may suggest dermatophytosis or even ectoparasitic involvement with fleas, *Cheyletiella* or scabies. A history of failure to regrow hair after clipping may suggest post-clipping alopecia (Box 11.3).

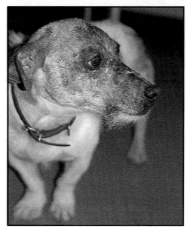

11.4   Focal alopecia on the face of a dog with *Trichophyton* infection.

Box 11.3: Post-clipping alopecia

Clinical presentation

Failure of hair growth occurs after clipping, usually for surgery or dematting, in clinically normal dogs. The clipped area remains unchanged for months, exactly as it was immediately after clipping, covered with fine stubble. Hair will grow back within 12 months in most cases but occasionally baldness will persist for up to 2 years. The problem can occur in any dog but is most commonly associated with plush-coated breeds, especially the Chow Chow and Siberian Husky.

Diagnosis

Diagnosis is based on history and clinical signs in a predisposed breed. Important differentials include endocrinopathies, especially hypothyroidism and hyperadrenocorticism. Specific tests to establish a diagnosis are not as reliable as clinical signs and progression of the disease. Histopathology of affected areas are similar to non-affected areas, both showing signs of catagen arrest.

Prognosis

Prognosis is good. Hair will grow back in all animals eventually.

Treatment options

No treatment is necessary.

Dermatological history

Pruritus

The presence of pruritus is an important clinical sign when deciding whether the hair loss has been self-inflicted due to trauma or whether hair is falling out.

Allowing the owner to grade their pet's level of pruritus on a scale of one to ten can give the clinician a clue to the relative discomfort of the animal. Severely pruritic dogs, particularly those with allergies and ectoparasitic disease, will generally have scores between five and ten. Non-pruritic animals have a score of one. Grading itch also allows a good assessment to be made of the animal's progress when a pruritic disease is treated, especially if the owner updates the veterinary surgeon by phone.

The areas to which pruritus is directed are also important. Scabies has a strong predilection for the extensor aspects of the joints and ear tips (Figure 11.5); atopic dogs often chew their feet.

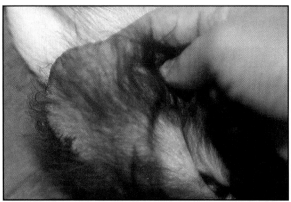

11.5   Focal alopecia with secondary crusting on the ear tip of a pruritic dog with sarcoptic mange.

Seasonal trends
Some diseases show a seasonal pattern of alopecia. Cyclical flank alopecia is a poorly understood hair cycle arrest alopecia. It is thought to be associated with changing photoperiod and hence usually shows a marked seasonal trend. Some animals lose focal areas of hair on their flanks in the winter months, and grow hair back as the day length increases in the spring. Other dogs follow an exactly opposite pattern, losing hair in the spring with regrowth in the autumn.

Hypersensitivity disorders commonly predispose to staphylococcal infection. The infective process, and hence the alopecia, may show a seasonal trend due to the underlying pathology, such as flea allergy or atopy. Pyoderma triggered by pollen allergies in an atopic dog may be worse from May to September. Flea allergy may be worse in the Autumn.

Response to therapy
Response to therapy may help to rule out specific conditions. For example, if appropriate miticidal therapy has been used then this may eliminate scabies from a list of potential differential diagnoses. If antibiotic, antifungal or glucocorticoid treatments have been prescribed, improvement or deterioration may be useful pointers. Many causes of alopecia, especially immune-mediated diseases such as alopecia areata and sebaceous adenitis, will improve on glucocorticoid therapy. Hypersensitivities uncomplicated by infection also respond well. Other diseases, such as demodicosis, dermatophytosis and staphylococcal folliculitis, may

show an initial response to glucocorticoid treatment due to its general anti-inflammatory activity, but will quickly become poorly responsive and deteriorate with continued glucocorticoid usage.

Physical examination
A thorough general physical examination is critical in all dermatological cases, even where the animal presents with a single area of alopecia. If focal alopecia in a mature dog is caused by infection or is an area of demodicosis then the dog is likely to have an underlying systemic disease. If that disease is hypothyroidism, then an examination may detect a bradycardia, or atrophic testicles. Both of these provide important diagnostic clues. Further details of a general examination are given in Chapter 2.

Dermatological inspection

Distribution of lesions
The distribution of the lesions is important (Figure 11.6). Bilaterally symmetrical alopecia has classically been associated with endocrine disease, especially hypothyroidism and hyperadrenocorticism. Follicular dysplasia and hair cycle arrest alopecias may present with identical signs. A general inspection of the hair coat may reveal whether the alopecia is a localized problem or an early manifestation of a more generalized disease. Follicular dysplasia may progress rapidly once the alopecia becomes apparent, but usually remains confined to the flanks. The coat on other areas of the body is usually good and hairs are not easily epilated.

In endocrine disease, alopecia may start on the flanks. If undiagnosed, it will progress to become generalized. The hair coat will be poor, lacking lustre often with associated seborrhoea. Hair is easily lost.

Alopecia areata (Box 11.4) usually causes alopecia on the face, as does *Trichophyton* infection. In both diseases the lesions are well demarcated and show no evidence of involvement of the rest of the body. Atopy and demodicosis can produce alopecia on the feet and face. The alopecia associated with uninfected atopy is apparent and is created by chewing. In demodicosis, true alopecia is caused by the follicular damage induced by the mites (Figure 11.7).

Apparent alopecia *versus* true alopecia

- In apparent alopecia, close examination of the area of hair loss reveals short stubbly hair. Attempts to pull out hair from the border of the lesion require some effort
- In true alopecia there is no stubble and hair can be easily epilated from the periphery.

Primary and secondary lesions
In follicular dysplasia, hair cycle arrest alopecia and endocrine disease there are often no accompanying lesions and the skin is not inflamed, unless complicated by secondary infection.

Pustules: Pustules are commonly seen in cases of pyoderma and in autoimmune skin diseases such as pemphigus. However pustules are not evident in all

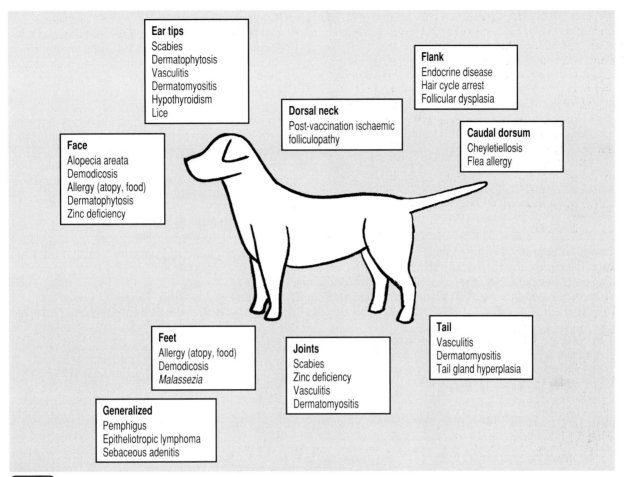

Ear tips
Scabies
Dermatophytosis
Vasculitis
Dermatomyositis
Hypothyroidism
Lice

Flank
Endocrine disease
Hair cycle arrest
Follicular dysplasia

Dorsal neck
Post-vaccination ischaemic
folliculopathy

Caudal dorsum
Cheyletiellosis
Flea allergy

Face
Alopecia areata
Demodicosis
Allergy (atopy, food)
Dermatophytosis
Zinc deficiency

Feet
Allergy (atopy, food)
Demodicosis
Malassezia

Joints
Scabies
Zinc deficiency
Vasculitis
Dermatomyositis

Tail
Vasculitis
Dermatomyositis
Tail gland hyperplasia

Generalized
Pemphigus
Epitheliotropic lymphoma
Sebaceous adenitis

11.6   Areas of predilection for canine focal alopecia of different origins.

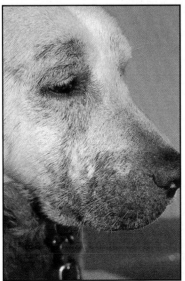

11.7   Focal alopecia with secondary hyperpigmentation on the face of a dog with adult onset demodicosis.

Box 11.4: Alopecia areata

Clinical presentation
This is a rare disease presenting with focal or multifocal patches of non-pruritic non-inflammatory alopecia. No sex or age predilection is recognized; Dachshunds may be predisposed. Lesions may occur at any site but the head, neck and trunk are often involved. Rarely, alopecia may be generalized. Hair regrowth can be spontaneous. Initial regrowth may be white, later reverting to original hair colour.

The pathogenesis is complex. Immunological damage to the anagen hair follicle is mediated by both anti-follicular autoantibodies and T lymphocytes..

Diagnosis
Microscope examination of hairs plucked from the periphery of alopecic areas reveals telogen, dysplastic and 'exclamation point' hairs (the end of the shaft tapers proximally). Definitive diagnosis is made from examination of a biopsy sample, though typical signs may be difficult to find. Multiple samples should be taken from the advancing edges of early lesions. Histopathology reveals peribulbar accumulations of mononuclear cells – the classical 'swarm of bees'.

Prognosis
The prognosis is good. Most patients recover spontaneously although it may take months to years.

Treatment options
Anecdotal evidence suggests that topical, intralesional or systemic treatment may be beneficial. Treatments used in man, in addition to glucocorticoids, include contact sensitizers, ciclosporin and photodynamic therapy. These therapies are unproven in dogs.

bacterial infections (Figure 11.8). In short coat folliculitis which typically produces patches of alopecia on the dorsum, the infective process rarely produces primary lesions. However the ease of epilation of hairs, accompanied by inflammation in the skin and the presence of follicular casts on the hairs suggest a follicular insult, possibly of an infectious nature.

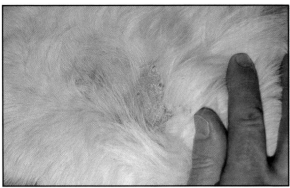

11.8 Focal alopecia on the dorsum of a dog with a superficial spreading pyoderma.

Follicular casts: Follicular casts are often identified on hair pluckings. Their presence might indicate follicular bacterial infection, but one should also consider demodicosis, dermatophytosis, sebaceous adenitis and hair cycle arrest alopecia.

Comedones: Comedones can be associated with alopecia secondary to demodicosis. They may also be seen with dermatophytosis, hyperadrenocorticism, hypothyroidism or long-term glucocorticoid usage.

Diagnosis

The approach to an apparent alopecia is very different to one for a true alopecia. The degree of pruritus present provides the single biggest clue as to whether hair is falling out or being pulled out. If this information cannot be gleaned from the owner or the history is thought to be unreliable, examination of hair pluckings gives an immediate indication. Pruritus can be clearly demonstrated if there is trauma to the hair tips on pluckings. Investigation at this stage should follow that outlined in Chapter 5 for an approach to pruritus. Where there is no evidence of damage to the hair tips then investigations should be directed to causes of follicular insult causing hair loss.

Skin scrapings and fungal cultures
Skin scrapings and fungal cultures should be obligatory in all cases of focal alopecia to rule out demodectic mange (see Chapter 21) and dermatophytosis (see Chapter 23).

Cytology
Where primary lesions are present, impression smears and pustule cytology may give an indication of an immune-mediated, neoplastic or infectious disorder.

Hair plucks
Hair plucks allow assessment of the stage of growth of the hair, and examination of the shaft as well as the hair tip.

- Telogen hair bulbs predominate in endocrine disease and often in hair cycle arrest alopecia
- Pigment incontinence may be visible in the hair shafts of dogs with colour-linked follicular dysplasia
- Typical 'exclamation mark' hairs are seen in alopecia areata
- Dermatophyte spores may be observed on the hair shafts of dogs with fungal infections. Staining with lactophenol cotton blue may highlight these
- Follicular casts are markers of a range of follicular disorders, particularly demodicosis, dermatophytosis, sebaceous adenitis and some endocrine diseases.

Endocrine function tests
Where the history and presenting signs are suggestive of a hormonal disorder, endocrine function tests are indicated (see Chapter 3).

Skin biopsy
Skin biopsy should never be performed as a substitute for more routine investigations. Biopsy samples should be obtained:

- When there are follicular casts but parasites and infectious agents cannot be demonstrated
- When there are high numbers of telogen hairs but endocrine function is normal
- When there is evidence of shaft defects, including pigmentary incontinence
- When a neoplastic lesion is suspected
- When disease has not responded to conventional therapy
- To establish a diagnosis where expensive or potentially dangerous drugs are to be used.

Samples for histopathology should be taken from a variety of sites. Early lesions should be sampled where possible, and biopsies should be taken from the middle as well as the periphery of expanding lesions. It is important to use a pathologist who is experienced in dermatohistopathology and to provide the pathologist with a full clinical history and potential differential diagnoses when submitting samples.

Further reading

Gross TL, Stannard AA and Yager JA (1997) An anatomical classification of folliculitis. *Veterinary Dermatology* **8,** 147–156

Paradis M (2000) Melatonin therapy for canine alopecia. In: *Kirk's Current Veterinary Therapy XIII,* ed. JD Bonagura, pp. 546–549. WB Saunders, Philadelphia

Scott DW, Miller WH and Griffin CE (2001) *Muller and Kirk's Small Animal Dermatology,* 6th edn, WB Saunders, Philadelphia

Stannard AA and Gross TL (1994) Non infectious folliculitis. *Proceedings of the 11th Annual Congress of the European Society of Veterinary Dermatology,* pp. 37–38a, Bordeaux, France.

Yager JA and Scott DW (1993) The skin and appendages. In: *Pathology of Domestic Animals, Vol 1,* 4th edn, ed. KVF Jubb, et al., pp. 550–551. Academic Press, San Diego

12

An approach to symmetrical alopecia in the dog

Manon Paradis and Rosario Cerundolo

Symmetrical alopecia in the dog is a frequent reason for veterinary consultation. The major cause of alopecia in the dog is self-trauma associated with pruritus, often caused by hypersensitivity or parasitism. If the alopecic dog presents a significant degree of pruritus, this should be investigated first (see Chapter 5). Alopecia due to infections such as dermatophytosis, demodicosis and bacterial folliculitis can be either pruritic or non-pruritic. In these instances, the hair may be physically damaged from licking, rubbing or scratching, or it may be more easily removed because of infection or inflammation within the hair follicle. Non-inflammatory alopecia in dogs is typically non-pruritic, and has several aetiologies. Although a large portion of these are due to endocrinopathies (hypothyroidism, hyperadrenocorticism, sex hormone imbalances), many are not, in spite of their 'endocrine pattern'.

The aim of this chapter is to provide the clinician with a clinical approach to the non-pruritic dog with symmetrical alopecia. For some of these disorders, the diagnosis is straightforward. However, for other disorders the final diagnosis can be more difficult to establish. Discussion is restricted to diseases of the endocrine glands and of the hair follicle units.

Differential diagnosis

Classification of the numerous disorders manifested clinically by symmetrical alopecia is difficult and debatable in part because of the significant overlap between categories. For example, entities such as canine recurrent flank alopecia and alopecia X can be grouped under genetically programmed acquired alopecia, endocrinopathies or follicular dysplasia. They are discussed in this chapter under endocrine disorders, since hormonal imbalance is at least part of the disorders. In addition, it is appropriate to dissociate them from other types of follicular dysplasia which have specific clinical presentations and histopathological changes.

Figure 12.1 shows an approach to the evaluation of non-pruritic symmetrical alopecia in dogs. For each case of symmetrical alopecia, a list of differential diagnoses should be established so that dermatological investigations can be selected on a rational basis.

Clinical approach

A complete history should be taken and a general physical examination conducted in order to detect any

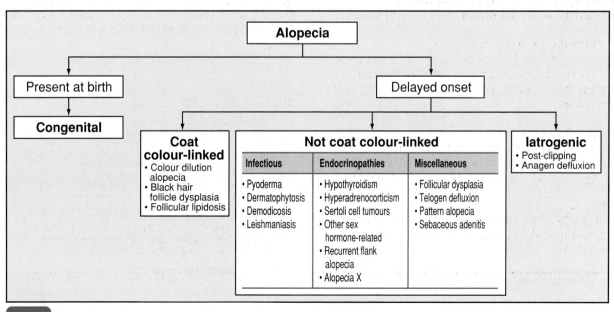

12.1 Evaluation of canine non-pruritic symmetrical alopecia.

abnormality present in other organs. A history of poly-uria–polydipsia, the presence of a pendulous abdomen or abnormal genitalia (testicular asymmetry or crypt-orchidism, vulvar enlargement) may greatly influence further tests to be carried out. The history and derma-tological examination should allow the clinician to rule in or out the presence of pruritus. If present, it should be investigated first, as described in Chapter 5. If pruritus is absent or minimal, then one should determine whether the pattern of hair loss is focal or symmetrical and diffuse. Skin scrapings and dermatophyte culture are routinely performed to rule in or out diseases such as demodicosis and dermatophytosis.

If alopecia is symmetrical and diffuse, one should look for the presence of inflammation and/or any pri-mary lesions such as papules and pustules. If active skin lesions are present, skin scrapings, skin cytology and dermatophyte cultures should be performed. If pruritus, inflammation or any other primary lesions are absent, the next most pertinent diagnostic procedure to perform will be influenced by age of onset, breed and sexual status.

Signalment and history

Consideration of the dog's age at the time of onset of alopecia, the rate of development of the alopecia, its spontaneous resolution or progression and the pres-ence of a cyclical pattern will help in compiling a list of differential diagnoses.

Age and time of onset

The onset of alopecia should always be related to the dog's age and any physiological and/or pathological event, management change or treatment.

Alopecia sometimes occurs a few weeks after phys-iological events, such as pregnancy and lactation, or pathological events, such as severe systemic disease, shock or surgery (e.g. telogen defluxion). Alopecia may also occur a few days after administration of cytotoxic agents such as methotrexate and cyclophos-phamide, or toxic substances, such as selenium, thal-lium and arsenic (e.g. anagen defluxion), although this is quite rare.

Failure of hair regrowth after clipping is suggestive of either hypothyroidism, hyperadrenocorticism or alo-pecia X. In Nordic breeds it is a common finding, as in these breeds the hair follicle cycle is longer than in other breeds.

Many disorders have an age at onset that is quite variable. Congenital alopecia is present at birth; demodicosis usually occurs before 1 year of age and hypothyroidism typically develops after 3 years of age. Hyperadrenocorticism occurs generally in middle-aged to old dogs.

Spontaneous remission

Spontaneous remission usually occurs in canine recur-rent flank alopecia, anagen and telogen defluxion, and post-clipping alopecia not secondary to endocrino-pathies. Although clinical signs in hyperadrenocorti-cism can initially wax and wane, alopecia usually does not regress spontaneously.

Breed

Certain breeds are predisposed to alopecic conditions such as hypothyroidism, alopecia X, pattern alopecia and canine recurrent flank alopecia. Figure 12.2 lists the breed predisposition to diseases presenting with symmetrical alopecia.

Coat colour

Coat colour may provide useful diagnostic information in pigment-related alopecia such as black hair follicular dysplasia, colour dilution alopecia and follicular lipid-osis. Careful evaluation of the coat may be required, as some dilute colours are subtle.

Sexual status

Sertoli cell tumours in dogs and hyperoestrogenism may also lead to alopecia. Lack of oestrous cycle may be seen in hypothyroidism or hyperadrenocorticism.

Further investigation

If the results of the above investigations have failed to produce a definitive diagnosis, further tests are neces-sary. These should be selected according to the index

Alopecia X	Alaskan Malamute, Chow Chow, Keeshond, Pomeranian, Poodle, Samoyed, Siberian Husky
Colour dilution alopecia (CDA)	Bernese Mountain Dog, Chihuahua, Chow Chow, Dachshund, Dobermann, Great Dane, Italian Greyhound, Newfoundland, Poodle, Miniature Pinscher, Saluki, Shetland Sheepdog, Schipperke, Silky Terrier, Staffordshire Bull Terrier, Whippet and Yorkshire Terrier
Follicular dysplasia (other than alopecia X, CRFA, BHFD and CDA)	Curly-coated Retriever, Dobermann, Irish Water Spaniel, Portuguese Water Dog
Hypothyroidism	Airedale, Beagle, Dobermann, Golden Retriever, Great Dane, Irish Setter, Old English Sheepdog
Hyperadrenocorticism	Boston Terrier, Boxer, Poodles
Pattern alopecia	Boston Terrier, Boxer, Chihuahua, Dachshund, Greyhound, Miniature Pinscher, Whippet
Recurrent flank alopecia (CRFA)	Airedale, Bearded Collie, Boxer, Bouvier des Flandres, English and French Bulldogs, Golden and Labrador Retrievers, Griffon Korthal, Schnauzer
Sebaceous adenitis	Akita Inu, Belgian Sheepdog, Border Collie, Chow Chow, English Springer Spaniel, German Shepherd Dog, Samoyed, Standard Poodle, Vizsla

12.2 Most common breeds predisposed to diseases presenting with symmetrical alopecia. (All of these conditions can also be seen in cross breeds.)

of suspicion. Haematology, biochemistry and urinalysis may be useful to evaluate the general health status of adult dogs with a permanent or recurrent alopecic condition or if a systemic disease, which may lead to alopecia, is suspected. Hormonal tests should be carried out if the clinical signs and results of blood and urinalysis suggest an endocrinopathy.

Endocrine alopecias

An endocrine aetiology should always be suspected in dogs with an adult-onset, bilateral, non-pruritic, symmetrical alopecia characterized by failure of hair regrowth after clipping, easily epilated hairs, cutaneous hyperpigmentation, presence of comedones, bacterial infections and/or the concurrent presence of systemic clinical signs (Figure 12.3). Once an endocrine aetiology is considered likely the clinician should investigate for hypothyroidism (Box 12.1), hyperadrenocorticism (Box 12.2 and Figure 12.4) or, in the intact male, Sertoli cell tumour (Box 12.3).

Other symmetrical alopecias that are believed to involve an endocrine aetiology include canine recurrent flank alopecia (Box 12.4) and alopecia X (Box 12.5).

Condition	Underlying pathology	Age of onset	Cutaneous signs apart from alopecia	Systemic signs	Laboratory findings	Diagnostic tests	Therapy
Hypothyroidism	Lymphocytic thyroiditis	Middle age	Myxoedema, seborrhoea	Lethargy, obesity	↑ Cholesterol	↓ total T4, ↓ free T4 ↑ TSH	Levothyroxine
Hyperadreno-corticism	Pituitary or adrenal neoplasia	Adult/old	Atrophic skin, calcinosis cutis, comedones, prominent cutaneous blood vessels	Polyuria, polydipsia, polyphagia, panting, muscle atrophy, myotonia, pot-belly, lethargy, testicular atrophy, abnormal oestrus	↑ Cholesterol, ↑ ALK, ↑ ALT, stress leucogram, isosthenuria	Abnormal cortisol response to ACTH stimulation, LDDS, HDDS; ↑ urinary C/C ratio; ultrasonography	Surgical: adrenalectomy, transsphenoidal hypophysectomy Medical: mitotane, ketoconazole, selegiline, trilostane
Hyper-oestrogenism in males	Sertoli cell tumour, seminoma, interstitial cell tumour	Adult	Hyperpigmentation, seborrhoea, linear preputial dermatosis, gynaecomastia	Behavioural disturbance: attractiveness of affected male to other males	Anaemia	↑ Basal oestrogen concentration	Surgical neutering
Hyper-oestrogenism in females	Ovarian cyst or functional neoplasia, exogenous oestrogen administration	Adult	Hyperpigmentation, enlarged vulva and nipples	Abnormal oestrus, aggressiveness and mounting behaviour towards other bitches	Anaemia	↑ Basal oestrogen concentration	Surgical neutering
Canine recurrent flank alopecia	Unknown	Adult	Hyperpigmentation	None	None	Skin biopsy	Melatonin
Alopecia X	Unknown	Adult	Hyperpigmentation, hair regrowth at the biopsy site	None	None	Abnormal 17-OHP response to ACTH stimulation	Trilostane Mitotane

12.3 Differential characteristics and treatment in endocrine alopecias.

Box 12.1: Hypothyroidism

Hypothyroidism is the most common canine endocrinopathy. However, due to the diversity of the clinical signs and to the lack of a perfect diagnostic test, hypothyroidism is also the most commonly misdiagnosed endocrinopathy in this species.

Pathogenesis

The most common cause of canine thyroid dysfunction is lymphocytic thyroiditis, which is genetically programmed (Scott-Moncrieff and Guptill-Yoran, 1999).

Thyroid hormones have a myriad of physiological effects and are necessary for normal cell metabolism. Receptors for these hormones have been identified in almost all tissues, where they increase the metabolic rate and oxygen consumption. They have catabolic effects on muscle and adipose tissue, stimulate erythropoiesis, and regulate cholesterol synthesis and degradation. Thyroid hormones are needed for the initiation of anagen hair follicles and regulation of the cornification process, sebaceous gland secretion and bacterial flora control.

Hypothyroidism occurs most commonly in mid- to large-sized purebred dogs, with an onset at between 3 and 8 years of age. Several breeds, including Dobermann, Golden Retriever, Irish Setter, Airedale, Great Dane, Old English Sheepdog, Borzoi and Beagle, are reported to be at increased risk.

continues ▶

Box 12.1: Hypothyroidism (continued)

Clinical signs

Hypothyroidism is characterized by a plethora of clinical signs affecting the skin and other organ systems:

- Common: thin, dry hair coat; seborrhoea; alopecia; lack of hair regrowth after clipping; weight gain/obesity; lethargy; weakness; hyperpigmentation
- Uncommon: pyoderma; facial myxoedema (tragic look); ceruminous otitis externa; ocular disorders; reproductive disorders; facial nerve paralysis; bradycardia; hypothermia.

However, none of the clinical signs is pathognomonic for hypothyroidism, and their appearance is generally gradual and insidious.

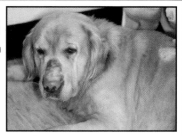

Golden Retriever with hypothyroidism, showing alopecia of the bridge of the nose, tragic face with myxoedema, and superficial pyoderma over the dorsum. (Courtesy of the Dermatology Unit, Royal Veterinary College.)

Congenital hypothyroidism is rare and results in disproportionate dwarfism (with epiphyseal dysgenesis), macroglossia, delayed dental eruption and cretinism, in addition to the usual clinical signs. In a clinical context, hypothyroidism is virtually non-existent in dogs under 2 years old.

Diagnosis

Of the numerous diagnostic tests currently available to evaluate thyroid function, no single test is optimal at present and hypothyroidism is still sometimes difficult to diagnose with confidence. Each test has its advantages and its limitations that should be known, and so far none can accurately confirm or rule out hypothyroidism in all cases. Readers are referred to Chapter 3 for more details about the diagnostic tests available.

When evaluating thyroid function in a dog, the clinician should:

- Select patients with clinical signs and age (over 2 years old) that are compatible with hypothyroidism
- Be aware of the several factors (mostly drugs and non-thyroidal illnesses) that can alter the test results and postpone thyroid evaluation until resolution of the illness or withdrawal of the drug, if possible
- Send the samples to a laboratory that has validated assays for dogs and has established reference values.

Definitive diagnosis of hypothyroidism can best be made by a combination of compatible clinical signs and abnormal specific thyroid test results, coupled with a successful long-term response to levothyroxine (T4) supplementation.

Thyroid function tests should be interpreted carefully and if there is discordance between the results of tests for total T4 and canine TSH, or the results are inconclusive, it is preferable to resubmit blood samples a few weeks to a few months later. Alternatively, one can perform additional tests to measure free T4 (by equilibrium dialysis) or anti-thyroglubulin antibodies (Dixon and Mooney, 1999). The TSH response test, although valuable in confirming a diagnosis of hypothyroidism, necessitates the use of bovine TSH which is no longer available for parenteral use. In the future a TSH stimulation test using recombinant human TSH may become more widely available (Sauvé and Paradis, 2000).

Measurement of anti-thyroglobulin antibodies, free T4 and canine TSH has been advocated for screening breeding stock of breeds at risk, e.g. Golden Retriever, Dobermann, Beagle and Borzoi (certification in North America), with the aim of ultimately eliminating heritable forms of thyroiditis.

Treatment

Successful response to levothyroxine supplementation is generally achieved but treatment of hypothyroidism is lifelong, therefore a definitive diagnosis is required before starting the therapy. Levothyroxine is administered orally, at the induction dose of 20 µg/kg bid (or 0.5 mg/m² bid) (Scott-Moncrieff and Guptill-Yoran, 1999). Lethargy can resolve within a few days, but it can take a few months for the hair coat to return to its normal appearance. After levothyroxine replacement therapy has been administered for 4–8 weeks or when all the clinical signs have resolved, a 'post-pill' serum total T4 concentration should be measured approximately 4–6 hours after administration to determine if adequate concentration of hormone is present in the blood. Typically, the authors aim for a total T4 value in the high normal range, or slightly above the normal range. Serum canine TSH concentration should normalize with appropriate therapy, though it is not the most useful parameter. At best, it can detect hypothyroid dogs that are undertreated, but the assay cannot distinguish between dogs that are adequately supplemented and those that are oversupplemented.

Thyrotoxicosis (PU/PD, weight loss, panting, nervousness, tachycardia) is rare in dogs, due to the rapid metabolism and renal and hepatic excretion of thyroid hormone. However, in most hypothyroid dogs, treatment can be reduced to once-a-day administration (20 µg/kg or 0.5 mg/m² sid) after an adequate clinical response is noted, without reduction in efficacy.

Due to the hereditary nature of this disorder, hypothyroid dogs should not be used for breeding.

Box 12.2: Hyperadrenocorticism (Cushing's disease)

Pathogenesis

Hyperadrenocorticism (HAC) is a common and well recognized disorder in dogs (Feldman, 1999). It may be either spontaneous or iatrogenic. Although many cases of HAC are caused by the administration of exogenous glucocorticoids, its occurrence has declined over the last decade due to better recognition and therapeutic approach of several disorders (e.g. allergies) that were historically controlled by relatively high doses and long-term use of glucocorticoids.

Approximately 85% of dogs with naturally occurring HAC suffer from pituitary-dependent HAC (PDH). The remaining 15% are due to an adrenocortical neoplasm (adenoma or adenocarcinoma) secreting excessive amounts of cortisol.

Spontaneous HAC occurs more frequently in middle-aged to older dogs, and some breeds such as the Dachshund, Boxer, Boston Terrier and Poodle are more at risk. Onset of clinical signs is insidious and slowly progressive.

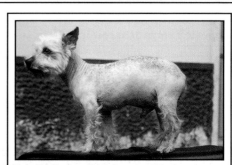

Yorkshire Terrier with pituitary-dependent hyperadrenocorticism, showing generalized hair loss and slightly pot-bellied appearance.

continues ▶

Box 12.2: Hyperadrenocorticism (Cushing's disease) (continued)

Clinical signs

- Very common: polyuria and polydipsia; polyphagia; abdominal enlargement; hepatomegaly; lethargy; muscle wasting; muscle weakness

- Common: symmetrical alopecia; skin hyperpigmentation; thin and hypotonic skin; obesity; muscular atrophy

- Uncommon: testicular atrophy in intact males; anoestrus in intact females; clitoral hypertrophy; comedones; panting; calcinosis cutis; bruising; facial paralysis.

Diagnosis

No single clinical sign, haematological or biochemical change is always present in each case of HAC and, worse, all of those changes can be seen in several other disorders. Therefore, before establishing a diagnosis of HAC several screening tests and diagnostic procedures must be performed in order to avoid misdiagnosing HAC and missing concomitant disorders. The diagnostic procedures that can be performed to confirm and localize HAC are outlined in Figure 12.4 and Chapter 3.

Among the tests available to confirm HAC, the low-dose dexamethasone suppression test (LDDST) and ACTH stimulation test are approximately 90–95% and 85% sensitive, respectively. Therefore, LDDST results will be normal in 5–10% of HAC patients and ACTH stimulation will be normal in about 15% of HAC patients. If the dog has the classic signs and laboratory abnormalities and no non-adrenal illness, one can be confident in the diagnosis of HAC. However, if non-adrenal illness is present, the LDDST has about a 50% false positive rate and ACTH stimulation has about a 15% false positive rate.

If an animal has been receiving any form of steroid, even topically, for weeks to months, either test can be altered due to feedback effects. The time needed for withdrawal and recovery of the pituitary–adrenal axis depends on the duration of treatment and form of steroid used.

Steroid therapy can cause clinical signs of HAC (iatrogenic) and can also cause atrophy of the adrenal cortex. This can be diagnosed by evaluating the lack of response to the ACTH stimulation test.

Urinary cortisol:creatinine ratio (UCCR) is essentially useful only to rule out HAC. Virtually 100% of dogs with spontaneous HAC have an elevated UCCR. However, most dogs with an elevated UCCR do not have HAC. If the UCCR is normal it is most likely the dog does not have HAC. If the ratio is elevated, a more specific test such as the LDDST or ACTH stimulation must be done to determine if HAC is truly present or not.

Tests available to differentiate between pituitary- and adrenal-dependent HAC in dogs are the high dose dexamethasone suppression test (HDDST) or an endogenous ACTH measurement and abdominal ultrasonography. About 75% of dogs can be differentiated using the HDDST. If the cortisol levels are suppressed, the diagnosis is PDH. If there is no suppression, then the dog could still have either form of HAC and an endogenous ACTH level should be submitted. If cortisol levels are not suppressed by the HDDST in a dog with confirmed HAC, the odds of pituitary-dependent *versus* adrenal-dependent HAC are 50:50.

Treatment

Several therapeutic options are available to treat HAC. In iatrogenic HAC, exogenous glucocorticoid should be withdrawn gradually until the hypothalamus–pituitary–adrenal axis is returned to normal.

Adrenalectomy

In adrenal neoplasm, adrenalectomy represents the treatment of choice.

Mitotane (op'-DDD)

Induction dose of 25–50 mg/kg/day orally every 24 hours, divided every 12 hours until effect (5–21 days; average 5–8 days). Then approximately 50 mg/kg once a week. Administer with food. Stop daily administration if: water intake decreases to < 60 ml/kg/24 h; partial or total anorexia, or lethargy, diarrhoea or vomiting occurs; cortisol concentration measured pre- and post-ACTH stimulation on day 8 or 9 of treatment is low/normal.

Side effects related to treatment and due to decrease in cortisol level below physiological needs are: lethargy, anorexia, weakness, vomiting and diarrhoea. If such side effects are encountered, mitotane must be stopped and a physiological dose of glucocorticoid (prednisolone 0.25 mg/kg/day orally) given for a week if needed. Prednisolone must be stopped at least 24 hours before measuring cortisol as it cross-reacts in the assay.

Dogs need to be re-evaluated periodically. An ACTH stimulation test may need to be performed every 3–6 months as the mitotane dose often needs to be increased during the first year of treatment.

Ketoconazole

Initiate therapy using 5–10 mg/kg daily for 10–15 days. Therapy must be continued using 10–15 mg/kg on a daily basis.

Selegiline

This drug is effective in a small number of dogs with pituitary-dependent HAC and in particular in those animals with a intermediate pituitary lobe neoplasia (Reusch *et al.*, 1999). It is used at 2 mg/kg/day.

Trilostane

The efficacy and long-term safety of this synthetic competitive (and reversible) inhibitor of 3ß-hydroxysteroid isomerase was recently evaluated for the treatment of canine HAC. Although this inhibitor of adrenal steroidogenesis does not seem potent enough to block cortisol biosynthesis in human patients with hypercorticolism, it showed promising results in dogs with hyperadrenocorticism (Ruckstuhl *et al.*, 2002). It also appeared to be quite safe and without the side effects seen with other therapies. It is used at a dose of 4–16 mg/kg/day. Trilostane is licensed for veterinary use in the dog in the UK – see the data sheet for more details.

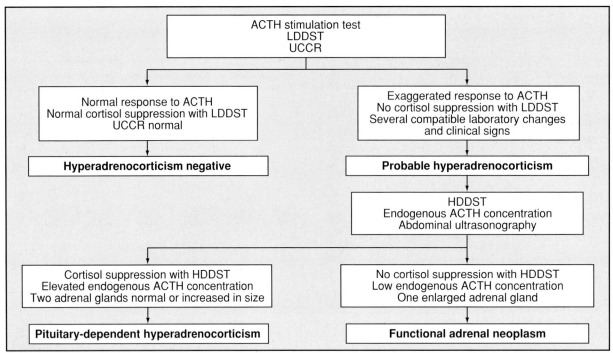

```
                    ACTH stimulation test
                         LDDST
                          UCCR
```

Normal response to ACTH	Exaggerated response to ACTH
Normal cortisol suppression with LDDST	No cortisol suppression with LDDST
UCCR normal	Several compatible laboratory changes and clinical signs

Hyperadrenocorticism negative   **Probable hyperadrenocorticism**

```
                          HDDST
            Endogenous ACTH concentration
              Abdominal ultrasonography
```

Cortisol suppression with HDDST	No cortisol suppression with HDDST
Elevated endogenous ACTH concentration	Low endogenous ACTH concentration
Two adrenal glands normal or increased in size	One enlarged adrenal gland

Pituitary-dependent hyperadrenocorticism   **Functional adrenal neoplasm**

12.4 Specific laboratory procedures to evaluate pituitary and adrenal function in suspected cases of canine hyperadrenocorticism. With a good ultrasound machine, skill and adequate abdominal echogenicity allowing good visualization of adrenal glands, it may not be necessary to perform diagnostic procedures such as HDDST or endogenous ACTH measurement. ACTH = adrenocorticotropic hormone; HDDST = high-dose dexamethasone suppression test; LDDST = low-dose dexamethasone suppression test; UCCR = urinary cortisol:creatinine ratio.

Box 12.3: Sertoli cell tumour and other sex hormone-related problems

Excesses, deficiencies and imbalance of sex hormones have been incriminated in a myriad of clinical syndromes in dogs. However, most dermatoses associated with sex hormones of gonadal or adrenal origin are uncommon and ill defined. Moreover, the existence of entities such as hypo-oestrogenism or oestrogen-responsive dermatosis in spayed female dogs is doubted by many dermatologists, and many of these cases might be canine pattern alopecia. Indeed, the vast majority of adrenalectomized and ovariectomized dogs maintained on only mineralocorticoids have normal skin and hair coats, indicating that sex steroids are not necessary for normal skin and haircoats in dogs.

Pathogenesis

Hyperoestrogenism may occur in males with a functional tumour of the testicle or in bitches with cystic ovaries, functional ovarian tumours or chronic exogenous oestrogen administration. Testicular neoplasia is common in dogs, especially in cryptorchid dogs, and Sertoli cell tumours are the most common type causing endocrine alopecia (seen in about one third of cases).

Clinical signs

Cutaneous changes in these syndromes include bilateral, symmetrical alopecia, variable hyperpigmentation and variable seborrhoeic skin disease. The affected male dog may have symmetrical alopecia, feminization, or both. The latter is characterized by pendulous prepuce, nipple enlargement and attraction of other male dogs. In females, hyperoestrogenism is manifested clinically by vulvar and nipple enlargement associated with oestrous cycle abnormalities such as prolonged oestrus and nymphomania.

Diagnosis

A palpable testicular mass, testicular asymmetry or cryptorchidism should suggest neoplasia in an intact male. Prostatomegaly (due to oestrogen-induced squamous metaplasia) and, less frequently, oestrogen-induced bone marrow depression can also occur. In bitches diagnosis is usually straightforward, especially if oestral and cutaneous changes are present.

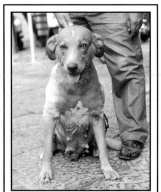

Crossbred dog with Sertoli cell tumour showing hair loss around the neck and the ventral part of the body. Gynaecomastia and pendulous prepuce are also evident.

Therapy

Bilateral castration, even if no testicular mass or asymmetry is palpable, is indicated, since the tumour may occur in a palpably normal scrotal testicle, although feminization is more likely with large tumours. Dogs should be examined carefully for metastasis prior to surgery, although it occurs in only 8% of cases. The therapy of choice in the bitch is ovariohysterectomy.

Box 12.4: Canine recurrent flank alopecia

Canine recurrent flank alopecia (CRFA) (formerly called seasonal flank alopecia, seasonal growth hormone deficiency, canine idiopathic cyclic flank alopecia or cyclic follicular dysplasia) is a recently recognized skin disorder of unknown aetiology. It is characterized by episodes of truncal hair loss that often occur on a recurrent basis. CRFA is most commonly seen in Boxers (may account for approximately half of all cases). Other breeds at high risk include English Bulldog, Airedale Terrier, Schnauzer (Miniature, Standard and Giant) and Griffon Korthal. Although CRFA seems to affect virtually any breed, this condition appears to be rare to absent in the plush-coat Nordic breeds, German Shepherd Dog and Cocker Spaniel. Dogs of either sex and of all reproductive status can be affected.

Pathogenesis

The cause of CRFA remains obscure. The high incidence in some breeds and the familial character of CRFA suggest a genetic influence. The seasonal nature and recurrence also suggest that photoperiod may be involved (Paradis, 1999). There is definitely a higher incidence of CRFA at higher latitude (around or north of the 45° parallel). In Australia and New Zealand, the onset of CRFA appears to be the reverse of what we see in the northern hemisphere (but during their short photoperiod season), supporting the importance of light exposure to this disorder.

Clinical signs

CRFA is characterized by a fairly abrupt onset of non-scarring alopecia, usually bilaterally symmetrical, with well demarcated borders and often markedly hyperpigmented alopecic skin. The alopecia is usually confined to the thoracolumbar region but occasionally this is seen in association with alopecia on the dorsum of the nose, base of the ears, base of tail and perineum.

Spontaneous regrowth of a normal pelage occurs in 3–8 months (range: 1–14 months) although some individuals have coat colour changes in previously affected areas (melanotrichia in Boxers; aurotrichia in Miniature Schnauzers). Hair regrowth may become less complete after several episodes in a few cases; it may even progress to an end-stage, permanent flank alopecia and marked hyperpigmentation.

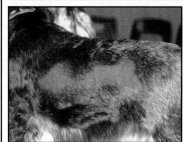

Approximately 20% of CRFA cases may have only one isolated episode of flank alopecia during their life. Most dogs, however, will develop recurrent alopecic episodes for years. Some dogs have an occasional year when the alopecia does not recur. The degree of alopecia is variable, with some dogs developing a virtually identical hair loss (size and duration) year after year, and other dogs developing larger areas and/or longer episodes of hair loss as years go by.

Miniature Schnauzer (2-year-old male) at first episode of CRFA.

The mean age at the onset of the first episode is approximately 4 years (range: 8 months to 11 years). In the northern hemisphere the majority of dogs have an onset of alopecia between November and March.

Diagnosis

For most cases of CRFA, the diagnosis is based on: history; clinical signs; rule out of hypothyroidism; and skin biopsies. Histopathological findings (such as 'witch's feet' or 'octopus-like hair follicles') are suggestive of, but not pathognomonic for, CRFA. In a dog presented at his first episode, other causes of alopecia such as endocrinopathies (hypothyroidism, hyperadrenocorticism) or other follicular dysplasias need to be ruled out. Hypothyroidism is an important differential diagnosis for CRFA. Moreover, hypothyroidism and CRFA can both occur in the same animal (Daminet and Paradis, 2000).

Treatment

The unpredictable course of CRFA and the spontaneous regrowth of hair render the evaluation of any therapeutic agent extremely difficult, whether used to prevent CRFA or to shorten an existing episode of alopecia. Oral melatonin, when available, can be administered before or preferably shortly after the onset of alopecia (Paradis, 1999). Its use as a preventive treatment is limited, considering that chance of recurrence is 60–70% in any given year. Dogs affected with CRFA appear healthy otherwise, and benign neglect is still a valuable therapeutic approach.

Box 12.5: Alopecia X

Alopecia X is the name several veterinary dermatologists are now using to refer to the following diseases:

- Pseudo-Cushing's
- Adult-onset growth hormone deficiency
- Hyposomatotropism of the adult dog
- Growth hormone-responsive alopecia
- Castration-responsive dermatosis
- Gonadal sex hormone dermatoses
- Sex hormone/growth hormone dermatosis
- Biopsy-responsive alopecia
- Adrenal sex hormone imbalance

- Congenital adrenal hyperplasia like-syndrome
- Lysodren-responsive dermatosis
- Follicular dysplasia of Nordic breeds (Woolly Syndrome)
- Siberian Husky follicular dysplasia (Woolly Syndrome)
- Follicular growth dysfunction of the plush-coated breeds
- Black skin syndrome of Pomeranians.

The diversity in proposed names is based, at least in part, upon the differences in endocrine evaluation results and/or clinical responses to various therapeutic modalities.

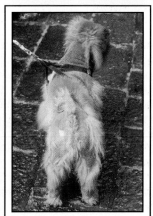

Pathogenesis

The aetiology of alopecia X remains obscure. A genetic predisposition to an unidentified hormonal imbalance is plausible, but a defect residing at the hair follicle level is also possible. If the problem is a primary disorder of the hair growth cycle, various stimuli (including different hormones) could draw hair follicles into anagen phase.

Chow Chow with alopecia X showing hair loss and hyperpigmentation around the neck, chest, rump and tail.

continues ▶

Box 12.5: Alopecia X (continued)

Clinical signs

Initially there is loss of primary hairs (with retention of secondary hairs) in the frictional areas (around the neck, caudomedial thighs and tail). Gradually, all hair is lost in those regions and eventually the truncal primary hairs are also lost, giving the remaining coat a puppy-like appearance. With time (several months to years) the secondary hairs become sparse, and hyperpigmentation of the exposed skin and/or colour change in the remaining hair coat may be seen. The head and legs are usually spared. A tendency to regrow hair at the biopsy site following skin biopsy or other external traumatic stimuli (skin scraping, sunburn, etc.) is a common finding in this syndrome.

Alopecia X is seen more often in young adults and more frequently in intact or neutered male dogs, but females can be affected. Breeds more at risk of developing this syndrome are the Nordic breeds and Poodles (see Figure 12.2).

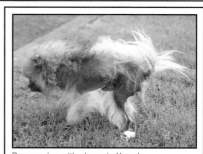

Pomeranian with alopecia X and hyperpigmentation over the trunk and tail.

Diagnosis

The diagnosis is based on history, physical examination findings, ruling out other diseases, skin biopsies and response to therapy. Histopathological examination of skin biopsies reveals non-specific changes consistent with endocrinopathies, however, the presence of excessive trichilemmal keratinization (flame follicles) is suggestive of this disorder.

A reproductive hormone panel before and following ACTH stimulation has been proposed (Schmietzel *et al.*, 1995). However, it may be expensive and it is performed in only a few specialized laboratories. More importantly, even when an abnormality is demonstrated, it does not seem to change the treatment approach or the outcome.

The differential diagnosis includes: hypothyroidism, hyperadrenocorticism (natural or exogenous), sex hormone imbalances due to functional gonadal neoplasms, telogen defluxion, sebaceous adenitis and other follicular dysplasias.

Treatment

Various medical and surgical treatments have been suggested. It is, however, important first to rule out hypothyroidism and hyperadrenocorticism. Castration is recommended as it often induces regrowth of hair which is either permanent or lasts for several months.

Hormonal supplementation with growth hormone, thyroxine, oestrogens, testosterone or melatonin have been used to stimulate hair regrowth with varying results.

Adrenolytic drugs such as mitotane have also been reported to be efficacious. Although the induction dose recommended is lower than for hyperadrenocorticism, the side effects and the possible hypoadrenocorticism associated with mitotane should be considered carefully before using it in affected animals.

Oral melatonin given at the rate of 3–6 mg bid–tid for up to 3 months may be effective in approximately 30–50% of the cases (Paradis, 1999). Trilostane has recently been reported to promote hair regrowth in Pomeranians and Miniature Poodles (Cerundolo *et al.*, 2001).

All of these forms of therapy may be associated with hair regrowth but the response is not predictable and there may only be a short-term effect. In any case benign neglect can be an option, since alopecia X appears to be only an aesthetic problem.

Non-endocrine alopecias

Differential characteristics and treatment of non-endocrine alopecias are summarized in Figure 12.5.

Follicular dysplasia and colour dilution alopecia are described in Boxes 12.6 and 12.7.

Congenital alopecia

The partial or total absence of hair at birth is a rare condition. Congenital alopecia is usually associated with other ectodermal defects such as absence of other epidermal appendages, anomalies of dentition and decreased tear production (Scott *et al.*, 2001). The condition has been reported occasionally in the Basset Hound, Beagle, Bichon Frisé, French Bulldog and Rottweiler. It is characteristic of some breeds selected for this pattern, such as the Abyssinian Dog, American Hairless Terrier, Mexican Hairless Dog and the Xoloitzcuintli. The Chinese Crested Dog is also affected by a congenital alopecia caused by a follicular dystrophy, which severely impairs hair growth.

Anagen defluxion

This is a rare condition caused by an abrupt cessation of mitotic activity in rapidly dividing hair matrix cells (anagen phase), usually associated with severe systemic disease or administration of cytotoxic medication (such as methotrexate or cyclophosphamide) or toxic substances (selenium, molybdenum, thallium and arsenic) (Scott *et al.,* 2001).

Clinical signs

A synchronous hair loss occurs within days to weeks of drug administration. It is usually multifocal and then becomes diffuse. The alopecia affects the trunk and occasionally the extremities. Hairs are easily epilated. The severity of alopecia may depend on the drug as well as the individual predisposition.

Diagnosis

The history of previous treatments or possible contact with toxic substances is suggestive. The trichogram shows anagen hair bulbs, often characterized by marked pigmentation and irregular hair shafts.

Treatment

There is no treatment for this condition but spontaneous resolution will occur if an offending drug is withdrawn.

Telogen defluxion

This is an uncommon condition in which the hair follicles go into premature rest. It is associated with

Condition	Underlying pathology	Age of onset	Cutaneous signs apart from alopecia	Systemic signs	Laboratory findings	Diagnostic tests	Therapy
Congenital alopecia	Ectodermal defect	At birth	None	Anomalies of dentition	None	Skin biopsy	None
Anagen defluxion	Sudden interruption of the anagen phase	Variable	None	Related to the severe systemic disease or to the cytotoxic therapy	Related to the underlying pathology	Trichogram	Withdraw offending drug
Colour dilution alopecia	Abnormality of melanization	< 1 year	Comedones, secondary pyoderma	None	None	Trichogram, skin biopsy	Melatonin?
Follicular dysplasia	Unknown	Variable	Secondary pyoderma	None	None	Skin biopsy	None
Pattern alopecia	Unknown	< 1 year	None	None	None	Skin biopsy	Melatonin?
Sebaceous adenitis	Unknown	Variable	Scaling	None	None	Trichogram, skin biopsy	Retinoids, essential fatty acids, moisturizers
Telogen defluxion	Synchronous arrest of the hair cycle	Variable	None	Only if systemic disease or physiological stress is present	None	Trichogram, skin biopsy	None, rapid resolution

12.5 Differential characteristics and treatment in non-endocrine alopecias.

Box 12.6: Follicular dysplasia

This is a group of heritable breed-specific hair coat abnormalities (Miller and Scott, 1995; Cerundolo *et al.*, 2000; Scott *et al.*, 2001).

Clinical signs
Focal or diffuse symmetrical alopecia occurs, usually affecting the dorsum and the flanks.

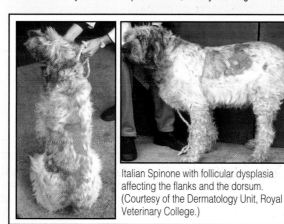
Italian Spinone with follicular dysplasia affecting the flanks and the dorsum. (Courtesy of the Dermatology Unit, Royal Veterinary College.)

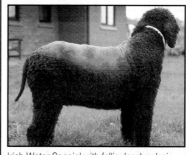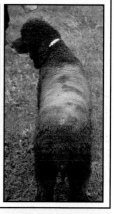
Irish Water Spaniel with follicular dysplasia affecting the dorsolateral part of the trunk. (Courtesy of the Dermatology Unit, Royal Veterinary College.)

Diagnosis
Breed predisposition and clinical signs are indicative of this condition. Histology of skin specimens shows varying degrees of follicular hyperkeratosis, melanin clumping and dysplastic hair follicles.

Treatment
No effective treatment is available. Sometimes changing the diet or supplementation with essential fatty acids may improve coat quality and reduce the severity of the alopecia. Secondary pyoderma should be treated with systemic antibiotics.

Box 12.7: Colour dilution alopecia (CDA)

This condition is caused by abnormalities in the anatomy and melanization of the pilosebaceous unit (Roperto *et al.*, 1995; Scott *et al.*, 2001). It has been reported in the blue colour dilution variant of several breeds (see Figure 12.2).

Clinical signs

Affected dogs show a progressive alopecia affecting only the dilute areas between 3 months and 3 years of age. Scaling and comedones with secondary bacterial infection are also present in affected areas.

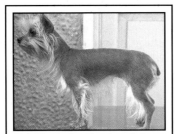

Yorkshire Terrier with colour dilution alopecia affecting the blue area of the body. (Reprinted from Roperto *et al.* (1995) with permission.)

Diagnosis

Breed predisposition and coat colour should suggest CDA. Trichogram shows hairs with structural abnormalities such as distortion and fracture. Large melanin clumps are seen along the hair shaft, causing distortion and fracture of the hair. Histological

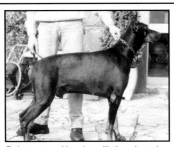

Dobermann with colour dilution alopecia, showing diffuse truncal hair loss.

examination of skin specimens from affected areas show abnormal melanin aggregates in the epidermal and follicular basal cells.

Differential diagnosis includes other inherited hair defects or demodicosis in young dogs, or endocrine disorders in adult dogs.

Treatment

Palliative therapy may be carried out with retinoids or essential fatty acids to improve hair and skin condition. Secondary pyoderma, often associated with scaling and follicular keratosis, should be treated with systemic antibiotics. Topical shampoos and moisturizers will also help to reduce the incidence of scaling.

stressful events such as pregnancy, parturition, lactation, severe systemic illness, marked febrile episodes, shock, surgery and various drugs (Scott *et al.*, 2001). The cause of hair loss is the synchronous premature progression from the anagen phase, through catagen, to telogen.

Clinical signs

Patchy to diffuse alopecia occurs within 2–4 months and affects the trunk. Hairs are usually easily epilated.

Diagnosis

The history of a metabolic stress and excessive epilation are suggestive. The trichogram shows telogen hairs with minimal or absent pigmentation.

Treatment

Specific therapy is not required, as hair regrowth occurs completely a few months after the cause of the metabolic stress has been resolved.

Pattern alopecia

Canine pattern alopecia (canine pattern baldness, CPA) is a relatively common disorder which may present with several different syndromes. It has been recognized in several short-coated breeds (Scott *et al.*, 2001).

Clinical signs

Various patterns of focal alopecia are present in affected dogs. Among these a pattern of progressive, symmetrical alopecia is localized on the postauricular regions, along the ventral neck, thorax, abdomen and on the caudomedial thighs (Figure 12.6). The hair loss starts around 6 months of age and gradually progresses over the following year, but remains restricted to the described areas. Affected areas often show multiple fine hairs.

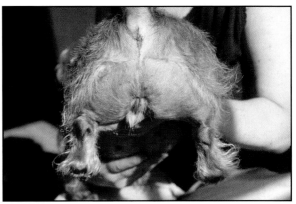

12.6 Dachshund with pattern alopecia affecting the caudal part of the thighs.

Diagnosis

The diagnosis is based on the history, the dermatological examination and exclusion of other diagnoses. Histopathological findings are characterized by miniaturization of hair follicles.

Treatment

This disease is just an aesthetic problem. No effective treatment has been reported, with the exception of melatonin; good results have been observed in several dogs treated with this drug (Paradis, 1999).

Sebaceous adenitis

Sebaceous adenitis is an idiopathic dermatosis whose cause and pathogenesis are unknown and which is characterized by a lymphocytic, granulomatous or pyogranulomatous inflammation involving the sebaceous glands, with their progressive destruction. The Standard Poodle is genetically predisposed to this disease (Dunstan and Hargis, 1995; Scott *et al.*, 2001).

Clinical signs

Various degrees of alopecia with severe scaling and crusting affect the head and trunk (Figure 12.7). The hair coat becomes dull, dry and brittle, with the presence of follicular casts, and is easily epilated.

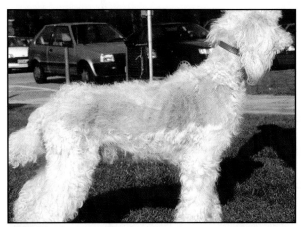

12.7 Standard Poodle with sebaceous adenitis. Hair loss is more evident over the trunk but hypotrichosis was present all over the body. (Courtesy of the Dermatology Unit, Royal Veterinary College.)

Diagnosis

The presence of follicular casts in a predisposed breed is usually suggestive of sebaceous adenitis. Histology of skin specimens shows variable degrees of sebaceous adenitis with complete absence of the glands in the late stage of the condition.

Treatment

The prognosis for improvement in coat condition is variable and, rarely, spontaneous remission occurs; dogs are otherwise healthy. Therapy may improve the coat quality but the destruction of the sebaceous glands is permanent. Various topical treatments such as antiseborrhoeic shampoos and propylene glycol, or systemic treatment such as ciclosporin, essential fatty acids, isotretinoin or etretinate have been recommended.

References and further reading

Cerundolo R (1999) Symmetrical alopecia in the dog. *In Practice* **21,** 350–359

Cerundolo R, Lloyd DH, McNeil PE *et al.* (2000) An analysis of factors underlying hypotrichosis and alopecia in Irish water spaniels in the United Kingdom. *Veterinary Dermatology* **11,** 107–122

Cerundolo R, Lloyd DH, Persechino A, Evans H and Cauvin A (2001) The use of trilostane for the treatment of Alopecia X in Pomeranians and miniature poodles. *Proceedings of the AAVD/ACVD Annual Meeting,* Norfolk, VA

Daminet S and Paradis M (2000) Evaluation of thyroid function in dogs suffering from recurrent flank alopecia. *Canadian Veterinary Journal* **41,** 699–703

Dixon RM and Mooney CT (1999) Canine serum thyroglobulin autoantibodies in health, hypothyroidism, and non-thyroidal illness. *Research in Veterinary Science* **66,** 243–246

Dunstan RW and Hargis AM (1995) The diagnosis of sebaceous adenitis in Standard Poodle dogs. In: *Kirk's Current Veterinary Therapy,* ed. JD Bonagura, pp. 619-622. WB Saunders, Philadelphia

Feldman EC (1999) Hyperadrenocorticism. In: *Textbook of Veterinary Internal Medicine, 5th edn,* ed. SJ Ettinger and EC Feldman, pp.1460-1488. WB Saunders, Philadelphia

Miller WH and Scott DW (1995) Follicular dysplasia of the Portuguese water dog. *Veterinary Dermatology* **6,** 67–74

Paradis M (1999) Melatonin therapy in canine alopecia. In: *Kirk's Current Veterinary Therapy XIII,* ed. JD Bonagura, pp. 546–549. WB Saunders, Philadelphia.

Reusch CE *et al.* (1999) The efficacy of L-deprenyl in dogs with pituitary-dependent hyperadrenocorticism. *Journal of Veterinary Internal Medicine* **13,** 291–301

Roperto F, Cerundolo R, Restucci B *et al.* (1995) Colour dilution alopecia (CDA) in ten Yorkshire terriers. *Veterinary Dermatology* **6,** 171–178

Ruckstuhl NS, Nett CS and Reusch CE (2002) Results of clinical examinations, laboratory tests, and ultrasonography in dogs with pituitary-dependent hyperadrenocorticism treated with trilostane. *American Journal of Veterinary Research* **63,** 506–512

Sauvé F and Paradis M (2000) Evaluation on thyroid function following stimulation with human recombinant thyrothropin in euthyroid dogs. *Canadian Veterinary Journal* **41,** 215–218

Schmietzel LP *et al.* (1995) Congenital adrenal-hyperplasia-like syndrome. In: *Kirk's Current Veterinary Therapy XII,* ed. JD Bonagura, pp. 600–604. WB Saunders, Philadelphia

Scott-Moncrieff JCR and Guptill-Yoran L (1999) Hypothyroidism. In: *Textbook of Veterinary Internal Medicine, 5th edn,* ed. SJ Ettinger and EC Feldman, pp. 1419–1429. WB Saunders, Philadelphia

Scott DW, Miller WH and Griffin CE (2001) *Muller and Kirk's Small Animal Dermatology, 6th edn.* WB Saunders, Philadelphia

Yager JA and Wilcock BP (1994) *Color Atlas and Text of Surgical Pathology of the Dog and Cat.* Mosby, London

13

An approach to facial dermatoses

Ewan Ferguson

The purpose of this chapter is to present a problem-oriented approach to the wide variety of dermatological diseases that present with a significant facial component. In some cases facial involvement is incidental but in others it is central to the pathological mechanism of the condition. Clinical signs may be confined to the face or may be widespread, involving many other areas. Conditions covered in this chapter include: those in which the face is the sole area involved; conditions where facial involvement is a predictable part of an overall pattern; and those where a facial distribution is of diagnostic significance. Conditions that have an essentially random distribution or where facial involvement is incidental will not be considered.

Facial dermatoses present with a combination of a limited number of principal clinical signs. Secondary clinical signs may also develop in characteristic patterns. Usually one of these clinical features dominates and this forms part of the basis for a problem-oriented approach to diagnosis.

Clinical presentations include:

- Pruritus
- Alopecia
- Pigmentary abnormalities
- Crusting and scaling
- Papules and pustules
- Swellings, nodules and draining tracts
- Ulceration
- Necrosis and fissuring

The head, face and ears include a number of unique anatomical structures and areas of skin with specialized functions. As a result, there are a variety of unique skin microenvironments present that have no counterpart elsewhere in the body. These microenvironments may show a distinct predilection towards specific dermatological conditions and therefore the distribution of clinical signs across this range of environments can be of immense diagnostic value. The distinct **anatomical zones** considered are:

- Nasal planum
- Lip folds
- Chin
- Muzzle
- Periorbital skin
- Preauricular skin
- Pinnae

The majority of diseases involving the face present with a **characteristic combination** of these two features – the anatomical zone affected and the clinical signs exhibited.

Differential diagnoses

Differentials for the clinical presentations affecting the facial region are shown in the tables that follow.

Clinical presentations

Pruritus

Facial pruritus is a common clinical presentation and may present as the sole clinical sign. However, it more commonly occurs in combination with more generalized pruritus or other clinical signs such as papules and crusts. It ranges from mild to severe and may be accompanied by considerable self-trauma. The presence or absence of more widespread involvement and other primary or secondary lesions is diagnostically significant (Figure 13.1).

Condition	Anatomical site						
	Nasal planum	Lip folds	Chin	Muzzle	Periorbital skin	Preauricular skin	Pinnae
Atopy Dietary intolerance	–	Erythema. Secondary pyodermas	Erythema, diffuse alopecia. Secondary *Malassezia* overgrowth and pyoderma common		Diffuse erythema, lichenification, hyperpigmentation (Figure 13.2). Diffuse secondary alopecia may develop over face but does not normally affect the pinnae.		
Contact allergy	Depigmentation, crusting, erythema		Erythema, papules, crusting, lichenification		Erythema, crusting and occasionally ulceration. Usually well demarcated and may be progressive if topical medications implicated		

13.1 Pruritic conditions affecting the face. (continues) ▶

Condition	Anatomical site						
	Nasal planum	*Lip folds*	*Chin*	*Muzzle*	*Periorbital skin*	*Preauricular skin*	*Pinnae*
Malassezia infection (Figure 13.2)	–	Erythema, alopecia lichenification. Pruritus may be intense	Less common but may cause diffuse erythema, alopecia		Erythema, seborrhoea, alopecia, lichenification, scaling, hyperpigmentation. May extend from existing ceruminous otitis		Erythema, otitis, lichenification, hyperpigmentation, pale or dark brown waxy cerumen
Demodicosis	–	Erythema, alopecia, follicular casting or comedones. May be well demarcated and focal or diffuse, especially when deep pyoderma present. Pruritus is usually mild but may be marked and is poorly responsive to conventional antipruritic therapy. Mites usually easy to demonstrate on scraping				Comedones, erythema, hyperpigmentation	Waxy, pale cream ceruminous otitis. Follicles often prominent as white 'freckling' due to follicular hyperkeratosis
Sarcoptic mange	–	Rarely	Rarely	Papules, scale, alopecia, excoriation. Often musty, 'mousy' odour. Widespread seborrhoea common. Mites often difficult to recover on scraping. Serological testing available for IgG antibodies against mite			Papular crusting of pinnal margins accompanied by scratch reflex and alopecia
Otodectes infestation	–	–	–	–	In severe cases may be found outside ear or in skin folds		Dry crumbly dark wax, pruritic otitis
Trombicula infestation	–	Rarely	–	–	Rarely	Erythematous papules, scaling, alopecia. Orange–red mites usually visible. Commonly found in Henry's pocket in the pinnal margin. Strictly seasonal	
Pyotraumatic dermatitis	–	Well defined erosions, exudation and crusting. Marked self-trauma	–	–	Erythema, excoriation, alopecia, erosions and exudation. Triggered by self-trauma. May be deeper involvement with pustules, papules, furunculosis, suggestive of *pyotraumatic folliculitis*		Erosions and crusting may affect base of pinnae

13.1 (continued) Pruritic conditions affecting the face.

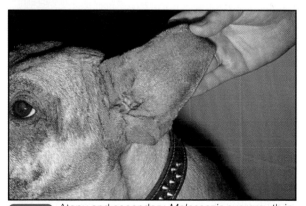

13.2 Atopy and secondary *Malassezia* overgrowth in a 5-year-old Rhodesian Ridgeback. There is marked lichenification and hyperpigmentation of the pinna and periorbital skin.

The clinical consequences of facial pruritus vary with species. Dogs usually attempt to relieve their pruritus through a combination of scratching and rubbing against environmental objects, including their owner. Cats are far more likely to scratch and are able to cause severe self-trauma very quickly. The rapidity with which secondary exudative lesions appear will often obscure the primary lesions making diagnosis more difficult. In such cases, particularly close attention should be paid to lesion margins and areas of recent involvement where the primary pathology is likely to be more apparent.

Alopecia

Hair cycle arrest is the most common cause of alopecia and is often associated with disturbances to the extrinsic control mechanisms as occurs in many endocrinopathies. However, these conditions tend to spare the head and are unlikely to be the cause of facial hair loss. More commonly, facial alopecia is associated either with inflammation or with metabolic or vascular compromise (Figure 13.3). The hair follicle is an extremely metabolically active tissue and if its nutritional and vascular demands are not met, growth and the hair cycle are affected. Ultimately, as happens in dermatomyositis, the follicle may be replaced entirely with less demanding tissue such as collagen.

Where alopecia is apparent, it is essential to determine whether there has been hair shaft damage – as would be consistent with pruritus and self-trauma – or a failure of hair shafts to be produced. Alopecia may also occur as an indirect effect of inflammatory mediators that lead to follicular arrest. Evidence of concurrent or preceding inflammation should be sought through close examination and in the history.

Evidence of interfollicular pathology may also provide valuable clues as to the pathogenesis of alopecia. Scaling and flaking are evidence of changes in epidermal turnover rates that may indicate keratinization abnormalities. Changes in follicular keratinization may be assessed by examining hair pluckings. Follicular casting, hair shaft pigmentary abnormalities or the presence of *Demodex* may be demonstrated.

Condition	Anatomical site						
	Nasal planum	Lip folds	Chin	Muzzle	Periorbital skin	Preauricular skin	Pinnae
Alopecia areata (Figure 13.4)	–	Well demarcated focal or multifocal patches, usually symmetrical, of total or near-total alopecia. Commonly around eyes and muzzle but may be generalized. May become hyperpigmented. Grossly non-inflammatory. Most affected animals recover spontaneously					Rarely involved
Pseudopelade	–	Well circumscribed non-inflammatory symmetrical areas of alopecia. Usually discrete but may be diffuse alopecia over the head and neck. May be scaly and hyperpigmented. Onychomadesis is usually present in cats. Pseudopelade has proved unresponsive to treatment to date					
Lymphocytic mural folliculitis	–	May have well defined focal areas of alopecia or diffuse alopecia. Scaling is variable. Best considered a reaction pattern that may be seen in a variety of diseases					
Demodicosis	–	Erythema, alopecia, follicular casting or comedones. May be well demarcated and focal to multifocal. Alopecia may be near total or diffuse, particularly when there is concurrent pyoderma				Comedones, erythema, hyperpigmentation and alopecia	Waxy otitis. Follicles often prominent as pale 'freckling'
Pattern alopecia Pinnal alopecia	–	–	–	–	–	Tardive condition producing diffuse alopecia with miniaturization of follicles. Temporal skin may be affected. Chronic cases may become hyperpigmented. Pinnal alopecia may be periodic in Siamese cats	
Dermatomyositis and ischaemic folliculopathy	Patchy depigmentation	Irregular patches of alopecia, scaling, erythema and crusting (Figure 13.5). May progress to scarring. Primarily affects collies and Shetland Sheepdogs, first appearing before 6 months of age					
Dermatophytosis	–	–	Annular areas of peripherally expanding alopecia, scale, crust and follicular papules and pustules. Hairs may be broken rather than absent. May show follicular hyperkeratosis and comedones. Aggressive lesions may show generalized seborrhoea, furunculosis and kerion formation				
Hyperadrenocorticism Hypothyroidism	–	–	–	–	–	–	Mild pinnal deformation and hair loss reported in cats
Traction alopecia	Generally confined to top of head. Well demarcated area of hair loss at site of the over-zealous application of grooming aids such as rubber bands. May lead to atrophic scarring and permanent hair loss						

13.3 Alopecic conditions affecting the face.

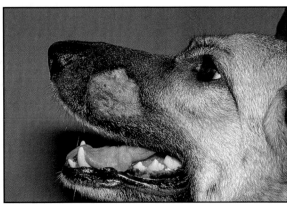

13.4 Alopecia areata in a 4-year-old German Shepherd Dog.

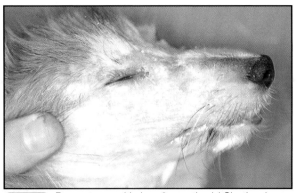

13.5 Dermatomyositis in a 9-month-old Shetland Sheepdog, showing widespread facial crusting and alopecia.

Pigmentary abnormalities

Normal pigmentation depends on the amount of eumelanin, phaeomelanin, carotene and trichochromes present in the skin and hair, and their distribution within the skin and adnexae. Lack of cysteine-containing proteins reduces the production of the red and yellow phaeomelanins. Inflammatory processes in the skin may lead to changes in pigmentation: cytokines such as interleukin-1 (IL-1), IL-6 and IL-7 inhibit melanogenesis, whilst leukotriene B4 upregulates melanin synthesis. It is therefore essential to obtain an accurate history as to the progression of lesions and to note whether pigmentary changes were preceded or accompanied by other dermatological changes (Figure 13.6).

Condition	Anatomical site						
	Nasal planum	*Lip folds*	*Chin*	*Muzzle*	*Periorbital skin*	*Preauricular skin*	*Pinnae*
Lupus erythematosus	Depigmentation, loss of rough cobblestone pattern, erosions, crusting, fissuring and inflammation	Erythema, depigmentation, erosions, crusting. May be punctate oral ulcers. May progress to alopecia. Pruritus variable. Scarring is a common sequel. Depigmentation of hair and skin common. Cases should be evaluated for systemic involvement. Cutaneous lesions exacerbated by ultraviolet light				Generally uninvolved	Crusting, scaling and alopecia
Uveodermatological syndrome (Vogt–Koyanagi–Harada syndrome)	Patches of depigmentation. May show erosion, crusting and scaling	Predilection for Chows, Samoyeds, Akitas. Dermatological changes preceded by granulomatous uveitis. Usually well demarcated areas of depigmentation and mild scaling. May progress to varying degrees of erosion, ulceration and crusting					
Vitiligo	Broadly symmetrical macular leucoderma and leucotrichia. May reverse spontaneously. Onset usually in young adults						
'Dudley nose'	Progressive depigmentation of nasal planum. Usually irreversible. No treatment	–	–	–	–	–	–
'Snow nose'	Incomplete, cyclic depigmentation, usually during winter months	–	–	–	–	–	–
Idiopathic hypopigmentation	Patchy depigmentation progressing to diffuse leucotrichia and a 'roan' coat. Seen in Newfoundlands	–	–	–	–	–	–
Lentigo simplex	Well circumscribed melanotic macules scattered over lips and nose. Seen in ginger cats. Macules enlarge gradually but are asymptomatic and do not transform to melanomas	–	–	Lentigines may be seen	–	–	
Nasal aspergillosis	Multifocal areas of ulceration, crusting and depigmentation	–	–	–	–	–	–

13.6 Pigmentary abnormalities affecting the face.

It is necessary also to determine whether pigmentary changes are diffuse or well defined, partial, scattered or total. Changes may be confined to hairs alone or skin pigment can be involved. Leucoderma and leucotrichia have been reported as an early sign of epitheliotrophic lymphoma. It should always be remembered that the retina contains melanin and may become involved, particularly when there is an immune-mediated attack directed at melanocytes.

Scaling and crusting

Scale is composed of loose sheets of cornified squames. Primary or secondary disturbances in keratinization result in diffuse scaling, which is rarely seen over the head. However, localized scaling as the result of focal inflammatory lesions is seen (Figure 13.7). These lesions may be confluent, giving a false impression of diffuse change. In contrast, crusts are formed from keratin, serum and cellular debris and suggest that there has been an exudative lesion present. This implies a wholly different pathomechanism from that which might be expected to produce scaling and it is therefore essential to be able to distinguish between these two processes and the lesions they create. As with many other areas, careful and detailed examination of the earliest lesions will greatly aid recognition of the true nature of the lesion.

Papules and pustules

Although *Staphylococcus intermedius* can be readily isolated from many facial lesions, straightforward pyoderma affecting the face and ears is relatively uncommon in the dog and extremely rare in the cat. A variety of other organisms, including many Gram-negative rods, can also be isolated. In many cases they will simply be opportunists and are unlikely to progress beyond the stratified layers of the epidermis. Pustules

Condition	Anatomical site						
	Nasal planum	Lips	Chin	Muzzle	Periorbital skin	Preauricular skin	Pinnae
Dermatomyositis	Depigmentation, scaling	Irregular patches of alopecia, scaling, erythema and crusting. May progress to scarring. Primarily affects collies and Shetland Sheepdogs, appearing before 6 months of age					
Zinc-responsive dermatosis	–	Primarily Siberian Huskies and Malamutes. Erythema progressing to alopecia, thick adherent yellowish scaling and crusting, exudation. Usually pruritic. In other breeds may be seen if zinc-deficient diet fed. Lesions also commonly occur over pressure points					
Vitamin A-responsive dermatosis	–	–	–	Primarily in Cocker Spaniels. Severe follicular hyperkeratosis leading to varying degrees of focal crusting, alopecia and follicular papules. Mild to moderate pruritus			
Idiopathic nasal hyperkeratosis	Dry verrucous feathered or ridges of keratin over dorsal nasal planum	–	–	–	–	–	–
Actinic damage	Erythema, crusting and hyperkeratosis	–	–	Poorly defined areas of erythema, hyperkeratosis and crusting. May progress to hyperkeratotic plaques or transform to squamous cell carcinoma			
Squamous cell carcinoma	Proliferative and ulcerative forms – see right	–	–	Proliferative form develops papillary masses, which damage and bleed easily. Ulcerative form develops shallow crusted ulcers, which deepen and become crater-like. Usually solitary lesions on the face			–
Dermatophilosis	–	Erythematous papules and pustules progressing to focal crusts. May develop into deeper lesions resulting in fistulae and granulomatous nodules		–	–	–	
Mosquito bite hypersensitivity (Figure 13.8)	–	–	–	Predominantly in cats. Seasonal. Outdoor access required. Erythematous papules/plaques often with ulcerated, crusted or necrotic appearance. Multiple lesions coalesce forming polycyclic alopecia and ulcerated patches			
Biting flies	–	–	–	Pruritus, papulocrustous dermatitis affecting thinly haired areas. Chronic changes include alopecia, crusting and fibrous nodules/plaques			
Idiopathic facial dermatitis of Persian cats	–	Crusty black exudates adherent to skin and distal hair shafts. Underlying skin is erythematous, and pyoderma or *Malassezia* overgrowth may occur. Initially non-pruritic but severe unresponsive pruritus eventually develops in many cases. Cause unknown. No consistently effective treatment recognized. Symptomatic management or euthanasia most common approaches taken					–
FeLV infection	–	Scaling, hyperplastic, crusting and erosive focal lesions. Moderate to severe pruritus reported. Biopsy required to confirm diagnosis. Most progress to show signs suggesting systemic illness such as anorexia and lethargy					
Leishmaniasis	Nasodigital hyperkeratosis/ hypopigmentation reported	–	–	Most commonly presents as a fine, silvery, exfoliative scaling dermatitis. May present as ulcerative or nodular dermatitis. Systemic signs are many and varied. Transmitted by biting flies, particularly sandflies. Zoonotic risk			–
Hereditary lupoid dermatosis of German Short-haired Pointer	–	–	–	Exfoliative, crusting and scaling lesions first appear on face at 6–36 months of age. May have a waxing and waning course. Poorly responsive to treatment. Uncommon. May be considered a breed variant of cutaneous lupus erythematosus			
Canine ear margin dermatoses	–	–	–	–	–	–	Idiopathic seborrhoeic scaling and follicular casting. May lead to painful fissuring. Symptomatic treatment only

13.7 Scaling and crusting disorders affecting the face.

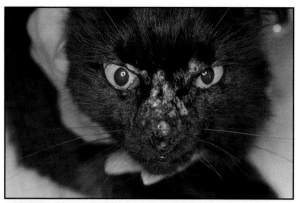

13.8 Mosquito bite hypersensitivity in a 6-year-old Domestic Shorthair, showing multifocal papulocrustous eruptions on the bridge of the nose.

are relatively easy to recognize although, being fragile, they tend to be transient. It is important therefore to recognize that pustules are normally followed by shallow erosions, crusts, collarettes and healing macules, which may show hyperpigmentation and scaling. The presence of any of these is compatible with pustular disease (Figure 13.9). Papules may progress to produce a similar range of lesions. Bullae tend to be deeper and produce ulcerative lesions (see later).

The contents of pustules are easily accessible for cytological examination and this technique should not be neglected. Deeper lesions should always be cultured to identify the organisms involved. Biopsy is often indicated to illustrate the reaction pattern present or to confirm a provisional diagnosis, particularly if autoimmune disease is suspected.

Condition	Anatomical site						
	Nasal planum	Lips	Chin	Muzzle	Periorbital skin	Preauricular skin	Pinnae
Pyoderma	Crusting, fissuring. Painful	Papules, pustules, crusts. Collarettes less commonly seen than in other areas. May be patchy or diffuse alopecia			Rare. Periorbital pyoderma frequently pruritic. Pustules in the pinnae are very unlikely to be bacterial in origin – consider pemphigus		
Furunculosis	–	Starts as superficial pyoderma. Deeper lesions produce haemorrhagic bullae, furunculosis, cellulitis and oedema. Periorbital furunculosis may develop in association with pruritus. Buried hair shafts may produce persistent granulomatous reaction, especially over chin				–	–
Mucocutaneous pyoderma	–	Symmetrical swelling and erythema of lips progressing to crusting/fissuring	–	–	–	–	–
Eosinophilic folliculitis and furunculosis	–	Typically young large/medium breeds. Onset acute, often peaks within 24 hours and episodes last 2–3 weeks. Papules, haemorrhagic blisters, nodules, plaques and varying degrees of ulceration, exudation and crusting. Pruritus and pain variable. Possibly arthropod-triggered				–	–
Juvenile cellulitis	–	Initially acute oedematous swelling of affected areas. Papules and pustules develop within 48 hours, progress to fistulae and drain and crust. Pustular otitis common. Lethargy, pyrexia, anorexia and joint pain may accompany dermatological disease				–	May develop pustular otitis
Feline/canine acne	–	In dog, not a true acne – simply a pyoderma variant. In cats – due to idiopathic keratinization defect causing comedones, crusts, papules and pustules. In severe cases, oedema, furunculosis and cellulitis may develop	–	–	–	–	–
Pemphigus foliaceus	Commonly leads to depigmentation	–	First lesions often on face and ears before other areas become involved and consist of erythematous macules which progress to pustules, crusts and collarettes. Scaling, erosions and alopecia may be present. Lesions may wax and wane and pain and pruritus are variable				
Sporotrichosis	–	–	Associated with puncture wounds. Multiple firm nodules and ulcerated plaques over face and pinnae. May show annular crusts and alopecia patches, may become verrucous. Nodules may ulcerate or develop draining tracts. Cats usually show persistent cellulitis and draining tracts on head. Potential zoonosis				
Vasculitis	–	–	Crusting dermatitis, principally over bridge of nose – pustules, papules and purpuric lesions due to vasculitis. Pruritus can be severe.				–

13.9 Papular and pustular disorders affecting the face.

Swellings, nodules and draining tracts

Lesions in this section fall broadly into two categories: solid lesions; and those containing a fluid (Figure 13.10). The unrivalled accessibility of dermatological lesions allows aspiration cytology not only to distinguish between these groups but also to make valuable early steps in making a definitive diagnosis (see Chapter 8). This is an opportunity that should never be ignored.

Condition	Anatomical site						
	Nasal planum	**Lips**	**Chin**	**Muzzle**	**Periorbital skin**	**Preauricular skin**	**Pinnae**
Abscess	–	–	Painful focal swellings, usually single, with variable degree of surrounding oedema. Rupture and drain leaving discharging sinuses. Alopecia of surface skin common. Most due to penetrative wounds contaminated by commensal organisms. Chronic or recurrent abscesses with granular pus may be due to a variety of other organisms. Culture is required for diagnosis			–	–
Mycobacterial granulomas	–	Single or multiple ulcers, abscesses, dermal or subcutaneous plaques and nodules. Lesions are usually non-healing and may discharge thick, malodorous yellow to green pus. Persistent draining sinuses may form. Anorexia, depression, weight loss, pyrexia and lymphadenopathy may be seen. Degree of systemic involvement and zoonotic risk varies with the species of *Mycobacterium* involved.					Pinnal nodules common in canine leprosy
Actinobacillosis	–	Single or multiple thick-walled abscesses discharging thick green to white pus with white nodules. Usually arise at site of bite or injury					–
Sporotrichosis	–	Multiple firm nodules and alopecic ulcerated plaques with crusted borders. Some lesions have verrucous appearance and may form draining tracts. Pain and pruritus rare and systemic signs usually absent although dissemination does occur, particularly in the cat. Zoonotic risk					
Cryptococcosis	Papules, nodules, ulcers, abcesses and draining tracts with the nose and lips involved in 20% of cases. 70% of cats show larger fluctuant swellings on bridge of nose or intranasal polyps. Association with exposure to pigeon droppings noted in most studies		–	–	–		Lesions often seen on pinnae in cats
Basal cell tumours	Single or multiple, firm, round, elevated and well circumscribed nodules, often alopecic, 1–2 cm in diameter. May be cystic, frequently ulcerated and melanotic. Benign forms are slow growing. Basal carcinomas may be seen in cats on the nasal planum and eyelids						–
Histiocytoma	–	Small well circumscribed firm benign nodules, often ulcerated. Common in the dog; rare in the cat. Fast-growing but resolve spontaneously in most cases. Pinnae and lips most common facial sites					
Systemic histiocytosis	Multiple epidermal or subcutaneous papules, plaques and nodules especially on the muzzle, nasal planum and eyelids. Surface or lesions may be erythematous and ulcerated. Seen principally in the Bernese Mountain Dog. May have fluctuating course or be rapidly progressive and fatal due to infiltration of multiple organ systems. Benign form confined to the skin is termed cutaneous histiocytosis and may present with lesions limited to nasal planum						
Mast cell tumours	–	In the cat, mastocytomas occur most commonly on the head and neck. Lesions may be multiple soft poorly demarcated, oedematous, pinkish masses or may be firm round well circumscribed white to yellow papules or nodules. Frequently pruritic and may ulcerate. Male and Siamese cats appear predisposed. A histiocytic variant is seen in young Siamese, with multiple pinkish papules and nodules primarily on the head and pinnae					
Plasmacytoma	–	Well circumscribed, raised smooth, firm to soft, pink to red dermal nodules. May be associated with multiple myeloma. Rare in the cat	–	–	–		Occasionally seen on pinnae
Papillomavirus infection	Single or multiple pedunculated or cauliflower-like nodules. May be firm to soft and are well circumscribed and alopecic. Other cutaneous lesions are described in other parts of the body						
Neuroendocrine tumours	–	Rare, solid, rapidly growing round nodules. May ulcerate. Most are solitary, malignant and metastasize – occasionally benign	–	–	–		Nodules my also see seen on ears (and digits)
Urticaria/ angio-oedema	–	Localized or generalized wheals, often erythematous with variable pruritus. May coalesce to form bizarre patterns or irregular plaques. Angioedema is characterized by larger oedematous swellings that commonly show some serum exudation			–		Urticaria may be seen on pinnae in some cases

13.10   Swellings, nodules and draining tracts affecting the face. (continues)   ▶

Condition	Anatomical site						
	Nasal planum	**Lips**	**Chin**	**Muzzle**	**Periorbital skin**	**Preauricular skin**	**Pinnae**
Dirofilariasis	–	Pruritic, ulcerative, nodular or papulocrustous dermatitis also affecting trunk and limbs					–
Tick infestation	–	–	–	–	–	Focal papules, crusts often with erythematous border. May progress to firm nodules. May be vectors for several important microbial diseases and cause a flaccid paralysis	
Spider bites	Local erythema surrounding bite site progressing to granulomatous nodules (*Latrodectus spp.*) or necrotic ulcers (*Loxosceles spp.*) Severe systemic reactions may occur					–	–
Insect stings and bites	–	–	–	Papules, often pruritic and crusting, progressing to erosive dermatitis. Nodular pinnal lesions may be seen which may become necrotic and ulcerate			
Caterpillar irritation	–	Sudden onset facial pruritus, oedema, urticaria or angio-oedema. Tongue may be swollen and ptyalism may be pronounced. Associated with the venomous bristles of the larvae of a number of Lepidoptera				–	–
Xanthoma	–	–	Multiple yellow to white papules, nodules or plaques – may be ulcerated. Surrounding skin is erythematous and lesions may be painful or pruritic. Associated with abnormality in lipid metabolism – lesions may also be seen on distal extremities, feet and bony prominences.				

13.10   (continued) Swellings, nodules and draining tracts affecting the face.

Ulceration

Ulcerative lesions, by definition, breach the epidermal basement membrane. They are comparatively rare, tending to arise through one of two processes: destruction of the epidermal layers; or cleaving of the epidermal layers and the formation of vesiculobullous lesions. The latter are readily identified if intact lesions are present but they are fragile and rupture easily. In general, vesiculobullous lesions are usually well circumscribed with adjacent skin being grossly normal. Destructive lesions, however, are often less well defined, more inflamed or crusted and tend to exhibit more aggressive gross pathology. The deep nature of the lesions leads to a greater risk of secondary infection, fluid loss and scarring.

Whatever the underlying pathomechanism may be, ulcerative lesions (Figure 13.11) cannot be treated lightly as many of the possible underlying conditions may be fatal. As the therapeutic protocols required to control some of the possible differentials are severe, confirmation of the diagnosis is necessary and this will usually require histopathological examination of representative biopsies. Cultures may be needed in other cases.

Condition	Anatomical site						
	Nasal planum	**Lips**	**Chin**	**Muzzle**	**Periorbital skin**	**Preauricular skin**	**Pinnae**
Pemphigus vulgaris	Vesicles and bullae progressing to erosions and ulceration, especially mucocutaneous junctions. Oral cavity involvement in up to 90%. Cutaneous lesions may occur elsewhere, particularly in axillae. Nikolsky sign may be present. Pruritus and pain variable. Lymphadenopathy and pyoderma seen. Animals may be depressed, anorexic and febrile. Biopsy required to confirm diagnosis. Prognosis guarded					–	Pinnae and ear canal lesions may be seen
Erythema multiforme	Erythematous macules, urticarial plaques, vesicles and bullae. Broadly symmetrical					–	–
Bullous pemphigoid	–	Oral and lip vesicles, bullae and ulcers seen in 33% of cases	–	–	Periorbital lesions may be seen	–	–
Epidermolysis bullosa	–	–	–	Multiple well defined erosive to ulcerative lesions, progressing to crusts, scarring and depigmentation, particularly over pinnae and bony prominences of face			
Candidiasis	–	Malodorous non-healing ulcers with superficial grey plaques and erythematous borders. Oral cavity and lips most commonly involved. Localized hyperkeratotic and crusted lesions reported on face, muzzle and pinnae. Pruritus variable and may be intense					

13.11   Ulcerative conditions affecting the face. (continues)   ▶

Condition	Anatomical site						
	Nasal planum	**Lips**	**Chin**	**Muzzle**	**Periorbital skin**	**Preauricular skin**	**Pinnae**
FeLV infection	–	Diffuse scaling, crusting and erosive lesions. Lips, perioral and preauricular skin and pinnae most commonly involved. Cats appear otherwise healthy but over time often become anorexic and lethargic					
Feline herpesvirus infection	Multifocal small ulcerative and necrotizing dermatitis, often with papular crusts. Usually in association with stomatitis or rhinotracheitis. May be generalized. Resolves spontaneously						
Poxvirus infection	–	–	–	–	Focal crusting and ulceration at bite wound may be followed by widespread macular/papular to nodular lesions, which rapidly crust and ulcerate. Lesions may scar and heal slowly over 3–4 weeks		
Eosinophilic ulcer	–	Well defined, firm raised red ulcerated lesions on upper lip. Pain and pruritus rare. Rarely, may transform to squamous cell carcinoma	–	–	–	–	–
Idiopathic ulcerative dermatosis of the Shetland Sheepdog	–	–	–	–	Multifocal vesicles and bullae. May coalesce and ulcerate to form large well demarcated ulcerated serpiginous lesions		

13.11 (continued) Ulcerative conditions affecting the face.

Necrosis and fissuring

Fissuring is usually seen as a secondary feature of hyperkeratosis and occurs due to the loss of flexibility of the skin surface. The pinnae and nasal planum are the regions most commonly affected (Figure 13.12). In the context of facial disease, necrosis usually occurs in association with vasculitis and is classifiable on the basis of the dominating inflammatory infiltrate, which may have some aetiopathogenic significance. The pathomechanism of some vasculitides is assumed to involve Type 3 hypersensitivity but it is likely that more complex mechanisms also play a role. Factors such as insect bites, dietary intolerance, neoplasia and connective tissue disorders have been associated with vasculitis (see Chapter 27).

Condition	Anatomical site						
	Nasal planum	**Lips**	**Chin**	**Muzzle**	**Periorbital skin**	**Preauricular skin**	**Pinnae**
Vasculitis	Erythema and purpura, plaques, papules and pustules, occasionally bullae. Hyperkeratosis, scaling, alopecia and hyperpigmentation common in slowly developing lesions. May see necrosis and crater-like ulcers. Lesions typically affect extremities but may be seen elsewhere. Extravasation of blood seen in acute lesions. Lesion pattern may follow vascular pathways						
Lupus erythematosus (Figure 13.13)	Depigmentation, loss of rough cobblestone pattern, erosions, crusting, fissuring and inflammation	Erythema, depigmentation, erosions, crusting. May be punctate oral ulcers. May progress to alopecia. Pruritus variable. Scarring is a common sequel. Depigmentation of hair and skin common. Cases should be evaluated for systemic involvement. Cutaneous lesions exacerbated by ultraviolet light			Generally uninvolved		Crusting, scaling and alopecia
Familial vasculopathy of the German Shepherd Dog	Nasal planum lesions may be seen	–	–	–	–	–	Reported in young GSD – autosomal recessive trait. Alopecia, crusts and ulceration of pinnae – usually also depigmentation and crusting of footpads, lethargy and pyrexia
Cold agglutinin disease (Figure 13.14)	–	–	–	–	–	–	Abrupt onset erythema, purpura, ulceration, pain, and necrosis of pinnae and other extremities. Usually precipitated by low temperatures

13.12 Necrosis and fissuring disorders affecting the face. (continues) ▶

Condition	Anatomical site						
	Nasal planum	*Lips*	*Chin*	*Muzzle*	*Periorbital skin*	*Preauricular skin*	*Pinnae*
Proliferative thrombovascular pinnal necrosis	–	–	–	–	–	–	Wedge-shaped lesions with central ulceration and scaly pigmented border. Progressive. Older lesions necrose, leading to deformation of pinnal margin
Feline auricular chondritis	–	–	–	–	–	–	Swollen, erythematous painful ears, usually curled and deformed. May be unilateral.

13.12 (continued) Necrosis and fissuring disorders affecting the face.

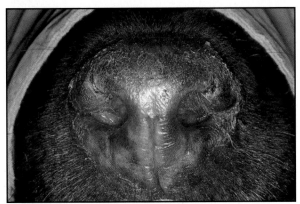

13.13 Discoid lupus erythematosus in a 3-year-old German Shepherd Dog. There is depigmentation, fissuring and loss of the normal 'cobblestone' pattern on the nasal planum.

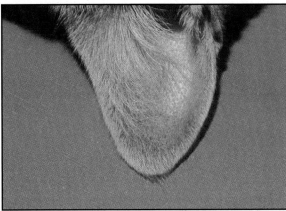

13.14 Cold agglutinin disease in an 8-year-old Domestic Shorthair, showing sharply demarcated purpura on the pinna and a necrotic ear tip.

Skin lesions typically occur in regions where the demand on the integument is greatest such as over bony prominences or at the extremities where blood supply is most easily jeopardised. Slowly developing lesions frequently become hyperkeratotic and hyperpigmented and tissue loss is slow and modified by concurrent healing processes. These lesions are often alopecic and scaling. Where the onset of vasculitis is rapid or severe, necrosis may precede the development of other lesions leading to a sharply demarcated border between lesional and nonlesional skin. Extravasation of blood may be seen. These are features, which are easily identifiable on close examination or may be elicited through careful history taking.

Further reading

Harvey RG, Harari J and Delauche AJ (2000) *Ear Diseases of the Dog and Cat*. Manson Publishing, London
Griffin CE, Kwochka KW and Macdonald JM (1992) *Current Veterinary Dermatology: The Science and Art of Therapy*. Mosby Year Book, St Louis
Wilkinson GT and Harvey RG (1994) *Colour Atlas of Small Animal Dermatology – A Guide to Diagnosis*. Manson Publishing, London

14

An approach to otitis externa and otitis media

Emmanuel Bensignor

Otitis is defined as an acute or chronic inflammation of the auditory canal. Depending on the depth of the disease, otitis can be classified as otitis externa (OE), otitis media (OM) or otitis interna (OI). Prognosis and treatment are different for each type of otitis.

OE is an inflammation of the external auditory canal and tympanic membrane. It is very common in dogs and cats: the incidence of OE has been reported as between 5–12% of consultations in dogs and up to 2% of cats referred to a dermatologist (Bensignor, 1999 ; Griffin, 1993, Scott et al., 2001).

OM has long been considered rare in dogs and cats. However, recent studies have shown that OM was very common in cases of chronic OE in dogs (up to 80% of cases), even if the tympanic membrane looked normal (Cole et al., 1998). The reasons for this are unclear, but it is suggested that in some instances the membrane can heal rapidly, thereby masking the depth of the infection. OM occasionally occurs after invasion of microorganisms from the nasopharynx or via the blood.

Dogs with pendulous and hypertrichotic ears and/ or with seborrhoea are predisposed to otitis. A retrospective study of 752 cases (Carlotti and Taillieu-Leroy, 1997) has shown that Poodles and Pyrenean Mountain Dogs are predisposed. In a prospective survey of 844 cases Bensignor et al. (2000) showed that Poodles and Labrador Retrievers may be at increased risk.

OE is usually not only a local phenomenon, but one manifestation of an underlying dermatosis. OE should be considered in a broader dermatological context, and it is essential to identify and treat all components of inflammation of the auditory canal. This requires a thorough diagnostic work-up, which should include a detailed history, a complete clinical examination (general, dermatological and otological) and diagnostic procedures, notably otoscopy, direct examination of the cerumen, cytology and bacteriology. Other diagnostic techniques may more rarely be needed (video-otoscopy, radiography, computed tomography, myringo-tomy – paracentesis of tympanic fluid, biopsy). If a thorough diagnostic work-up is not done and only symptomatic treatment is administered, some cases may resolve but most will recur.

Treatment involves cleaning and the use of topical medications. Systemic therapy is rarely needed in OE but should be considered in OM. In every case, treatment of an underlying disease is mandatory.

Differential diagnosis

Otitis externa can usually be diagnosed easily by the clinician: erythema of the pinna and/or the auditory canal, associated with excessive production of cerumen and/or pus, resulting in pruritus and/or pain are typical. Face rubbing, scratching, head shaking, sharp pain and/or bad smell are very characteristic features of OE.

However, it must be remembered that otitis is not a diagnosis but rather a pattern of cutaneous disease. As many cases of OE are not primary, but linked to an underlying disease, a large number of potential aetiological factors must be considered. The underlying disease should be diagnosed and treated to resolve the OE and prevent relapse. Underlying factors (Figure 14.1) may be classified as follows (Griffin, 1993):

- Predisposing factors, which increase the risk of OE
- Primary factors, which directly induce OE

Predisposing factors
Conformation of the ear
Humidity
Inappropriate cleaning
Hypertrichosis
Predisposition to seborrhoea
Irritant treatments

Primary factors
Atopy
Ectoparasites
Keratinization disorders
Pyoderma
Autoimmune dermatosis
Foreign bodies
Tumours

Secondary factors
Yeasts
Bacteria

Perpetuating factors
Epidermal and sebaceous hyperplasia
Ulceration
Otitis media

14.1 Differential diagnosis and aetiological factors of otitis externa.

- Secondary factors, which do not typically create disease in normal ears but aggravate it
- Perpetuating factors, which are related to a change in anatomical structure or disruption of the physiological function of the ear.

In chronic cases, more than one factor is present.

Primary factors

Atopy
Atopy is the most common cause of otitis externa in dogs. It should be emphasized that some cases of atopy may present only with OE. Food allergy or intolerance may also be responsible for OE in dogs and cats. Over 20% of food-allergic dogs start with OE alone, and ear disease is present in 80% of food allergic dogs. Contact allergy is far less common, but inappropriate use of ear products containing potential irritants or allergens may be responsible for this disease. These irritant reactions often go misdiagnosed.

Ectoparasites
Ectoparasites should always be considered as a primary cause of otitis externa. *Otodectes cynotis* is particularly important. It is a psoroptid mite characterized by long legs with unjointed projections and suckers. The mites live on the surface of the skin, particularly in the auditory canal, and feed on epidermal debris and tissue fluids. They irritate the ear epithelium and generate an allergic reaction in susceptible hosts. *O. cynotis* infestation may represent 7–10% of cases of OE in dogs and up to 50% of cases in cats. It is very contagious.

Other parasites may rarely be responsible for OE in dogs and cats (e.g. *Demodex* spp., *Otobius megnini*).

Keratinization disorders
Keratinization disorders (primary or secondary to, for example, endocrinopathies) may be responsible for changes in glandular activity and overproduction of cerumen. This predisposes to OE.

Autoimmune disease
Rarely, cases of autoimmune OE will appear. Usually cutaneous signs are limited to the pinnae. Superficial and deep pemphigus, and cutaneous or systemic lupus, have been described in association with OE.

Foreign bodies
Foreign bodies must be considered in cases of acute unilateral otitis, particularly in dogs with pendulous and hypertrichotic ears. Generally, grass awns and seeds are involved. Some cases of chronic bilateral ear disease may also be due to grass awns.

Tumours
Tumours of the ear are relatively uncommon, but should be suspected whenever chronic OE does not respond to appropriate therapy. Tumours may be benign (papilloma, sebaceous adenoma, benign ceruminoma, fibroma) or malignant (squamous cell carcinoma, sebaceous carcinoma, malignant ceruminoma, fibrosarcoma, mastocytoma). In general, ear tumours are more

common but less malignant in dogs than in cats (McKeever, 1993). Ear polyps are seen exclusively in cats. They represent an inflammatory reaction and are not true neoplasms. They may be very extensive, invading the middle ear, the eustachian tube and the nasopharynx (McKeever, 1993).

Secondary factors
Bacteria or yeasts are very frequently isolated in otitis externa in dogs and cats. These microorganisms should, however, always be considered secondary to the inflammatory disease, and are therefore best considered secondary factors. A true idiopathic infectious OE is extremely rare in dogs and cats. The microorganisms commonly encountered in normal ears (*Enterobacter* sp., *Staphylococcus* sp., *Malassezia* sp.) are part of the normal flora of the external ear canal (Kiss, 1997). Where there is inflammation or an altered microclimate, they may colonize the ear canal and amplify the disease. Bacteria most often isolated from the ears of dogs with OE are *Staphylococcus intermedius*, *Streptococcus* sp. and *Pseudomonas* sp. or *Proteus* sp. Infection with *Pseudomonas* sp. often causes severe purulent OE. This is very refractory to treatment and needs a thorough work-up (Box 14.1).

Box 14.1: *Pseudomonas* otitis

Clinical presentation
Pseudomonas spp. are recovered from 0.4% of normal ears, and from 20% of otitic ears. *Pseudomonas* otitis is more common in recurrent cases for which there has been long-term treatment with antibiotics (August, 1988). *Pseudomonas* spp. are responsible for very serious OE and OM, with pain and copious amounts of exudate (most often yellow pus). Extensive ulceration of the ear canal epithelium is also frequently encountered.

Establishing the diagnosis
Diagnosis is by demonstrating rods on cytology, followed by culture.

Prognosis
Prognosis should always be guarded, as multiple antibiotic resistance is common. *Pseudomonas* otitis should always be considered as a therapeutic challenge, necessitating frequent re-evaluations and long periods of treatment. Antibiotic sensitivity testing should always be performed prior to therapy. Cost of therapy is also a concern.

Treatment options
Treatment necessitates frequent cleaning (with disinfectants such as povidone–iodine or chlorhexidine) and antibiotics. Due to the pain and frequent ulceration, in-clinic cleaning under sedation is often indicated.

Pseudomonas spp. are usually sensitive to polymyxin B. Ticarcillin has been found to be useful and injectable amikacin and fluoroquinolones are also valuable. Tobramycin ophthalmic drops are another option. Aluminium acetate and acetic acid are helpful as they decrease the pH. Acetic acid 2% solution is lethal to *Pseudomonas* within 1 minute of contact.

Malassezia pachydermatis is commonly isolated in canine or feline OE. In the cat other species (*M. sympodialis* and *M. globosa*) have been demonstrated in the external ear canal but it is unclear whether they are pathogenic. *Malassezia* otitis (Box 14.2) is very common but, as with bacterial disease, it is often secondary to an underlying, mainly allergic, dermatitis. It should also be remembered that some

Box 14.2: *Malassezia* otitis

Clinical presentation

Malassezia otitis is very common in dogs, often occurring secondary to an allergy. Cerumen is often moist, brown and accompanied by an unpleasant smell. However, it may be dry and black, as in ear mite infestation, or mimic pus. Pruritus is often severe.

Establishing the diagnosis

Demonstration of yeasts on microscopic examination of cytological samples is simple, but it is more difficult to assess their pathogenicity as ear canals of normal dogs may be colonized by yeasts. The author considers that finding more than 5–10 yeasts per high power field (x1000) is suggestive of *Malassezia* otitis and justifies antifungal treatment.

Prognosis

Prognosis is good if an underlying factor is diagnosed and corrected. Otherwise, recurrence is likely. Some cases of OM may be due to *Malassezia* sp., and here the prognosis is more guarded.

Treatment options

Many antifungal drugs are available. Topical azole derivatives (clotrimazole, miconazole) are very effective against *Malassezia* sp. These drugs should be applied once or twice a day for 10–14 days until the infection has cleared. For cases of *Malassezia* OM, the use of systemic medications in association with topical treatment may be needed. Ketoconazole (10 mg/kg/day) and itraconazole (5 mg/kg/day) are very effective.

cases of dermatophyte-related OE have been described in cats, without any other dermatological lesion. A fungal culture of the cerumen may therefore sometimes be indicated.

Perpetuating factors

Perpetuating factors are mainly linked to a modification of the anatomy of the external ear canal, which prevents healing. Epidermal hyperkeratosis and acanthosis are associated with the dermal fibrosis and oedema, and apocrine gland hyperplasia seen in chronic cases of OE. They cause thickening of the skin and stenosis of the canal lumen, which inhibit effective cleaning and application of topical medication, perpetuating secondary infections.

Undiagnosed otitis media could be the principal cause of chronic otitis. OM has been reported to be present in about 16% of cases of acute OE and up to 83% of chronic cases (Cole *et al.*, 1998 ; Scott *et al.*, 2001). Furthermore, recent studies have shown that OM should be looked for routinely in cases of chronic otitis even if no rupture of the tympanic membrane can be seen. Pus in the tympanic bulla can be the source of chronic infection and topical antibiotics cannot penetrate deep enough into the ear canal. Pro-inflammatory toxins and debris may constantly be released from this area. These cases of OM have therapeutic implications, not only because they will need systemic treatment, but also because it has been demonstrated that the microbial flora in the external ear canal are different to those in the tympanic bulla: a mixed infection (yeasts and bacteria) is often present in the external canal whereas a *Pseudomonas* infection is particularly common in the tympanic bulla (Cole *et al.*, 1998). Differences in bacterial sensitivity to common antibiotics, depending on the depth of infection, also seem to be the rule.

Clinical approach

History

Taking the history is the first step in the investigation of otitis (Figure 14.2).

Age of onset
Young animals predisposed to ectoparasites, notably *Otodectes cynotis*   Adult animals prone to allergic otitis externa   Old animals predisposed to tumours or autoimmune dermatoses
Development of signs and seasonality
Acute episode of unilateral otitis: suggestive of a foreign body   Recurrent bilateral OE occurring every spring: suggests allergic otitis   Gradually developing unilateral OE: suggestive of neoplastic process
Evidence of contagion
Often (but not always) noted in ear mite infection
Environment
Presence of foreign bodies   Excessive humidity (swimming dogs)   Aeroallergens   Free roaming animals prone to otoacariosis
Viral status
Chronic OE in cats often linked to feline leukaemia virus or feline immunodeficiency virus infection   Herpesvirus infection in cats may trigger facial dermatitis with OE, or generalized erythema multiforme with frequent ear involvement
Prior therapies
Trauma induced by poor cleaning technique by the owner (use of cotton buds)   Use of inappropriate treatment (e.g. alcohol, ether)   Allergic reactions to neomycin or glucocorticoids may occur

14.2 Important aspects of history in the otitis case.

Clinical examination

General examination

A general clinical examination should be carried out initially, looking for neurological signs (vestibular or labyrinthic syndrome, facial paresis), secondary to OM and OI. For cats with suppurative OE, testing for retroviruses is essential. It is also important to examine the pharynx and larynx carefully to detect nasopharyngeal polyps. The clinician should be aware that some paraneoplastic disease may be accompanied by OE. Finally, some cancers may be associated with OE (e.g. mast cell tumour, Figure 14.3).

Dermatological examination

As otitis is usually a local manifestation of an underlying dermatosis, it is necessary to check the patient for other skin lesions. This will help to determine the aetiology (e.g. cheilitis and pododermatitis might suggest atopy).

Auricular examination

The pinnae and entrances to the ear canals should be carefully examined before moving on to the external canals. The healthier ear must always be examined

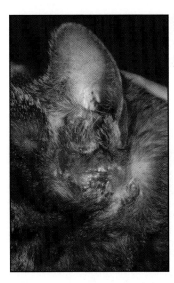

14.3 Invasive mast cell tumour of the external ear canal of a cat.

first. After palpating to evaluate pain, thickening and ossification of the ear canal, the presence of cerumen or pus is noted. This allows the clinical distinction between erythematoceruminous otitis externa (ECOE) and suppurative otitis externa (SOE) (Carlotti, 1994). ECOE is characterized by erythema and black or brownish cerumen (Figure 14.4). In SOE (Figure 14.5), a lot of pus is present, and a 'squelching' noise and pain are often noted when palpating the ear. Although the type of discharge is suggestive of the aetiology (e.g. dry black cerumen in cases of ear mite infection, moist brown discharge for *Malassezia* otitis, yellow exudate in cases of *Pseudomonas* otitis), this can be misleading. For instance, it has recently been demonstrated that dry black exudate in dogs is usually associated with *Malassezia* otitis (Bensignor *et al.*, 2000).

An otoscopic examination of the external ear canal is the next step. A standard otoscope with cones of various lengths, diameters and shapes is necessary. Veterinary devices are preferred, as cones designed for human ears are too short for use in dogs and cats. Recently video-otoscopic devices (fibre-optic video-enhanced otoscopes) have become commercially available. These machines permit the ear canal to be examined more clearly than classic otoscopes (Figure 14.6). Nervous animals may need to be sedated, not only to allow visualization but also to avoid trauma, as potentially harmful instruments will be introduced into the ear canal. The auroscopic examination is aimed at detecting foreign bodies and inflammatory changes (lichenification, stenosis, oedema, erosions/ulcerations, dermal calcification, ceruminous hyperplasia, tumours). It should always allow the visualization of the tympanic membrane (Figure 14.7). This appears in normal ears as a concave translucent membrane, with a dorsal, white, thick, well vascularized pars flaccida and a ventral semi-transparent pars tensa. Any rupture of this membrane (small tear or total destruction) indicates OM. It is always advisable to keep a record of lesions, to enable a good follow-up.

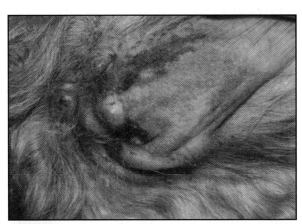

14.4 Erythematoceruminous otitis externa.

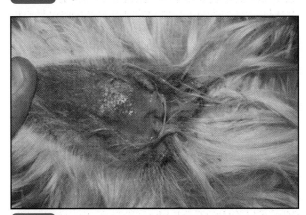

14.5 Suppurative otitis externa.

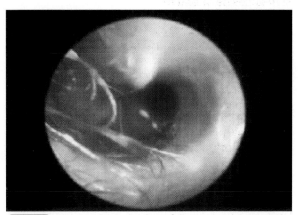

14.6 Video-otoscopic view of the external ear canal in a normal dog.

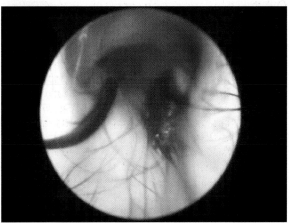

14.7 Video-otoscopic view of the tympanic membrane in a normal dog. Note the hairs.

When a large amount of cerumen, debris or pus is present, it may be impossible to perform a thorough otoscopic examination. In these cases, cleaning is necessary. However, this cleaning procedure should only be performed after initial complementary examinations (see below).

Further investigation

Figure 14.8 shows a practical approach to otitis externa and otitis media.

Direct microscopy

Direct microscopic examination of the cerumen for the presence of parasites is carried out. The cerumen is sampled with a curette or swab and is diluted in chloral lactophenol or liquid paraffin. Observation at a magnification of X40 is usually adequate to detect parasites (*Otodectes cynotis* (Figure 14.9), *Demodex* spp. or larvae of the tick *Otobius megnini*). This procedure must be completed even if there is little cerumen present, particularly in cats.

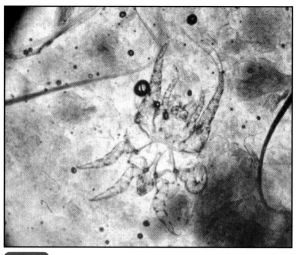

14.9   *Otodectes cynotis* in lactophenol.

Cytology

Magnifications of X400 and X1000 allow cytological examination of the cerumen for the presence of bacteria and yeasts. *Malassezia* spp. may be identified

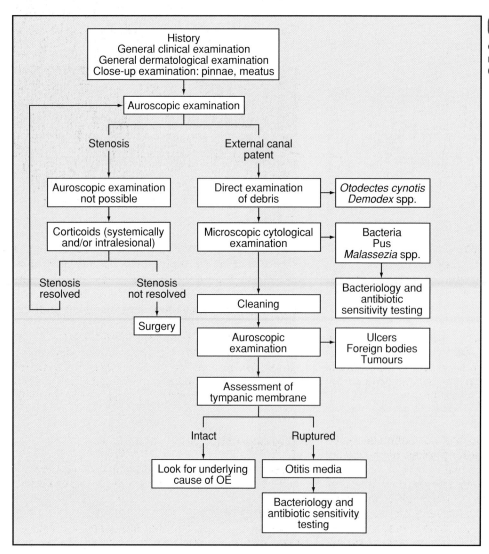

14.8   A practical approach to otitis externa and otitis media. (Adapted from DN Carlotti.)

History
General clinical examination
General dermatological examination
Close-up examination: pinnae, meatus
↓
Auroscopic examination
├─ Stenosis
│   ↓
│   Auroscopic examination not possible
│   ↓
│   Corticoids (systemically and/or intralesional)
│   ├─ Stenosis resolved
│   └─ Stenosis not resolved
│   ↓
│   Surgery
│
└─ External canal patent
    ↓
    Direct examination of debris → *Otodectes cynotis* *Demodex* spp.
    ↓
    Microscopic cytological examination → Bacteria Pus *Malassezia* spp. → Bacteriology and antibiotic sensitivity testing
    ↓
    Cleaning
    ↓
    Auroscopic examination → Ulcers Foreign bodies Tumours
    ↓
    Assessment of tympanic membrane
    ├─ Intact
    │   ↓
    │   Look for underlying cause of OE
    └─ Ruptured
        ↓
        Otitis media
        ↓
        Bacteriology and antibiotic sensitivity testing

(Figure 14.10). It is difficult to assess the pathogenic role of these yeasts as they may be recovered in the ear canals from healthy dogs and cats. Cocci must be distinguished from rods as this may indicate a *Pseudomonas* sp. infection, which is difficult to treat and will need antibiotic sensitivity testing. Degenerated neutrophils are present in SOE, and phagocytosis of bacteria can often be observed (Figure 14.11).

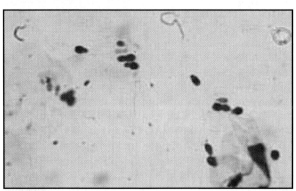

14.10 Cytology of ear exudate, showing *Malassezia pachydermatis* stained with Diff-Quik®.

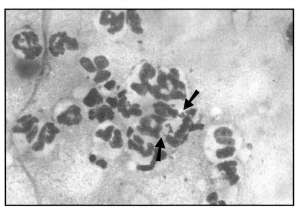

14.11 Cytology of ear exudate, showing bacterial cocci (arrowed) within neutrophils. (Diff-Quik®). (Courtesy of D. Pin)

Bacteriological culture
Bacteriological culture accompanied by antibiotic sensitivity testing is indicated in chronic or recurrent cases of SOE, when prior appropriate topical and/or systemic antibiotic therapy has not been effective. It is also indicated when rods have been demonstrated, and in OM. This is because therapy will be long-term for these cases, and multiple antibacterial resistance is often encountered with *Pseudomonas* spp. A sterile swab should be inserted through the sterile cone of an auroscope attachment, to prevent contamination.

Ear Cleaning
If the tympanic membrane has not been visualized previously, a thorough cleaning (often necessitating sedation) should be carried out.

Non-ototoxic diluted cleansers should be used and the ear canal flushed until a clear liquid is obtained. Retrograde cleaning with an enema bag or suction device is ideal. A feeding tube attached to a syringe filled with saline and passed through a surgical otoscope

cone down the canal is a useful alternative. The solution is infused then aspirated back out with the debris. Care must be taken to direct the tip of the tube ventrally to the tympanic membrane to avoid causing vestibular syndrome or deafness after cleaning. The process should be repeated until the ear is completely clean. Auroscopic examination should then allow evaluation of the canal wall and the patency and transparency of the tympanic membrane.

Paracentesis
In cases of OM, or when OM is strongly suspected, paracentesis followed by cytology and bacteriology should be performed. However, this procedure is not easy, and it should ideally be done with the aid of a video-otoscope. Referral to a trained veterinary dermatologist may be advisable.

Imaging techniques
It is possible to perform radiography or CT scanning of the tympanic bullae (Figure 14.12). This should be carried out in all cases of chronic otitis externa and where there is an invasive tumour of the ear canal.

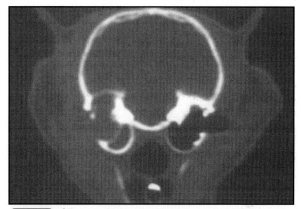

14.12 CT scan demonstrating destruction of the ear canal and otitis media in a cat. (Courtesy of F.Delisle)

Biopsy
If a tumour, or an autoimmune dermatosis is suspected, biopsies are indicated. They are best performed under video-otoscopic control, or by passing endoscopic biopsy forceps through the otoscope cone.

Investigation of underlying disease
It is essential to look for an underlying disease to explain the inflammation of the ear canal. The choice of complementary examinations depends on the suspected cause (e.g. intradermal tests, elimination diet).

Therapeutic principles

These recommendations reflect the author's current point of view. The list of products cited is not exhaustive.

Cleaning
Cleaning is an important step in the effective management of OE, as pus and inflammatory debris can

inactivate some medications and reduce the access of topical therapies. The owner must be instructed how to clean the ears effectively. The procedure must be repeated two to three times a week until the ear canal is free of cerumen, pus and debris. Cleaning agents should be non-irritant. Various ceruminolytic agents exist (dioctyl sodium sulphosuccinate, calcium sulphosuccinate, carbamide peroxide, propylene glycol). For ECOE a lipid solution is preferred, whereas for SOE an aqueous solution is better. A number of products are available. Some may be ototoxic and should be avoided if the tympanic membrane is ruptured.

The solution is flushed into the ear canal, and a gentle massage helps dissolve the debris. Thereafter the animal is let free, and will shake its head. The ear canal is then dried with absorbent paper. The use of cotton swabs is not recommended.

Topical therapy

Topical therapy is the cornerstone of treatment. It should be directed towards the cause of the disease (e.g. acaricidal treatment in case of otoacariosis, antifungal treatment for *Malassezia* otitis, antibiotics for SOE). The use of products containing more than three different agents should be avoided, as the concentration of each active ingredient is decreased in such preparations.

A number of different products are licensed for use in dogs and cats. They should be applied in a clean external canal, and the supplier's instructions should be followed. In general, for acute cases of OE, 7–14 days of therapy are needed. This may be longer (up to 4 weeks) for chronic cases. Care must also be taken to ensure that the agents in these preparations are not ototoxic if the tympanic membrane is ruptured.

Acaricidal treatments

Various ear treatments containing lindane, rotenone, pyrethroids or avermectins are available. These products should be applied at least twice a week for 3 consecutive weeks as eggs are usually not sensitive to the acaricidal effects of therapy. Acaricides that are not systemically absorbed must also be applied on the body as some *Otodectes* can survive out of the ear canals and be responsible for reinfestation. In-contact animals must be treated, because they can act as a source of recontamination.

Antibiotic therapy

Antibacterial agents are indicated when infection is present. Selection depends on the type of bacteria demonstrated on cytology, and on the results of sensitivity testing. Neomycin, gentamicin and polymyxin B are excellent first choice antibiotics. Recently, topical fluoroquinolones have been used successfully in severe cases of OE. A product containing enrofloxacin is available on the US market and one containing marbofloxacin in Europe. These products may be considered second choices, as development of resistance may be an issue.

Silver sulfadiazine 1% is very effective for the treatment of infection with *Pseudomonas* sp. Ticarcillin is also an option for very refractory cases.

Antifungal therapy

Numerous agents are available for the treatment of *Malassezia* otitis. These include nystatin, thiabendazole, pimaricin, miconazole and clotrimazole. Silver sulfadiazine is effective against *Malassezia*.

Anti-inflammatory therapy

Glucocorticoids are present in nearly every commercial topical anti-inflammatory preparation available for dogs and cats. Glucocorticoids decrease inflammation, pruritus, erythema, exudation and tissue proliferation, and help promote drainage and ventilation. As the anti-inflammatory effect depends on the type of steroid used, care should be taken carefully to evaluate the risk:benefit ratio of these substances. Although iatrogenic Cushing's syndrome following auricular treatment is extremely rare, some cases of atrophy and some pro-infectious effects have been described. Systemic absorption may also occur. The more potent steroids (betamethasone valerate, fluocinolone acetonide) should, therefore, be used for no more than a few days, after which treatment should be switched to less potent corticosteroids. Some authors, however, use fluocinolone acetonide for the long-term management of allergic OE.

Others

Local anaesthetics may be useful for pain relief.

Acetic acid and vinegar have been used in *Pseudomonas* sp. infection, to reduce the pH of the external ear canal and to destroy the bacteria. As these solutions are very acidic and potentially irritant, their use is debatable.

Instructions for owners

Client education should form an important part of the therapeutic plan. Most owners will not apply the treatment correctly if they are not first told how to do it. A veterinary surgeon or nurse should apply the first treatment at the clinic, carefully explaining to the owner how to do it effectively (e.g. hold the pinna in one hand and apply the tube into the canal; press the bottle or the tube once or twice; gently massage the canal to allow the product to diffuse; wipe away the excess solution with cotton wool).

Systemic treatment

Avermectins

For otoacariosis, the clinician can use systemic avermectins. Selamectin is available as a spot-on formulation and licensed for use in cats with *O. cynotis* infestation (two applications 1 month apart). Injectable ivermectin (0.2–0.4 mg/kg s.c., two injections 10–14 days apart) is also very effective but should be avoided in sensitive breeds (Collies, Old English Sheepdog, Shetland Sheepdog) and in young animals. Ivermectin is not licensed for use in dogs and cats and it is essential to obtain informed consent from owners before starting therapy.

Antibiotics

Systemic antibiotics are used in OM. Antibiotic selection should be based on the results of sensitivity testing. Antibiotics which concentrate in pus are required. Treatment must be given for long periods (up to several months).

Glucocorticoids

For stenotic ear canals, or when hyperproliferative tissues invade the external ear canal, the use of systemic glucocorticoids is indicated for a few days, until the canal is opened and topical therapy may be used. Prednisolone at 0.5–1.0 mg/kg/day and methylprednisolone (0.4–0.8 mg/kg/day) are usually effective. In rare cases, it is also possible to inject corticosteroids locally, directly into the ear canal. Multiple small injections are made as deep as possible in the canal. This procedure is usually painful and requires sedation. These treatments must not be given for more than a few days as a suppurative otitis is usually present. If no clinical response is seen within 2 weeks of anti-inflammatory therapy, surgery is indicated.

Surgery

Surgery is rarely indicated in OE. Generally, thorough diagnostic investigation, cleaning procedures and appropriate medical treatment will allow a cure. Recurrences are often linked to an unrecognized and untreated underlying disease.

However, about 50% of OM cases need surgery (Rogers, 1988). Total ablation of the external auditory canal associated with ventral bulla osteotomy is usually the only way to obtain a cure (Bradley, 1988). Neither partial ablation nor lateral wall resection w' successful in most cases.

Treatment of the underlying disease

This is the most important aspect of the treatment of chronic OE or OM. Treatment clearly depends on the diagnosis (see above).

Follow-up

Regular re-examinations should be scheduled until the otitis has cleared. At each visit, otoscopic and cytological examinations are required. The condition should not be considered cured until clinical examination shows no abnormality and no inflammatory cells are detected.

References and further reading

August JR (1988) Otitis externa: a disease of multifactorial etiology. *Veterinary Clinics of North America: Small Animal Practice* **18,** 731–742

Bensignor E (1999) Dermatoses de l'oreille externe. In: *Encyclopédie Vétérinaire, Dermatologie, 3300,* p. 11. Elsevier, Paris

Bensignor E, Legeay D and Medaille C (2000) Etude prospective sur les otites externes du chien adulte en France. *Pratique Médicale et Chirurgicale de l'Animal de Compagnie* **35,** 405–414

Bradley RL (1988) Surgical management of otitis externa. *Veterinary Clinics of North America: Small Animal Practice* **18,** 813–819

Carlotti DN (1994) Otite externe du chien et du chat. In: *Encyclopédie Vétérinaire, Dermatologie, 3300,* pp.1–6. Elsevier, Paris

Carlotti DN and Taillieu-Leroy S (1997) L'otite externe chez le chien: étiologie et clinique, revue bibliographique et étude rétrospective portant sur 752 cas. *Pratique Médicale et Chirurgicale de l' Animal de Compagnie* **32,** 243–257

Chickering WR (1988) Cytologic evaluation of otitic exudates. *Veterinary Clinics of North America: Small Animal Practice* **18,** 773–782

Cole LK, Kwochka KW, Kpwalski JJ *et al.* (1998) Microbial flora and antimicrobial susceptibility patterns of isolated pathogens from the horizontal ear canal and middle ear in dogs with otitis media. *Journal of the American Veterinary Medical Association* **212,** 534–538

Griffin CE (1993) Otitis externa and otitis media. In: *Current Veterinary Dermatology: The Science and Art of Therapy,* ed. CE Griffin *et al.,* pp. 245–264. Mosby Year Book, St Louis

Kiss G (1997) New combinations for the therapy of canine otitis externa. 1. Microbiology of otitis externa. *Journal of Small Animal Practice* **38,** 51–56

McKeever P (1993) Otitis externa. In: *Manual of Small Animal Dermatology,* ed. PH Locke *et al.,* pp. 131–140. BSAVA Publications, Cheltenham

Prélaud P (1999) Dermatites Allergiques du Chien et du Chat. Masson, Paris

Rogers KS (1988) Tumors of the ear canal. *Veterinary Clinics of North America: Small Animal Practice* **18,** 859–868

Roth L (1988) Pathologic changes in otitis externa. *Veterinary Clinics of North America: Small Animal Practice* **18,** 755–764

Scott DW, Miller WH and Griffin CE (2001) *Muller and Kirk's Small Animal Dermatology, 6th edn.* WB Saunders, Philadelphia

15

An approach to pododermatitis

Stephen D. White

Pododermatitis is best defined as any inflammatory skin disease involving the feet. Depending upon the aetiology, pododermatitis may exist concurrently with the same disease process elsewhere on the body or it may be the sole pathology present. Abnormalities in walking are obvious to owners, and a small animal may not be presented for veterinary care until the dermatitis affects the feet, even though the disease may have been present previously, on other parts of the skin or internally.

Pododermatitis is a frequently encountered syndrome in small animal practice and there are many causes. While some aetiologies result in multiple types of lesions, the clinician will find it useful to classify cases based on clinical appearance:

- Interdigital erythema
- Alopecia without pruritus
- Crusted/fissured foot pads
- Sloughing foot pads
- Nodular disease
- Claw disease.

Differential diagnosis

Interdigital erythema

This is the most common clinical presentation of pododermatitis. The most common aetiologies are atopic dermatitis and food allergy (see Chapter 18). These are often complicated by secondary infections caused by either *Staphylococcus intermedius* or *Malassezia pachydermatis* (see Chapters 22 and 24). Demodicosis may also present with erythema.

Alopecia without pruritus

This is uncommon, but is often associated with dermatophytosis, demodicosis and ischaemic folliculopathy (see Chapter 27).

Crusted or fissured footpads

These are most often caused by pemphigus foliaceus (see Chapter 26) or metabolic diseases such as zinc-responsive dermatosis, superficial necrolytic dermatosis, feline paraneoplastic alopecia secondary to pancreatic adenocarcinoma, thymoma-associated erythema multiforme (see Chapter 28) or idiopathic footpad hyperkeratosis (Box 15.1). When the crusts exfoliate or the fissures widen, the lesions may progress to frank ulcers.

Box 15.1: Footpad hyperkeratosis

Clinical presentation
Footpad hyperkeratosis occurs in dogs usually by the age of 6 months. The entire surface of the pad is involved. The keratin may be verrucous, grooved, ridged or feathered. The pads of large breed dogs may become fissured and painful. There is a predisposition in the Dogue de Bordeaux, Kerry Blue and Irish Terriers (Paradis, 1992; Binder *et al.*, 2000; Scott *et al.*, 2001). There are no other skin lesions.

Diagnosis
Diagnosis is based on histopathology, which shows epidermal hyperplasia and marked diffuse orthokeratotic hyperkeratosis. Canine ichthyosis may also cause such lesions but this is a congenital disease which involves large areas of the body.

Prognosis
The prognosis is fair. The disease may be controlled with continual treatment.

Treatment
Therapy is palliative and involves trimming away non-viable keratotic tissue, and the use of a keratolytic topical, such as a salicylic acid gel.

Sloughing footpads

Sloughing footpads are most commonly caused by vasculitis and/or an ischaemic dermatopathy (drug-related or idiopathic) (see Chapter 27); alternatively, cutaneous lymphoma may infiltrate the epidermis and cause a similar clinical picture.

Nodular diseases

Nodular diseases of the foot are often thought to be neoplastic (benign or malignant). However they may also be the result of a folliculitis (pyoderma, *Demodex* or dermatophyte) which has ruptured through the wall of the follicle and become a furunculosis. Systemic fungal diseases, when involving the skin, frequently present as nodules.

Nodules may also result from sterile pyogranulomas (Box 15.2), excess collagen production as in nodular dermatofibrosis (Box 15.3) or a depositional process involving deposits of xanthomatous (lipid) or mineral (calcinosis cutis) material.

Claw disease

This has a variety of aetiologies, and is discussed at length in Chapter 16.

Box 15.2: Sterile granuloma

Clinical presentation
Sterile granulomas involving the feet have been seen in several breeds, especially the English Bulldog, Great Dane, Boxer and Dachshund. Clinical signs are nodular lesions (Figure 15.B2.1). A seeming variant of this disease is seen primarily in German Shepherd Dogs and consists of draining tracts usually occurring immediately proximal to the metacarpal or metatarsal pads (Figure 15.B2.2).

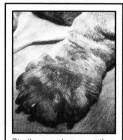
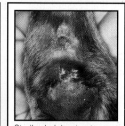

Sterile granulomas on the foot of a 10-year-old male Dachshund.

Sterile draining tract proximal to the carpal pad in a 5-year-old male German Shepherd Dog.

Diagnosis
Diagnosis is based both on histopathology, which shows a pyogranulomatous, nodular to diffuse dermatitis which tends to track the appendages, and culture, which is negative for bacteria and fungal organisms.

Prognosis
Prognosis is fair to good with prolonged treatment.

Treatment
Prednisone or prednisolone at a dosage of 1 mg/kg every 12–24 hours is usually effective to induce lesion regression. Some dogs may respond to niacinamide and tetracycline (500 mg of each drug/dog tid; if the dog weighs less than 10 kg, 250 mg/dog of each drug should be used). Some dogs may be tapered off corticosteroids entirely, while others will need to be on a long-term, alternate day, low-dose regimen.

Box 15.3: Nodular dermatofibrosis syndrome

Clinical presentation
Nodular dermatofibrosis syndrome is seen in German Shepherd Dogs and occasionally other breeds (White *et al.*, 1998). Cutaneous lesions are firm nodules with a pitted ('orange skin') appearance (Figure 15.B3.1). These are often seen on the distal extremities, but may be generalized in distribution. The nodules are associated with the presence of renal cystic disease: this may be in the form of benign renal epithelial cysts, renal cystadenomas or cystadenocarcinomas. The cysts are found in both kidneys.

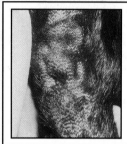

Nodules of dermatofibrosis in a 9-year-old male neutered Labrador Retriever x Gordon Setter crossbred dog. (Reproduced from White *et al.*, 1998, with the permission of Blackwell Publishers/Blackwell Science Ltd/Polity Press.)

Diagnosis
Histological study of the nodules reveals dense collagen fibrosis. This finding in association with the presence of renal cystic disease (best confirmed by ultrasonography) is diagnostic. Occasionally the nodules will occur prior to the renal cysts becoming large enough to be diagnosed by ultrasonography, so scanning should be repeated at 6-month intervals if the disease is suspected.

Prognosis
While the prognosis is serious, some dogs with benign renal cysts have survived for 5 years or more after diagnosis.

Treatment
There is no known treatment for the renal cystic disease. The cutaneous nodules may be removed if interfering with locomotion. This is not routinely advised, as the distal extremities do not lend themselves easily to the extensive reconstructive surgery required to remove the nodules. Other clinicians have suggested intralesional corticosteroid injections; the author has not found these to be effective.

Clinical approach

A thorough history and physical examination are vital in the diagnosis of a pododermatitis.

History
Questions for the owner may be divided into various categories (diseases listed are those most relevant to the preceding question(s)):

The environment
- Rough or unsanitary housing; consider trauma, contact irritants, hookworms, *Pelodera*
- Hunting dogs
- Other pets involved
- If a cat, what type of material is used in the litter box? The author has seen cases of both eosinophilic granuloma and plasmacytic pododermatitis (Box 15.4) due to the use of heavily perfumed/chemically treated 'anti-odour' cat sand; these resolved within 4 weeks of changing to a different cat sand, or to paper-based litter.

History of the lesions

- Seasonal: atopic dermatitis
- Response to previous antibiotics: pyoderma
- Response to previous corticosteroids: allergies, irritants, sterile pyogranuloma, autoimmune diseases (if high doses used)
- Lesions elsewhere on the body
  - Axilla, face: atopic dermatitis or food allergy
  - Dependent or ventral areas of the body: contact irritant or allergen, hookworms, *Pelodera*
  - Mucocutaneous junctions: autoimmune disease, superficial necrolytic dermatitis, zinc-responsive dermatosis, thallium poisoning, leishmaniasis, demodicosis
  - Otitis externa: *Malassezia* dermatitis
- Diet: consider generic dog food dermatoses
- Other medical problems
- Travel history: the pet may have contracted an infectious disease not native to the practice area.

Box 15.4: Plasmacytic pododermatitis

Clinical presentation

Plasmacytic pododermatitis is a rare idiopathic cause of foot pad swelling and ulceration in cats. The initial condition is a soft, nonpainful swelling of the footpads, which may progress to crusts, ulceration and granulation tissue. Ulceration may lead to pain and lameness. The digital pads, metacarpal or metatarsal pads may all be involved (Taylor and Schmeitzel, 1990).

Diagnosis

Confirmation is by biopsy, which reveals a diffuse dermatitis with a massive plasma cell infiltration. This disease may be associated with FIV infection, and affected cats should be tested for this virus.

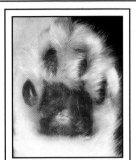

Plasmacytic pododermatitis in a 9-year-old female spayed Domestic Shorthair cat. Note swollen ('puffy') metacarpal footpad.

Prognosis

Prognosis is variable, dependent on response to treatment.

Treatment

The best mode of therapy is still undetermined. Some cases will regress spontaneously.

Litter tray

The type of sand used in the litter tray should be changed.

Doxycycline

A recent report (Bettenay et al., 2001) documented a favourable

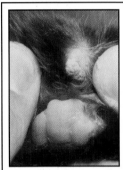

Plasmacytic pododermatitis in a 7-year-old female spayed Himalayan cat. Note crust on digital pad.

response to doxycycline 10 mg/cat sid for 3–4 weeks. This would seem to be the first treatment modality to try, because of its lack of both expense and side effects.

Prednisolone

Prednisolone at 4.4 mg/kg sid has not always been beneficial (Guaguère et al., 1992).

Gold therapy

Gold therapy using the gold salt aurothioglucose has also been reported (Medleau et al., 1982). A suggested regimen is 1 mg/kg i.m. once weekly until the disease is well controlled, typically 4–16 weeks. Once the disease is well controlled, the frequency of injections is decreased to ideally once a month. Potential adverse reactions are thrombocytopenia, anaemia and renal disease (glomerulonephropathy). Sometimes the thrombocytopenia is preceded by eosinophilia. Cats on gold salts should be monitored with periodic (ideally once monthly) complete blood and platelet counts and urine protein assessments.

Surgery

Surgical removal has been reported to be effective (Guaguère et al., 1992).

Physical examination

Physical examination should include:

- A thorough search for lesions elsewhere on the body
- Palpation of lymph nodes
- Determination of how many feet are involved.

The triad of pedal alopecia with scale and claw abnormalities is especially suggestive of dermatophytosis.

'Fox-red' salivary staining may be associated with any pruritic disease that causes the dog to lick at the feet; however it is most commonly associated with atopic dermatitis or food allergy, with or without secondary staphylococcal and/or *Malassezia* infection.

Laboratory tests

Skin scrapings

Skin scrapings for ectoparasites should be superficial and deep (for *Demodex*) (see also Chapters 3 and 21).

Difficulty in scraping the feet with a sharp scalpel can be avoided by substituting a medical grade spatula. This instrument is sharp enough to draw blood (signifying a deep skin scrape) but dull enough that any sudden movement by the animal will not result in an iatrogenic wound.

Dogs with long-standing pododemodicosis may have too much fibrosis to enable the mites to be found with a deep skin scraping. Long-term cases of pododermatitis, particularly those resulting in thickening or deformation of the foot, should always be biopsied to rule out demodicosis.

Cytology

Skin scrapings should be taken for cytology (for *Malassezia* and *Staphylococcus* infections) (see also Chapter 3). Exudate around the claw bed should be gently scraped and examined. Brownish exudates frequently contain *Malassezia* organisms.

Cytology is performed on any exudate or pustule contents (see Chapter 3).

Fungal culture

Fungal culture is performed, especially for dermatophytes (see Chapters 3 and 23).

Other tests

Dependent upon history and physical examination, other tests might include:

- CBC, serum enzyme panel, urinalysis if systemic disease present or suspected
- Feline leukaemia virus and feline immunodeficiency virus tests in a cat with suspected plasmacytic pododermatitis
- Faecal examination for hookworms
- Biopsy for histopathology, possibly for bacterial culture or for immunopathology
- Instituting a limited allergen diet
- Intradermal or serological testing for atopic dermatitis
- Ultrasonography of kidneys if dermatofibrosis/ cystic renal adenoma/adenocarcinoma syndrome (see Chapter 28) is suspected (White et al., 1998).

The author generally approaches skin-scrape-negative cases in the dog by classifying them as either with or without nodules/fistulas or abnormal foot pads. Those with these lesions should be biopsied for histopathology and bacterial or fungal cultures performed. Those without these lesions tend to be pruritic and allergic in nature. In the cat, pedal dermatosis is relatively rare and the author biopsies all cases.

Do not hesitate to biopsy footpads! Under general anaesthesia, a 4 mm biopsy punch is used and the wound closed with a cruciate suture. For cats, the owners should substitute paper for sand in the litter box for 2 weeks.

Treatment

Successful therapy of pedal dermatoses is dependent upon pursuing a definite diagnosis. In the author's practice, most pododermatitis in the dog is caused by allergies, *Malassezia*, pyoderma, demodicosis or pemphigus, roughly in that order. While treatment of the various diseases which may cause pododermatitis is covered at length in their respective chapters, the following are a few thoughts relevant to the author's experience in the treatment of pododermatitis.

Pyoderma

Therapy for pyoderma involves long-term (6 weeks or more) antibiotics, ideally based on culture and sensitivity. If culture reveals the isolation of several species of bacteria with differing sensitivities, an antibiotic should be chosen that is effective against the (almost inevitably isolated) staphylococcal species. In recurrent cases, underlying allergic diseases, hypothyroidism or hyperadrenocorticism may be suspected. If these tests reveal no abnormalities, bacterins may be used. Some cases will need life-long antibiotics. A gradual reduction in frequency of administration of the antibiotic may be attempted once clinical remission is achieved.

Phytopododermatitis

Various species of plants have awns that can cause lesions if lodged interdigitally. These lesions may appear as ulcerations, proliferative nodules, swellings or draining tracts. Animals usually present with lameness. Diagnosis may be evident on physical examination, although exploration and/or biopsy of the draining tracts with demonstration of plant material on histopathological examination may be necessary to confirm the diagnosis. Removal of solitary plant material is the preferred therapy. If multiple microscopic splinters or

spines are involved (such as a pet who falls into a cactus bed), long-term oral low-dose prednisolone (1 mg/kg every 24–48 hours) may relieve clinical signs, as has been reported in man. Eventually the corticosteroids may be discontinued.

Superficial necrolytic dermatitis

As an ancillary treatment to systemic therapy for superficial necrolytic dermatitis, the author has found that applying corticosteroid ointment or cream to the affected feet (after resolving any secondary infections) seems to relieve discomfort. The product may be applied to both the footpad and the haired skin areas, initially every 24 hours, then upon improvement on an as needed basis.

References and further reading

Bettenay SV, Mueller RV, Dow K *et al.* (2001) Feline plasmacytic pododermatitis – a prospective study of a novel treatment using systemic doxycycline. Brief Communications, *Proceedings of the 16th Annual American Academy of Veterinary Dermatology and the American College of Veterinary Dermatology Meeting*, Norfolk, Virginia

Binder H, Arnold S, Schelling C *et al.* (2000) Palmoplantar hyperkeratosis in Irish Terriers: evidence of autosomal recessive inheritance. *Journal of Small Animal Practice* **41**, 52–55

Brennan KE and Ihrke PJ (1983) Grass awn migration in dogs and cats: a retrospective study of 182 cases. *Journal of the American Veterinary Medical Association* **182**, 1201–1204

Guaguère E, Hubert B and Delabre C (1992) Feline pododermatoses. *Veterinary Dermatology* **3**, 1–12

Kunkle GA, White SD, Calderwood-Mays M *et al.* (1993) Focal metatarsal fistulas in five dogs. *Journal of the American Veterinary Medical Association* **202**, 756–7

Medleau L, Kaswan RL and Lorenz MD (1982) Ulcerative pododermatitis in a cat: immunofluorescent findings and response to chrysotherapy. *Journal of the American Animal Hospital Association* **18**, 449–451

Paradis M (1992) Footpad hyperkeratosis in a family of Dogues de Bordeaux. *Veterinary Dermatology* **3**, 75–78

Scott DW, Miller WH and Griffin CE (2001) *Muller and Kirk's Small Animal Dermatology 6th edn*, pp 935–936. WB Saunders Company, Philadelphia

Taylor JE and Schmeitzel LP (1990) Plasma cell pododermatitis with chronic footpad hemorrhage in two cats. *Journal of the American Veterinary Medical Association* **197**, 375–377

White SD (1989) Pododermatitis. *Veterinary Dermatology* **1**, 1–18

White SD, Rosychuk RAW, Shultheiss P *et al.* (1998) Nodular dermatofibrosis and cystic renal disease in three mix-breed dogs and a boxer. *Veterinary Dermatology* **9**, 119–126

16

An approach to diseases of claws and claw folds

Danny W. Scott

The claws and claw folds can be affected in conjunction with other areas of skin in numerous canine and feline dermatoses. However, dogs and cats rarely present with claw and claw fold abnormalities as their *only* manifestation of dermatological disease. Such dogs and cats account for less than 3% of dogs and cats examined at the university hospital at Cornell University.

Certain terms are used specifically when describing claw and claw fold abnormalities (Figure 16.1). More than one of these abnormalities may be seen in the same claw or in different claws of the same animal. Other abnormalities include excessive keratinous and/or waxy deposits on claws, staining of claws and an abnormal claw growth rate. Varying degrees of lameness, pain on touch or palpation, pruritus and regional lymphadenopathy may be present.

Paronychia is characterized by inflammation of the paronychial skin and claw fold, and may show varying degrees of erythema, oedema, oozing, crusting, scaling, alopecia, necrosis, erosion, ulceration, hyperpigmentation and lichenification. Occasional animals will also manifest varying combinations of pyrexia, depression, lethargy and inappetence, depending on the associated cause (especially immune-mediated disease and severe infections).

Diseases of the claw and claw fold are seen with equal frequency in the dog. However, in the cat, diseases of the claw fold are much more common than diseases of the claw.

Differential diagnosis

A wide variety of disorders are associated with claw and claw fold diseases in dogs (Figure 16.2) and cats (Figure 16.3). Animals can present with abnormalities of: one claw, multiple claws on one paw, or multiple claws on multiple paws. Animals with *asymmetrical* claw or claw fold disease (one or multiple claws on one paw) are likely to have infections (bacteria, fungi), trauma, or neoplasia as aetiological factors. Animals with *symmetrical* problems (multiple claws on multiple paws) are likely to have immune-mediated, metabolic, genetic, nutritional or viral (feline leukaemia virus (FeLV), feline immunodeficiency virus (FIV)) disorders.

Asymmetrical disorders
Asymmetrical claw and claw fold infections are usually bacterial (especially *Staphylococcus intermedius*

Term	Meaning
Anonychia	Absence of claws (usually congenital)
Brachyonychia	Short claws
Leuconychia	Whitening of the claws
Macronychia	Unusually large claws
Micronychia	Unusually small claws
Onychalgia	Claw pain
Onychauxis (hyperonychia)	Simple hypertrophy of claws
Onychia (onychitis)	Inflammation somewhere in the claw unit
Onychocryptosis (onyxis)	Ingrown claw
Onychodystrophy	Abnormal claw formation
Onychogryposis	Hypertrophy and abnormal curvature of claws
Onycholysis	Separation of claw structure at distal attachment and progressing proximally
Onychomadesis (onychoptosis)	Sloughing of claws
Onychomalacia (hapalonychia)	Softening of claws
Onychomycosis	Fungal infection of claws
Onychopathy (onychosis)	Disease or abnormality of claws
Onychorrhexis	Fragmentation and horizontal separation in claw lamellae at the free edge
Onychoschizia (onychoschisis)	Splitting or lamination of claws, usually beginning distally
Pachyonychia	Thickening of claws
Paronychia (perionychia)	Inflammation or infection of claw folds
Platonychia	Increased curvature of claws in long axis
Trachyonychia	Lustreless, longitudinally ridged, rough-surfaced claws

16.1 Terminology for claw and claw fold disorders.

Bacterial infection
Secondary to trauma

Fungal infection
Dermatophytosis
Malassezia
Candida
Blastomyces
Cryptococcus
Geotrichosis

Parasitic disease
Demodicosis
Hookworm dermatitis
Ascarids

Protozoal disease
Leishmaniasis

Viral disease
Distemper

Trauma
Physical
Chemical (salt, fertilizer)
Acquired arteriovenous fistula

Immune-mediated diseases
Lupoid onychodystrophy
Systemic lupus erythematosus
Pemphigus vulgaris
Pemphigus foliaceus
Bullous pemphigoid
Vasculitis
Adverse drug reaction (including vaccines)
Cryoglobulinaemia

Metabolic diseases
Hypothyroidism
Hyperadrenocorticism
Necrolytic migratory erythema (via predisposition to bacterial and fungal infections)
Acromegaly (macronychia, rapid growth and onychogryposis)

Genetic diseases
Epidermolysis bullosa
Dermatomyositis
Primary seborrhoea
Linear epidermal naevus
Anonychia
Supernumerary claws

Neoplasia
Squamous cell carcinoma

Miscellaneous disorders
Nutritional deficiencies (including lethal acrodermatitis and zinc-responsive dermatoses)
Thallotoxicosis
Ergotism
Idiopathic onychodystrophy
Idiopathic onychomadesis

16.2 Causes of claw and claw fold disorders in dogs.

Bacterial infection
Secondary to trauma and viral infections

Fungal infection
Dermatophytosis
Malassezia
Candida
Sporothrix
Cryptococcus

Parasitic disease
Demodicosis

Viral disease
FeLV and FIV infections: via predisposition to bacterial and fungal infections

Trauma
Physical
Acquired arteriovenous fistula

Immune-mediated diseases
Pemphigus vulgaris
Systemic lupus erythematosus
Vasculitis
Adverse drug reaction (including vaccines)
Cryoglobulinaemia
Eosinophilic plaque (allergy)

Metabolic diseases
Diabetes mellitus (bacterial and fungal infections)
Hyperadrenocorticism (bacterial and fungal infections)
Hyperthyroidism (rapid growth)

Genetic disease
Epidermolysis bullosa

Neoplasia
Especially squamous cell carcinoma and metastatic lung carcinoma

Miscellaneous disorders
Nutritional deficiencies
Disseminated intravascular coagulopathy
Idiopathic onychodystrophy

16.3 Causes of claw and claw fold disorders in cats.

in dogs) and of presumed traumatic origin (bite wound, blunt injury, tearing, overzealous pedicure). Asymmetrical onychomadesis and onychodystrophy are usually traumatic or infectious in origin. Traumatic and infectious claw and claw fold diseases are especially common in hunting and racing dogs. Dermatophytosis (onychomycosis) is a rare cause of asymmetric claw disease in dogs and cats (Scott and Miller, 1992a,b). Acquired arteriovenous fistulae result from penetrating wounds, blunt trauma or postsurgical complications of onychectomy. Disease (persistent or recurrent oedema and bacterial paronychia) often appears weeks to months following the initial injury, and may be accompanied by palpable thrills, pulsating blood vessels and continuous machinery murmurs in the area of the fistula.

Squamous cell carcinoma is the most common neoplasm affecting the claw. Older animals, especially large breed, black dogs (Labrador Retriever, Standard Poodle, Giant Schnauzer, Bouvier de Flandres), present with a swollen, painful paronychial area on one digit (Figure 16.4). Secondary bacterial paronychia is common, as are eventual onychodystrophy and onychomadesis.

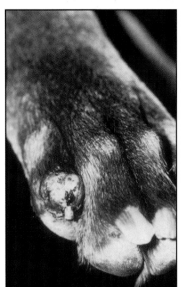

16.4 Subungual squamous cell carcinoma in a Weimeraner. The paronychial skin of the affected skin is swollen, erythematous and ulcerated, and the claw is dystrophic. (Reproduced from Scott, Miller and Griffin (2001) with permission of WB Saunders.)

Symmetrical disorders

Symmetrical claw fold disorders are most commonly due to bacterial paronychia associated with:

- Concurrent metabolic disorders: hyperadrenocorticism, hypothyroidism (Figure 16.5), diabetes mellitus, necrolytic migratory erythema
- Immunosuppression: FeLV (Figure 16.6), FIV
- Immune-mediated disease (Figure 16.7): especially pemphigus foliaceus.

Malassezia paronychia and onychia are characterized by red–brown discoloration of paronychial hairs and claws, erythematous paronychial skin, accumulation of yellowish-brown waxy material in the claw fold and pruritus.

Symmetrical claw disease is most commonly associated with immune-mediated diseases (especially lupoid onychodystrophy (Box 16.1) and pemphigus

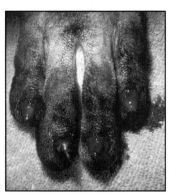

16.5 Symmetrical haemopurulent staphylococcal paronychia and onychomadesis in a hypothyroid dog.

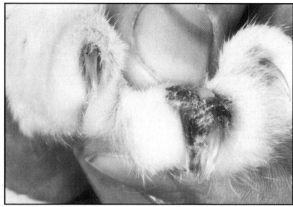

16.6 Symmetrical bacterial paronychia (*Escherichia coli*) in an FeLV-positive cat.

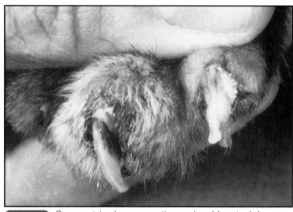

16.7 Symmetrical suppurative, mixed bacterial paronychia (*E. coli* and *Enterococcus* sp.) in a cat with systemic lupus erythematosus. (Reproduced from Scott, Miller and Griffin (2001) with permission of WB Saunders.)

foliaceus (Figure 16.8)). Variable claw abnormalities (onychodystrophy, onychomalacia, onychorrhexis, onychogryposis, onychomadesis) have been reported in association with canine primary seborrhoea, canine distemper, leishmaniasis, severe ascarid infestation, hookworm dermatitis, nutritional deficiencies, thallotoxicosis and ergotism.

Ulcerative, destructive lesions of the claw fold are seen in aged cats as a result of metastasis from usually asymptomatic bronchiogenic or squamous cell carcinomas of the lung. Usually, multiple digits of multiple paws are affected, but occasionally multiple digits on one paw or one digit only are affected.

Dry, brittle claws can be the result of dehydration, such as is seen with excessive exposure to water, mud, soaps and cleansers, and in warm, dry environments.

'Idiopathic' symmetrical onychodystrophy (variable degrees of onychomalacia, onychorrhexis, onychoschizia, and onychogryposis) has been reported, especially in Dachshunds, Siberian Huskies and very old ('senile') dogs. 'Idiopathic' symmetrical onychomadesis has been reported, especially in German Shepherd Dogs, Whippets and English Springer Spaniels. It must be emphasized that onychobiopsy was apparently not performed in these dogs. Therefore, these dogs could have had any number of the aforementioned specific disorders.

Box 16.1: Canine symmetrical lupoid onychodystrophy

Symmetrical lupoid onychodystrophy has been reported in dogs aged 1–10 years, with no apparent sex predilection (Rosychuk, 1995; Scott *et al.*, 1995; Vicek *et al.*, 1997; Bergvall, 1998; Lower *et al.*, 1999; Mueller *et al.*, 2000; Scott *et al.*, 2001). Although all breeds and crossbreeds can be affected, German Shepherd Dogs and Rottweilers appear to be predisposed. Lupoid onychodystrophy is the most common cause of symmetrical claw disease in dogs.

Pathogenesis

Lupoid onychodystrophy is *not* a single disease, but rather an immune-mediated cutaneous reaction pattern with probably several different aetiologies. These include adverse food reactions and adverse drug reactions (including vaccinations) (Mueller *et al.*, 2000; Scott *et al.*, 2001). Many cases are currently idiopathic (Scott *et al.*, 1995; Bergvall, 1998; Lower *et al.*, 1999). The apparent predilection for certain breeds (Scott *et al.*, 1995; Mueller *et al.*, 2000) and the occurrence in siblings (Vicek *et al.*, 1997) indicates that genetic predisposition may be important in some cases.

Clinical presentation

Affected dogs typically begin with onychomadesis of one claw on one or more paws (Figure 16.B1.1). However, within 2–10 weeks all claws on all paws are usually affected. Observant owners will note a 'brown line' or 'bruising' (subungual haemorrhage) prior to the sloughing of affected claws. In about 50% of the cases, lameness and pain on palpation are evident. Regrowth is characterized by short, misshapen, dry, soft, brittle, often crumbly and discoloured claws. Some dogs develop secondary bacterial paronychia. Affected dogs are usually otherwise healthy.

Diagnosis

The diagnosis is confirmed by onychobiopsy via onychectomy (Scott *et al.*, 1995). Histological examination reveals a hydropic and/or lichenoid interface onychitis (Scott *et al.*, 1995). In view of these histopathological findings, the drug and vaccination history should be carefully reviewed, and a novel antigen diet could be considered.

Treatment

Many cases respond to omega-6/omega-3 fatty acids (Rosychuk, 1995; Scott *et al.*, 1995; Vicek *et al.*, 1997; Bergvall, 1998; Lower *et al.*, 1999).

Symmetrical lupoid onychodystrophy in a Bearded Collie.

The combination of tetracycline (or doxycycline) and niacinamide is also frequently effective, and may be effective when omega-6/omega-3 fatty acids have failed (Rosychuk, 1995; Scott *et al.*, 2001). The dosage of tetracycline and niacinamide is 250 mg of each, tid orally for dogs weighing < 10 kg, and 500 mg of each, tid orally for dogs > 10 kg (Scott *et al.*, 2001).

Systemic glucocorticoids (prednisone or prednisolone at 2 mg/kg orally sid) and large doses of vitamin E (400 IU orally bid) have also been reported to be effective (Scott *et al.*, 2001). Medically refractory cases should be given a novel antigen diet (Mueller *et al.*, 2000).

Dogs with lupoid onychodystrophy typically relapse when therapy (including novel antigen diets) is stopped (Mueller *et al.*, 2000; Scott *et al.*, 1995).

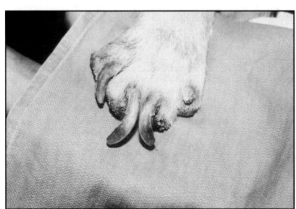

16.8 Symmetrical onychodystrophy in an Akita with pemphigus foliaceus. Three claws demonstrate onychogryposis, and the other is short, brittle, and soft (onychomalacia and onychorrhexis).
(Reproduced from Scott, Miller and Griffin (2001) with permission of WB Saunders.)

Clinical approach

As the causes of claw and claw fold disease are numerous, a wide variety of diagnostic tests or procedures may be needed. These are determined on the basis of history and physical examination findings. A thorough drug history, including vaccinations, is important, especially in dogs and cats with symmetrical claw or claw bed disease. Claw disease may occur 2–8 weeks following vaccination (Boord *et al.*, 1997; Scott *et al.*, 2001).

Cytology

Cytological examination is very helpful in establishing the presence of:

- Bacterial or fungal infection (suppurative to pyogranulomatous to granulomatous inflammation, degenerate neutrophils, phagocytosed microorganisms). Bacterial culture and sensitivity testing (see Chapters 3 and 22) and fungal culture (see Chapters 3 and 23) are not commonly performed
- *Malassezia* infection (more than four yeast per X400 microscopic field)
- Pemphigus diseases (non-degenerate neutrophils and/or eosinophils and numerous acantholytic keratinocytes)
- Neoplasia.

Material from within the claw fold or under the claw should be obtained for evaluation.

Skin scrapings and hair samples

Skin scrapings and plucked hairs from paronychial skin can be examined for parasites and dermatophytes, respectively.

Biopsy

Biopsy is the only way of confirming a diagnosis of certain claw diseases, such as lupoid onychodystrophy, pemphigus, pemphigoid and neoplasia.

Submission of a sloughed or avulsed claw is almost never of any diagnostic benefit (except for the rare case of onychomycosis). The claw bed is best visualized when the third phalanx is removed with the intact claw and the entire structure is sectioned longitudinally. Some owners are hesitant to have this done. A technique for onychobiopsy without onychectomy has been described (Mueller and Olivry, 1999). This author finds surgical amputation more reliable. When affected, the dewclaw is often the preferred claw to remove. As is the case with all skin biopsy specimens, claw and paroncyhial skin should be sent to someone with expertise in dermatopathology, be they a pathologist or dermatologist. Intrakeratinocyte vacuoles, intraepithelial and dermoepidermal clefts, pseudospongiosis and apoptotic keratinocytes are common features of normal canine and feline claw specimens and must not be mistaken for pathological changes (Mueller *et al.*, 1993; Scott and Foil, 1998).

Radiography

Radiography is indicated in animals wherein neoplasia and systemic fungal diseases are suspected: both to assess possible local bone involvement and to evaluate the thorax for possible metastatic or primary tumours or granulomas.

Ancillary tests

Laboratory evaluations such as haemogram, chemistry panel, urinalysis, antinuclear antibody titre, thyroid hormone concentrations and bacterial and fungal cultures are very low-yield tests in the diagnostic work-up of claw and claw fold disease.

Therapeutic principles

Prognosis is most accurately established and therapy is most accurately employed when a specific diagnosis is made. Because normal canine claws grow at an average rate of 0.8–1.9 mm per week, it is often 3–4 months before a convincing response to treatment is seen. It may take a year before a completely normal claw is achieved (Boord *et al.*, 1997; Scott *et al.*, 2001). If the claw bed has been sufficiently damaged by the disease process, focal or total claw abnormalities may be permanent.

Infections

Infections must be treated aggressively with appropriate antimicrobial agents, often for several weeks to months: appropriate antibacterials for bacteria (see Chapter 22), and appropriate antifungals for dermatophytosis (see Chapter 23) and *Malassezia* (see Chapter 24). Idiopathic, recurrent bacterial paronychia in dogs, or that associated with FeLV/FIV infections in cats, may require long-term antibiotic therapy (Scott *et al.*, 2001).

Immune-mediated disorders

Immune-mediated disorders (especially pemphigus, pemphigoid, lupus erythematosus, and vasculitis) may require aggressive treatment with potent immunomodulatory drugs such as systemic glucocorticoids, azathioprine, chlorambucil, aurothioglucose, pentoxifylline, or ciclosporin (see Chapters 26 and 27). Lupoid onychodystrophy has been reported to respond to omega-6/omega-3 fatty acids, tetracycline (or doxycycline) and niacinamide, systemic glucocorticoids, large doses of vitamin E and novel antigen diets (see Box 16.1) (Bergvall, 1998; Lower *et al.*, 1999; Vicek *et al.*, 1997).

Other treatments

When onychodystrophy leads to onychoschizia, onychalgia and secondary infections, prophylactic trimming and filing of the claws and frequent application of human acrylic nail cement products can be very helpful (Verde and Basurco, 2000).

Anecdotal reports indicate that gelatin (10 grains orally bid for Dachshunds; 1 gm/kg orally sid) or biotin (5 µg/kg orally sid) may be effective in some dogs with 'idiopathic' onychodystrophy or brittle claws (Rosychuk, 1995). Anecdotal reports also suggest that pentoxifylline (10 mg/kg orally bid) may be effective in some dogs with 'idiopathic' onychomadesis.

In animals with chronic, medically refractory claw disorders, or in large dogs wherein the chronic administration of certain therapeutic agents would be economically infeasible, onychectomy is a reasonable and effective therapeutic option.

References and further reading

Bergvall K (1998) Treatment of symmetrical onychomadesis and onychodystrophy in five dogs with omega-3 and omega-6 fatty acids. *Veterinary Dermatology* **9**, 263–268

Boord MJ *et al.* (1997) Onychectomy as a therapy for symmetrical claw and claw fold disease in the dog. *Journal of the American Animal Hospital Association* **33**, 131–138

Lower K *et al.* (1999) A Shetland Sheepdog with crusty, deformed toenails. *Veterinary Medicine* **94**, 860–864

Mueller RS *et al.* (1993) Microanatomy of the canine claw. *Veterinary Dermatology* **4**, 5–11

Mueller RS and Olivry T (1999) Onychobiopsy without onychectomy: description of a new biopsy technique for canine claws. *Veterinary Dermatology* **10**, 55-59

Mueller RS *et al.* (2000) Diagnosis of canine claw disease - a prospective study of 24 dogs. *Veterinary Dermatology* **11**, 133–141

Rosychuk RAW (1995) Diseases of the claw and claw fold. In: *Kirk's Current Veterinary Therapy, 12th edn*, ed. JD Bonagura, pp. 641–647. WB Saunders, Philadelphia

Scott DW and Miller WH (1992a) Disorders of the claw and claw bed in cats. *Compendium on Continuing Education* **14**, 449–457

Scott DW and Miller WH (1992b) Disorders of the claw and claw bed in dogs. *Compendium on Continuing Education* **14**, 1448–1458

Scott DW *et al.* (1995) Symmetrical lupoid onychodystrophy in dogs: a retrospective analysis of 18 cases (1989–1993). *Journal of the American Animal Hospital Association* **31**, 194–201

Scott DW and Foil CS (1998) Claw diseases in dogs and cats. In: *Advances in Veterinary Dermatology*, ed. KW Kwochka *et al.*, vol. 3, pp. 406–408. Butterworth-Heinemann, Oxford

Scott DW, Miller WH and Griffin CE (2001) *Muller & Kirk's Small Animal Dermatology, 6th edn*, pp. 94–1374. WB Saunders, Philadelphia

Verde MT and Basurco A (2000) Symmetrical lupoid onychodystrophy in a crossbred pointer dog: long-term observations. *Veterinary Record* **146**, 376–378

Vicek T *et al.* (1997) Symmetrical lupoid onychodystrophy in two sibling Rottweilers. *Veterinary Pathology* **34**, 507

17

An approach to anal sac diseases

David H. Scarff

Disease of the anal sacs is a common reason for presentation of dogs to a veterinary surgeon (Anderson, 1984), though it is uncommon in cats. Little is known of the aetiology or pathogenesis and the approach is therefore somewhat symptomatic, often ending with surgical removal of the sacs. This chapter will detail a diagnostic approach based upon current knowledge, and will include a brief discussion of anal furunculosis (perianal fistula) in the dog.

The anal sacs

Anatomy and physiology

The anal sacs of the dog are paired cutaneous diverticula situated either side of the anus. They lie between the external anal sphincter muscle and the rectum. They are connected to the outside by a short duct which opens lateral to the anus. These structures form a reservoir for the malodorous secretions of the apocrine and sebaceous gland lining the sacs. The anal sacs are not to be confused with the perianal (hepatoid) glands or the circumanal glands.

The material which collects in the anal sacs in the dog is a mixture of sebaceous and apocrine secretions, together with desquamated cells from the stratum corneum of the skin lining them. The apocrine glands are situated around the fundus of the sac, whereas the sebaceous glands surround the duct (Anderson, 1984).

The anal sacs release their contents during defecation, when the sac is squeezed by the external anal sphincter against the faecal mass in the rectum. It is likely that the sac secretions play a role in social behaviour in the dog and cat.

There is considerable variation in the colour, consistency and odour of secretions from normal anal sacs, from black to green, from watery to viscid.

Microbiology

The normal flora of the anal sacs has been examined (Halnan, 1976b). In the healthy dog, the most common isolates were micrococci, *Escherichia coli*, *Streptococcus faecalis* and *Staphylococcus* spp. Fungal cultures were not performed. In another study, 46% of normal anal sacs were demonstrated to contain *Malassezia pachydermatis* (Hajsig *et al.*, 1985).

Differential diagnosis

The differential diagnosis in the dog and cat must include all conditions that can cause pruritus of the caudal trunk, tail base or perineum, together with those conditions that result in fistulae or subcutaneous swellings in the perianal region (Figure 17.1).

Presentation	Differential diagnosis
Caudal pruritus	Flea bite hypersensitivity Adverse food reaction Atopic dermatitis Cheyletiellosis Perineal intertrigo (skin fold disease) Tail fold intertrigo Vulval fold intertrigo Anal sac infection Anal sac impaction
Perianal swelling	Anal sac abscess Anal sac neoplasia Perineal hernia Perianal (hepatoid) neoplasia
Perianal sinus/fistula	Ruptured anal sac abscess Anal furunculosis

17.1 Differential diagnosis of anal sac disease.

Clinical approach

The clinical approach to anal sac disease does not differ from that for most dermatoses. History-taking, thorough clinical examination and diagnostic tests are all important for successful diagnosis and management.

History

History-taking must focus on the presenting signs, together with gathering information about possible concurrent disease.

If the presenting sign is caudal pruritus, then owners must be questioned about:

• Flea control
• Owner lesions – fleas and *Cheyletiella*
• Pattern of disease – is there concurrent pruritus of the face or feet, suggesting atopic dermatitis?

- Dietary history – important if there is any likelihood of concurrent allergic disease
- Breed of dog – important if tail fold intertrigo is suspected
- Whether the dog 'scoots' (rubs its anus on the ground); if the animal does not, then has it ever? Scooting is highly suggestive of anal disease, but some dogs with significant anal sac disease never scoot
- Licking the anal region. Cats are able to lick the anal region, and do so regularly. Owners may be unable to distinguish excessive licking from what is normal.

With the presence of perianal fistulation or sinus formation, the breed of dog is important. The overwhelming majority of dogs with anal furunculosis (perianal fistula; Box 17.1) are German Shepherd Dogs or their crosses.

Previous anal sac disease is important; in a dog with a chronic history of anal sac impaction (Box 17.2), anal sac abscess (Box 17.3) is more likely.

Box 17.1: Anal furunculosis (perianal fistula)

Pathogenesis
Immune-mediated disease (possibly genetic).

Clinical presentation
German Shepherd Dog is the most commonly affected breed. All ages may be affected.

Presentation includes dyschezia, tenesmus, blood on stools, frequent licking of the perineum. Area may be painful to examine.

On examination perianal sinus formation is noted (true rectocutaneous fistulae are rare).

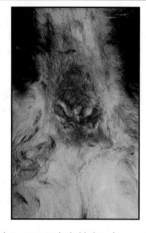

Treatment
Treatment includes either medical therapy or surgical ablation of affected tissue.

Medical therapies include ciclosporin, topical tacrolimus, antibiotics, and steroids if there is concurrent colitis.

Management of concurrent illness including hypothyroidism, colitis or dietary sensitivities is important.

Surgical treatment entails removal of *all* affected tissue, and anal sacs if involved. Complete anal resection with rectal pull-through may be necessary in severe cases.

Box 17.2: Anal sac impaction

Clinical presentation
Underlying causes include soft stools and obesity. Small breeds are over-represented.

Clinical signs include scooting, and self-trauma to perineal and tail base region. Anal sacs may be difficult to express. Expressed material is thick and flocculant.

Treatment
Treatment includes regular emptying of the anal sacs. Surgical removal is indicated if condition is recurrent.

Box 17.3: Anal sac abscess

Clinical presentation
Clinical signs include pain in the perineal region and a discharging sinus or perianal mass. Examination of the discharge reveals inflammatory cells and bacteria. The condition may follow anal sac impaction.

Treatment
Usually responds to a short course of appropriate systemic antibiotics. In the German Shepherd Dog, anal sac abscess may progress to perianal sinus.

If the problem is recurrent, then anal sac removal is indicated, once the abscess has healed.

Anal sac neoplasia is often associated with paraneoplastic signs: polyuria and polydipsia may occur due to pseudohyperparathyroidism. In the presence of such a history, blood samples should be examined for haematology and serum biochemistry to include urea and calcium levels.

Examination
Examination of the dog or cat requires the following:

- Systemic examination (concurrent disease, suitability for future surgery)
- Dermatological examination (allergic, endocrine or parasitic disease)
- Assessment of perineum (sinus or fistula, intertrigo)
- Assessment of tail and vulval folds if present
- Careful palpation of anal sacs (present? thickened? mass present?)
- Careful expression of anal sacs and collection of contents (difficult to express?)

Following the history and clinical examination a differential diagnosis list may be narrowed, and a diagnostic plan drawn up. Should there be signs compatible with allergic, endocrine or parasitic skin disease, then these should be pursued.

Diagnostic tests

Gross and microscopic examination
The first diagnostic test in all cases of anal sac disease is the gross and microscopic examination of the anal sac contents (Figure 17.2). Whilst the nature of the anal sac contents may be suggestive of a type of disease, only the presence of haemorrhagic discharge is always abnormal.

From the microscopic examination it is possible to assess relative numbers of bacterial types. Gram-positive cocci, Gram-negative rods and large Gram-positive rods (anaerobes) may be seen, together with yeasts. *Malassezia* yeasts may be present in large numbers in diseased sacs, especially in the presence of *Malassezia* dermatitis elsewhere.

Bacterial culture
Bacterial culture of the contents of diseased glands has revealed a number of organisms: essentially those

Gross appearance of contents	Microscopic appearance	Interpretation
Watery brown material	Desquamated cells, few bacteria or yeasts; no inflammatory cells	Normal
Thick, waxy material ± clumps	Aggregates of keratinized material, few bacteria or yeasts	Anal sac impaction
Purulent, malodorous exudate ± haemorrhage	Toxic neutrophils +++, many bacteria	Acute infection, abscess
Watery to creamy brown–green	Bacteria ± yeasts; some inflammatory cells	Chronic infection

17.2 Interpretation of gross and microscopic appearance of anal sac contents.

found in normal glands together with diptheroids, *Pseudomonas* sp., *Proteus* sp. and *Clostridium welchii*. Should bacterial culture be required, it is important to attempt to limit contamination of samples by faecal flora by careful sample collection and rigorous antisepsis. Anal sac infection is discussed in Box 17.4.

Box 17.4: Anal sac infection

Aetiology
Underlying causes probably include allergy and endocrine disease; also iatrogenic damage from expression.

Clinical presentation
Clinical signs include scooting and perineal/caudal trunk pruritus. Anal sacs are usually easy to empty but may have thickened walls. Infection also occurs in the cat.

Examination of contents reveals bacteria or yeasts ± inflammatory cells.

Treatment
Treatment options include flushing, topical antibiotics, systemic antibiotics or antifungal treatment, or surgical removal. If sacs are removed, an open technique is preferable, as ductal remnants may be the cause of continued pruritus.

Biopsy

If a perianal mass is detected, then biopsy material may be taken using either fine needle aspiration or a Trucut needle.

Radiography

If a malignancy is suspected, then radiographic assessment of the local and regional lymph nodes (especially in the sublumbar region) must be performed.

Therapeutic approach

The therapeutic approach to anal sac disease is determined by the specific disease entity present. Options include topical and systemic drugs, and surgery.

Topical therapy

Since the anal sac is a pouch of skin, any infection in the lumen of the sac is essentially on the skin surface. For this reason topical therapy is sometimes more effective than systemic treatment.

Topical therapy in this instance means the instillation of antibacterial and/or anti-inflammatory products into the anal sac, by means of a nasolacrimal cannula or cat catheter. The choice of therapy depends upon the nature of the problem, and the organisms demonstrated. Products suggested include sterile saline, antibiotic preparations (metronidazole or clindamycin), antiseptics (povidone–iodine or chlorhexidine solutions) or antibiotic/steroid preparations. In the USA, ointments combining neomycin and thiostrepton are frequently used. If anal sac impaction is a problem, then ceruminolytic agents may be used. Treatments may have to be repeated, and recurrence of disease is still a possibility.

Systemic therapy

The use of systemic antibacterial or antifungal agents may be necessary in cases of acute infection or abscess. Identification of possible causative organisms is important, as anaerobes or yeasts require specific treatment. Drugs commonly used include clindamycin, metronidazole and amoxicillin/clavulanate. Treatment should be continued beyond clinical cure, and microscopic examination of anal sac contents to assess efficacy of treatment is important. Again, recurrence is commonplace, and may indicate the need for surgical removal of the anal sacs.

Surgery

Surgical removal of anal sacs is indicated if medical therapy fails, or if recurrence is frequent in the absence of manageable underlying disease. If perianal masses are present, their removal will often necessitate removal of the ipsilateral anal sac, as damage to the sac may lead to recurrent abscessation or sinus formation.

There have been many techniques described for the surgical removal of anal sacs. It must be emphasized, however, that the filling of the sacs with caustics such as phenol or silver nitrate is *never* indicated.

The two techniques now commonly employed are closed and open removal.

Closed anal sac removal

A closed technique for the removal of anal sacs has been used for many years now, and some surgeons will use no other procedure.

1. Anaesthetize the patient. Clip and prepare the perineum for surgery.
2. Empty the anal sacs and refill with a heated gel. The gel hardens to define the extent of the sacs.
3. A purse string suture may be placed to avoid faecal contamination of the surgical site.
4. Make a curved incision over the palpated distal portion of the sac.

5. Use blunt dissection to isolate the sac and duct, taking care not to damage the nervous supply to the external sphincter.
6. Place a ligature on the duct and remove the sac.
7. Repair the wound.

The advantages of this technique are the lack of damage to the external sphincter muscle and the avoidance of damage to the anal canal. Disadvantages include the leaving of some anal sac duct and possible damage to local nerves. Should a hole be made in the sac, the filler gel can escape and make the surgery more difficult.

Open anal sac removal

A 'lay-open' technique for anal sac removal has been described more recently, and has gained favour with many surgeons. This technique is quicker than the one described above, and results in complete removal of all anal sac and ductal tissue. It is important to allow the dog to empty its rectum prior to surgery, as it is not possible to place a purse string suture.

1. Anaesthetize the patient. Clip and prepare the perineum for surgery. A swab placed in the rectum may prevent leakage of faecal material during surgery.
2. Make an incision along the duct and into the sac: either place a probe into the duct and cut on to it; or insert one blade of straight Metzenbaum scissors into the duct.
3. Make an incision medial to the duct and lift the whole duct away from the anal canal.
4. Grasp the distal open wall with a pair of tissue forceps and free the sac from underlying tissue by blunt and sharp dissection.
5. Repair the wound, taking care to appose the cut ends of the external sphincter muscle.

The advantages of this technique are speed and the ease of identifying whether the whole sac has been removed. A disadvantage is that the external sphincter muscle is cut and takes some time to regain normal function. This does not lead to incontinence, but occasional faeces may be dropped in the first days after surgery.

This technique is also suitable for anal sac removal in the cat.

Neoplasia

If an anal sac mass is present, then the extent of the removal depends upon the biopsy results. If there is distant spread, then removal is inappropriate.

References and further reading

Anderson RK (1984) Anal sac and its related dermatoses. *Compendium on Continuing Education for the Practicing Veterinarian* **6**, 829–837

Hajsig M, Tadic V and Lukman P (1985) *Malassezia* dermatitis in dogs: significance of its location. *Veterinaski Archiv* **55**, 259–266

Halnan CRE (1976a) The diagnosis of anal sacculitis in the dog. *Journal of Small Animal Practice* **17**, 527–535

Halnan CRE (1976b) The frequency of occurrence of anal sacculitis in the dog. *Journal of Small Animal Practice* **17**, 537–541

Halnan CRE (1976c) Therapy of anal sacculitis in the dog. *Journal of Small Animal Practice* **17**, 685–691

Halnan CRE (1976d) The experimental reproduction of anal sacculitis. *Journal of Small Animal Practice* **17**, 693–697

Harvey CE (1974) Incidence and distribution of anal sac disease in the dog. *Journal of the American Animal Hospital Association* **10**, 573–577

Jones RL, Godinho KS and Palmer GH (1994) Clinical observations on the use of oral amoxycillin/clavulanate in the treatment of gingivitis in dogs and cats and anal sacculitis in dogs. *British Veterinary Journal* **150**, 385–388

Mason IS (1995) Anal sac disorders. In: *Handbook of Small Animal Dermatology*, ed. K Moriello and IS Mason, pp. 269–271. Pergamon Press, Oxford

Nesbitt GH (1989) Anal sacculitis. *Veterinary Reports* **1**, 4

Pappalardo E, Martino P and Noli C (2002) *Proceedings of the 17th Meeting of the AAVD*, p.28

Robson D, Barton G, Bassett R and Lorimer M (2002) *Proceedings of the 17th Meeting of the AAVD*, p.36

18

Atopy and adverse food reaction

Ralf S. Mueller and Hilary Jackson

Atopy is defined as an inherited predisposition to develop a type I hypersensitivity to environmental allergens. Historically, the allergens were presumed to be inhaled, but it is more likely that allergens are absorbed percutaneously and bound to epidermal Langerhans' cells. Presentation of these allergens by the Langerhans' cells to T cells leads to a preferential activation of Th2 cells that secrete cytokines favouring the production of allergen-specific IgE antibodies. These IgE antibodies are bound to the surface of circulating basophils and tissue mast cells. When allergens cross-link the surface-bound IgE antibodies, a degranulation of the cells with subsequent release of inflammatory mediators occurs. Preformed mediators stored in the granules include histamine, heparin and proteolytic enzymes, but synthesis and release of other mediators such as prostaglandins and leukotrienes also occur at the time of degranulation. Erythema and pruritus, typical features of allergic disease, occur. Allergen-specific IgGd antibodies have been implicated in the pathogenesis of atopic dermatitis, as they bind to mast cell surfaces, but their exact role in this disease is unclear. Strong breed predilections and limited breeding trials showed atopic dermatitis to be a genetically programmed disease. A further factor involved in the pathogenesis may include the magnitude of allergen exposure, particularly in puppyhood.

The term adverse food reaction encompasses immunological and non-immunological reactions to elements in the diet. The exact pathogenesis is currently unknown. For practical purposes it is useful to consider atopic dermatitis, adverse food reaction and flea allergy dermatitis as potentially co-existing problems (Figure 18.1).

According to the allergic threshold principle, pruritus from several concurrent skin diseases may 'add up'. Every animal has an individual pruritic threshold below which clinical signs are not evident. In an animal with bacterial pyoderma secondary to atopy as well as concurrent flea bite hypersensitivity, some of the pruritus is caused by the pyoderma, some by the atopic dermatitis (AD) and some by flea bites. It may not be necessary to treat all the factors contributing to pruritus to reduce the level to below the threshold. Management of flea allergy dermatitis and secondary pyoderma in a dog with atopic dermatitis may be sufficient to render the animal comfortable. Thus, it is of extreme importance for the management of atopic dermatitis to minimize the pruritus by addressing all the compound-

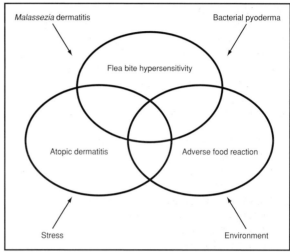

18.1 Factors influencing pruritus of allergic patients.

ing concurrent or secondary pruritic skin diseases such as flea bite hypersensitivity, food intolerance, *Malassezia* dermatitis or bacterial pyoderma.

Clinical approach

Atopic dermatitis is one of the most common skin diseases in the dog and the second most common hypersensitivity in the cat. Atopic dermatitis should be included in the differential diagnoses of any dog with pruritus or pyoderma and any cat with miliary dermatitis, eosinophilic granuloma, non-inflammatory alopecia or pruritus.

History

- The presenting complaint for most atopic dogs will be pruritus, although recurrent pyoderma completely responsive to antibiotics may also be due to atopic dermatitis. Owners often do not consider face rubbing or foot licking signs of pruritus and need to be questioned specifically about various forms of pruritus
- Clinical signs of canine atopic dermatitis begin typically during young adulthood, between 1 and 3 years of age, although atopic dermatitis may occasionally occur in animals as young as 3 months or as old as 12 years

- Initially, seasonal pruritus is most commonly reported, although this may vary with the climate and environment the patient lives in. However, owners commonly report an increasingly longer period of pruritus every year and after a few years many dogs are affected perennially
- Response to glucocorticoids at anti-inflammatory doses is seen in the vast majority of patients with atopic dermatitis without secondary infection. Glucocorticoids will decrease inflammation and pruritus in most patients initially, but a repeated good response indicates a high likelihood of allergic skin disease
- Certain dog breeds are predisposed to atopic dermatitis (Figure 18.2). These breed predispositions may vary from area to area (for example, German Shepherd Dogs are predisposed to atopic dermatitis in Europe and Australia, but not in the United States)
- Feline atopic dermatitis may affect cats of any breed or sex. Miliary dermatitis has been reported to occur more commonly in younger cats, but in general atopic disease may occur at any age in the cat.

Boston Terrier
Boxer
Bull Terrier
Cairn Terrier
Dalmatian
English Bulldog
German Shepherd Dog
Golden Retriever
Jack Russell Terrier
Labrador Retriever
Lhasa Apso
Pug
Scottish Terrier
Shar Pei
Schnauzer
Shih Tsu
West Highland White Terrier

18.2   Breed predilections for canine atopic dermatitis.

Physical examination

Dog

Salivary staining, alopecia, erythema, lichenification and erosions are seen on predilection sites (Figures 18.3 and 18.4); greasy and moist or scaly skin and otitis externa (Figure 18.5) are commonly present. Unilateral otitis externa due to atopic dermatitis has been seen. Atopic rhinitis and conjunctivitis may occur concurrent to dermatological signs or individually. Acral lick dermatitis (Figure 18.6) or pyotraumatic dermatitis ('hot spots') may also be due to atopic dermatitis. Clinical signs of secondary bacterial and/or yeast infection, such as papules, pustules, epidermal collarettes and crusts, are commonly present (Figure 18.7).

Interdigital areas
Carpal/tarsal regions
Face
Ears
Perianal area
Inguinal area
Ventral abdomen
Axillae

18.3   Sites of predilection for canine atopic dermatitis.

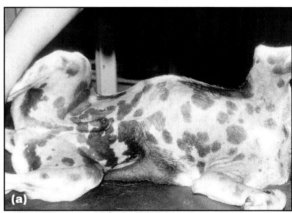

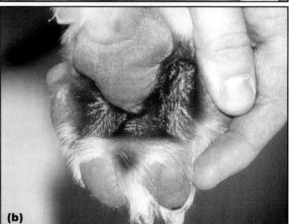

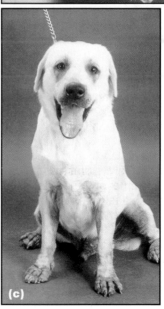

18.4   Canine atopic dermatitis. (a) Ventral erythema of the axillae, abdomen and groin in a crossbred dog. (b) Interdigital erythema in a 3-year-old female spayed Labrador Retriever. (c) A 3-year-old male Labrador Retriever with typical clinical features: note involvement of the paws, ventral abdomen and periorbital areas. Alopecia is secondary to self-trauma.

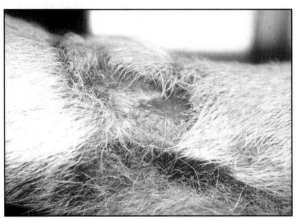

18.5 Chronic otitis externa in a 5-year-old Cocker Spaniel.

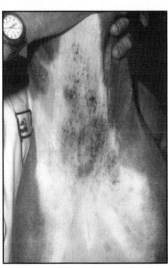

18.6 Focal acral lick dermatitis of the left foreleg of a 7-year-old German Shepherd bitch.

18.7 Bacterial folliculitis of the ventral neck in an atopic 3-year-old female spayed Boxer.

Adverse food reaction in the dog presents as non-seasonal pruritus or recurrent pyoderma with possible concurrent gastrointestinal signs, but no age or sex predilections are reported. The disease often mimics canine atopic dermatitis. Response to gluco-corticoid therapy can be variable. Gastrointestinal signs are often mild and may not be included in information volunteered by the owner. Intermittent vomiting, diarrhoea and borborygmus (rumbling bowel sounds) may occur.

Cat

Atopy is a possible aetiology for a number of cutaneous reaction patterns. Miliary dermatitis (Figure 18.8a), non-inflammatory alopecia (Figure 18.8b) and all lesions of the eosinophilic granuloma complex (Figure 18.8c) may be associated with feline atopic dermatitis. More details on eosinophilic granulomas are given in Chapter 32. Feline atopic dermatitis may cause pruritic dermatitis with severe self-trauma, particularly of the head and neck, and subsequent alopecia, erosions, ulcers and crusting in more severe and chronic disease.

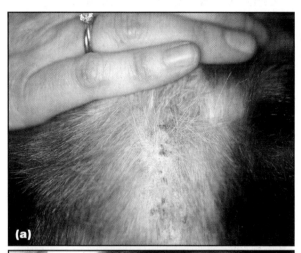

(a)

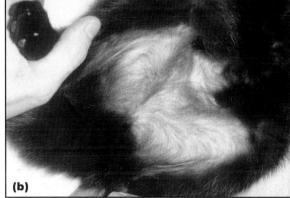

(b)

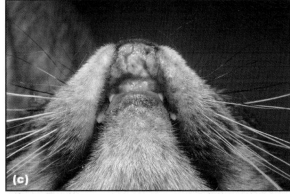

(c)

18.8 Feline atopic dermatitis: (a) Miliary dermatitis in an 8-year-old female spayed Siamese. (b) Non-inflammatory alopecia of the ventral abdomen of a Domestic Shorthair. (c) A 2-year-old Domestic Shorthair with an indolent ulcer of the upper lip.

Diagnosis

Atopy

The diagnosis of atopic dermatitis in small animals is usually based on history, physical examination and ruling out differential diagnoses. Willemse (1986) adapted major and minor criteria accepted for human atopic dermatitis for use in veterinary medicine (Figure 18.9). These criteria can be used as a guideline for the diagnosis of canine atopic dermatitis. An approach to the pruritic dog is outlined in Figure 18.10 and an approach to miliary dermatitis is given in Figure 18.11.

Differential diagnosis of canine atopic dermatitis

Adverse food reaction can present identically to non-seasonal atopic dermatitis in the dog and cat and must be included as a differential diagnosis of every animal with perennial symptoms. The only way to rule out adverse food reaction at present is an elimination diet, described in more detail below.

Scabies, flea bite hypersensitivity, bacterial pyoderma, *Malassezia* dermatitis and cheyletiellosis may all mimic atopic dermatitis. Diagnosis and treatment of these diseases is discussed in more detail in other chapters.

Contact allergic or irritant dermatitis may mimic atopy. Typically, non- or sparsely haired areas such as the inguinal area, the axillae, and/or the scrotum are involved. In short-coated dogs such as Bull Terriers or Boxers, the palmar/plantar interdigital spaces may also be affected. In dogs with pendulous pinnae, the inside of the pinna may be affected if the patient lies on its side and that surface is in direct contact with a contact allergen. Contact allergy may also be caused by medications.

Differential diagnosis of feline atopic dermatitis

Miliary dermatitis may be caused by a wide variety of diseases. Most commonly, it is due to flea bite hypersensitivity and a thorough flea control trial is mandatory in every patient with miliary dermatitis.

Adverse food reaction may also lead to miliary dermatitis and an elimination diet is currently the only diagnostic tool to rule out this disease.

Ectoparasites such as *Notoedres cati*, *Cheyletiella blakei* or *Otodectes cynotis*, dermatophytosis, bacterial infection and, in rare cases, pemphigus foliaceus and mast cell tumours may present in a similar way to miliary dermatitis and are discussed in more detail elsewhere in this book. The eosinophilic granuloma complex and non-inflammatory alopecia may be caused by flea bite hypersensitivity, adverse food reaction or atopic dermatitis. For more detail the reader is referred to other chapters.

Major criteria (at least three of which should be present)
Pruritus
Typical distribution (facial and/or digital involvement or lichenification of the flexor surfaces of the tarsal joint and/or the extensor surface of the carpal joint)
Chronic or chronically relapsing dermatitis
Individual or family history of atopy and/or presence of breed predisposition

Minor criteria (at least three of which should be present)
Onset of symptoms < 3 years of age
Facial erythema and cheilitis
Bilateral conjunctivitis
Superficial staphylococcal pyoderma
Hyperhidrosis
Positive skin test reactions to environmental allergens
Elevated allergen-specific IgE
Elevated allergen-specific IgGd

18.9 Major and minor diagnostic criteria for atopic dermatitis in the dog (adapted from Willemse, 1986).

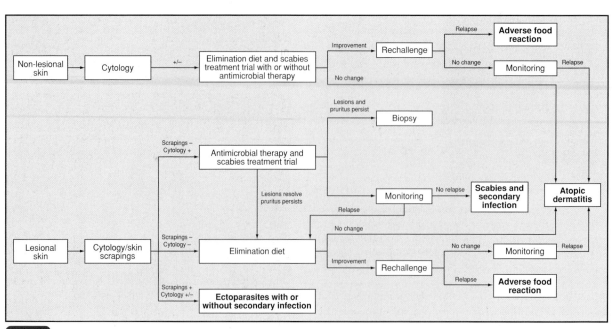

18.10 Approach to the pruritic dog.

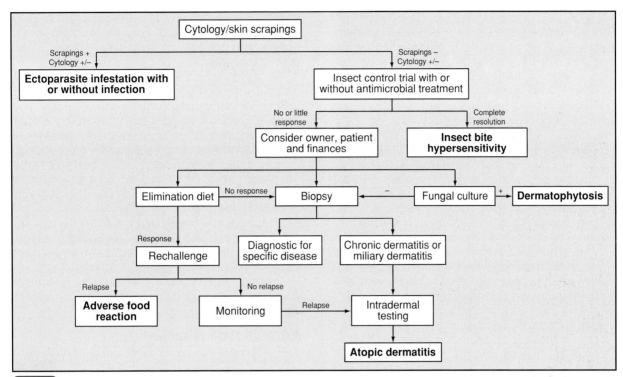

18.11 Approach to the cat with miliary dermatitis. (From Mueller, 2000, with permission)

Head and neck pruritus is most commonly caused by an adverse food reaction, atopic dermatitis and ectoparasites such as *Otodectes cynotis* and *Notoedres cati*. Otoscopic examination, microscopic examination of otic debris, skin scrapings and trial therapy may be used to rule out ectoparasites.

Allergy testing

Once atopic disease is diagnosed by history, clinical examination and ruling out relevant differential diagnoses, offending allergens may be identified with either intradermal testing or serum testing for allergen-specific IgE. Decreasing allergen exposure may be achieved in some patients, although typically only with limited benefits. Animals with increased pruritus during or directly after walks are more likely to be allergic to pollens. If the pruritus is predominantly present indoors, housedust mites are more likely. Thus, the predominant purpose for allergy testing is to allow the formulation of a patient-specific allergen extract used for immunotherapy or allergy shots. Implications, costs, adverse effects and prognosis need to be discussed in great detail with the owner before considering any form of allergy testing. Details of allergy testing are discussed below and in Chapter 3 but, at present, intradermal testing is considered the test of choice for the identification of allergens involved in atopic dermatitis by most dermatologists, serum testing for allergen-specific IgE is accepted as a second-best solution.

Intradermal testing: In preparation for intradermal testing, it is important to observe the withdrawal times for various anti-inflammatory drugs that may interfere with skin test reactivity (Figure 18.12).

Medication	Withdrawal time
Glucocorticoids:	
Single injectable depot preparations	6–8 weeks
Short-term oral glucocorticoids (< 4 months)	4 weeks
Long-term oral glucocorticoids	6–12 weeks
Topical glucocorticoids (ear or eye medications, ointments or creams)	2 weeks
Antihistamines	2 weeks

18.12 Withdrawal times of various medications prior to intradermal testing.

Animals are sedated and placed in lateral recumbency, an area on the lateral chest is clipped and a number of allergens, a negative control (typically saline solution) and a positive control (typically histamine), are injected intradermally. Relevant allergens will bind to allergen-specific IgE on the surface of intradermal mast cells, cross-link these receptors and lead to mast cell degranulation and formation of an erythematous wheal (Figure 18.13). After 15–25 minutes the reactions

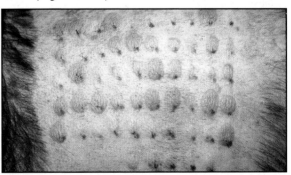

18.13 Skin test with numerous positive reactions in a 5-year-old male collie cross.

are evaluated and compared to the negative and positive control. Based on their diameter, induration and erythema, a score from 0 to 4 is assigned (0 being determined by the negative, 4 by the positive control). The severity of the reactions does not necessarily correlate with the severity of the clinical signs.

Negative intradermal tests in atopic patients may occur for several reasons:

- Although selection of allergens for skin testing aims at choosing the most relevant allergens for the local environment and thus identifies the vast majority of atopic patients, it is limited by availability of allergens, lack of knowledge about dog- and cat-specific allergens and financial constraints. Thus, the patient may be allergic to allergens not included in the test
- Withdrawal periods for anti-inflammatory agents may not have been observed or may have been too short for the particular patient
- Due to constant exposure to certain allergens and subsequent constant degranulation of mast cells, there may not be enough intact, 'loaded' mast cells present to cause a strong wheal and flare reaction to these allergens in the height of the allergy season. The ideal time for intradermal testing in atopic patients with seasonal clinical signs is shortly after the end of the allergy season for that particular patient
- Some atopic patients consistently lack positive reactions on skin testing and will show positive reactions on serum testing for allergen-specific antibodies. The reason for this is not currently known
- Severe stress theoretically may cause release of sufficient endogenous glucocorticoids to inhibit skin test reactions.

'False-positive' skin test reactions are less common and may occur due to cross-reactivity of allergens. An example is the reported cross-reactivity of housedust mites with scabies antigen, leading to false-positive reactions against dust mite antigen in dogs with scabies. Subclinical atopic dermatitis may cause positive reactions on skin tests of clinically normal dogs, which may be under their pruritic threshold at the time of testing. Irritant or true false-positive reactions may also occur. Carefully ruling out differential diagnoses for atopic dermatitis and thus skin testing of clinically atopic patients is the best assurance against false-positive skin test reactions.

Serum testing: Various companies around the world offer serum testing for allergen-specific IgE. Enzyme-linked immunosorbent assays (ELISA) and radio-allergosorbent tests (RAST) are offered; the results of ELISA tests seem to be more reproducible. With newer technology and tests based on monoclonal anti-IgE antibodies, the false-positive reactions so commonly seen some years ago have become fewer. Tests evaluate either individual allergens or grouped allergens (e.g. several individual grass pollens in one group). The authors do not recommend results of the latter as a base for formulation of allergen-

specific immunotherapy, as allergens not involved in the patient's disease may be included in the vaccine and potentially lead to new allergies in this particular patient.

Negative serum test results in atopic patients may occur due to allergen selection or inherent patient factors. Interference of anti-inflammatory drugs, particularly glucocorticoids, varies depending on the serum test used. Some tests are extremely sensitive and will not show positive reactions after glucocorticoid therapy, others seem to be less influenced by it. Negative results due to drug interference seem to be more common in patients on long-term therapy with glucocorticoids even at low doses.

'False-positive' results will be due to either subclinical atopic dermatitis, inherent problems of the assay or cross reactivity of allergens and seem to be more common than in skin testing.

It is even more important to perform a meticulous diagnostic work-up prior to serum testing than prior to intradermal testing.

Adverse food reaction

The only reliable way of diagnosing adverse food reaction in the dog and cat is to feed a novel protein diet for a minimum of 6 weeks (see Chapter 3). A reduction in pruritus should occur during this period.

Dogs

In the majority of cases improvement should be noted after 4–6 weeks on a strict novel protein diet (Figure 18.14). However, sometimes it may be necessary to extend the diet to 8–10 weeks to demonstrate significant improvement. Many therapeutic and prophylactic agents now contain flavours, and care should be taken to replace them with a non-flavoured alternative.

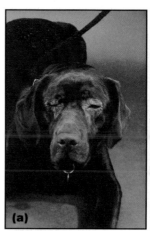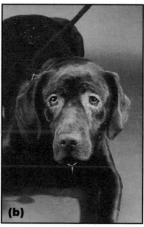

18.14 (a) A 10-month-old female spayed Labrador Retriever with adverse food reaction. Clinical signs are facially orientated. (b) The same dog after 4 weeks on a hypoallergenic diet trial.

The selected diet should be based on a protein to which the animal has had little or no exposure previously. For the normal healthy adult dog an unsupplemented single protein and carbohydrate diet can be fed without complications for the duration of the trial but must be balanced for long-term feeding. The incidence of dogs reported in the literature that have tolerated a home-cooked diet but not the commercial equivalent (implicating the additives or a difference in protein processing) is very small. Feeding a commercial hypoallergenic diet is usually easier for the client. During the trial no table scraps must be fed. If dogs are used to treats, then the treats given during the diet trial must be in line with the ingredients of the diet. For example, if duck with potato is fed, then treats may include grilled pieces of duck meat. Duck jerky may be produced by drying duck meat in the oven at low temperatures of 75–85°C for 3–4 hours. Grilled potatoes may also be given as treats. Thus, feeding habits do not need to be changed dramatically and client compliance increases, yet the animal still receives only the selected protein and carbohydrate source.

Hydrolysate diets are a new generation of veterinary diets with an indication for use in the animal with gastrointestinal or cutaneous hypersensitivities. The theoretical advantage of these diets is that a novel protein need not be utilized since the dietary protein has been hydrolysed to peptides that are smaller than those required to provoke an immune response. Due to few data on their performance at the time of writing, they cannot be recommended as an initial choice for a novel protein diet trial.

Cats

The same principle of feeding a novel protein diet followed by the demonstration of a relapse of clinical signs on challenge applies (Figure 18.15). However, cats have specific nutritional requirements and the feeding of an unsupplemented home-cooked diet for more than 4 weeks can result in nutritional deficiences.

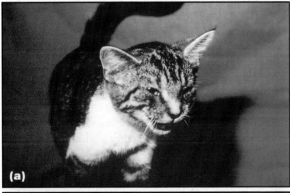
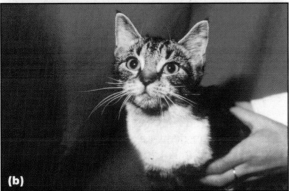

18.15 (a) A 5-month-old female spayed Domestic Shorthair with adverse food reaction. (b) The same kitten after 10 weeks on a hypoallergenic diet trial.

Cats refusing a diet for several days may be prone to hepatic lipidosis and thus early compliance is much more important than in dogs.

If an improvement is perceived during or towards the end of the diet trial then the presumptive diagnosis should be confirmed by challenge with previously fed food items. The patient may have atopic dermatitis and the diet trial may have been initiated coincidentally with a change in season, or the improvement might be attributable to concurrent therapeutics such as flea control or topical shampoo therapy. Finally, hypoallergenic diets often result in an improved plane of nutrition particularly in respect to essential fatty acid therapy.

The most straightforward way to confirm the diagnosis is to challenge with the previous diet and treats. This should be mixed with the test diet (approximately 20%). Pruritus and/or gastrointestinal signs should occur within a few hours to, at the most, 2 weeks of this challenge. Then the animal may either be maintained on the hypoallergenic diet provided it is balanced for long-term feeding or it may be challenged with individual allergens such as beef, chicken, fish, wheat, corn and milk. The advantage of this latter option is that the animal need not be maintained on an expensive prescription diet if the identity of the offending allergens is known. Most affected animals are allergic to more than one dietary allergen.

Management and therapeutics

The client has two major options. In patients with atopic dermatitis, the disease may be further characterized by identifying offending allergens with intradermal testing or serum testing for allergen-specific IgE (see above). This allows formulation of allergen-specific immunotherapy, currently the only treatment modality specific for atopic disease. It also occasionally may provide clues for limiting the exposure to involved allergens. The other option is symptomatic anti-pruritic therapy without specific knowledge of allergens involved in the disease.

In patients with adverse food reaction, a sequential rechallenge with individual proteins, as described above, will often identify the offending food ingredient(s), which then need to be avoided. An alternative is to continue long term with a commercial diet that is well tolerated by that particular patient without determining which ingredient of the original food was responsible for the clinical signs.

Allergen-specific immunotherapy ('allergy shots')

Hyposensitization (also called desensitization or allergy vaccination) involves subcutaneous injection of relevant allergens at intervals and in increasing concentrations (induction period), until the target maintenance dose is reached. This dose is administered on a regular basis as needed by the patient. The success rate of this therapy varies between 50% and 80% in most studies. Improvement is not expected for the first few months of therapy. Allergy shots should be administered for a minimum of 1 year before treatment is considered ineffective and discontinued.

Allergens

The allergen extracts need to be selected carefully, with consideration of the previous history and likely allergen exposure. The veterinary surgeon who formulates the allergen extracts needs to consider factors such as local allergen distribution and pollination times. The general practitioner is advised to contact veterinary dermatologists or medical allergists for advice at the outset.

- Aqueous allergens are used most commonly and require small doses but frequent administration
- Emulsion allergens (allergens in propylene glycol, glycerin or mineral oil) are slowly absorbed and require the least number of injections
- Alum-precipitated allergens are an intermediate form only rarely used in the USA or Australia, but used commonly in Europe.

Schedules

Immunotherapy schedules vary greatly among practising allergists. Typically, subcutaneous injections are given every other day to once weekly. Maintenance doses are reached after 1–4 months with the various regimens.

'Rush' immunotherapy has been reported recently, where induction doses are given every 30 minutes and maintenance is reached after the first day. Animals should be under constant supervision during 'rush' immunotherapy and the authors do *not* recommend this protocol for cats with atopic dermatitis. Advantages of 'rush' immunotherapy include a shorter induction period and an easier schedule for owners. Clinical studies evaluating its efficacy are currently being undertaken.

Typical maintenance therapy uses 1 ml of extract subcutaneously every 1–3 weeks. Owners may be educated to give the injections and also need to be aware of possible side effects, particularly anaphylactic shock.

Anaphylactic shock

Anaphylactic shock occurs rarely but is an **emergency necessitating immediate veterinary attention**.

Owners giving injections should be requested to:

- Administer injections during the normal business hours of their local veterinary surgeon
- Monitor their pet for the first 30 minutes after allergen injections
- **Immediately** visit the veterinary surgeon if swelling, wheals, vomiting, diarrhoea or respiratory problems occur during that time.

Animals with a history of such a reaction should be pretreated with antihistamines or glucocorticoids 2–3 hours prior to administration of the allergen extract. It is recommended that the first few subcutaneous injections are administered at a veterinary hospital. Anaphylactic shock or an anaphylactoid reaction does not typically necessitate cessation of immunotherapy.

Monitoring

Monitoring atopic patients on immunotherapy is essential, and regular phone contacts or revisits are strongly recommended. If the patient deteriorates on therapy, diagnosis and (if needed) treatment of possible secondary bacterial or yeast infections are very important.

Deterioration without infection necessitates a change in the injection protocol, particularly if the increased pruritus is seen directly after allergen injection. Depending on the individual patient, the same dose of allergen may be repeated until there is no more increased pruritus after the injection, or the dose of the allergen may have to be decreased and future increases may have to occur in smaller increments. Similarly, increased pruritus before the injection of allergen extract that subsides afterwards may indicate the need for more frequent injections.

Response

A significant improvement on immunotherapy is not expected until several weeks to months into therapy. Owners tend to get frustrated in this initial period and often need to be encouraged to continue therapy despite an apparent lack of response. To avoid owner frustration, concurrent symptomatic therapy is frequently necessary. The patient should always show mild residual pruritus to allow judgement of the vaccine efficacy. If the patient's pruritus disappears completely, symptomatic therapy should be decreased until either mild pruritus is present again or the patient is exclusively maintained with allergen-specific immunotherapy.

Remission and relapse

Once a patient is in remission on allergy shots only, the frequency of the injection may be decreased slowly until mild pruritus recurs or injections are given every 2 months for a whole year without any recurrence of clinical signs. At that time, owners may decide to continue the therapy indefinitely or try to discontinue the allergy shots. A small number of dogs will stay in long-term remission after some years of immunotherapy, but relapses are also possible.

Decreasing the allergen load

Decreasing the amount of allergen the patient is exposed to has been attempted in human and veterinary medicine and has been particularly effective in humans sensitive to housedust mites. Unfortunately, clients may invest a lot of effort and money with no apparent result. However, some patients may benefit from the measures described below.

Typically, patients allergic to indoor antigens such as housedust mites have symptoms perennially, are worse during periods of prolonged indoor confinement and better when taken on camping trips or being boarded in kennels or hospitals. A decrease in housedust mite allergens may be achieved with various methods:

- Vacuuming frequently typically worsens the situation as antigens are too small to be kept in the vacuum bag and are dispersed through the air. However, those vacuum cleaners with HEPA or electrostatically charged microfilters perform well
- The major reservoirs for housedust mites are carpets, upholstered furniture and mattresses and pillows. Plastic encasings for mattresses and

pillows are available and may be particularly useful if the animal sleeps on or in close proximity to these. Removing carpets and replacing with wooden floor boards, tiles or linoleum will greatly reduce the number of housedust mites

- There is evidence that environmental flea control measures such as insect growth regulators or sodium borate applied to carpets may reduce the number of housedust mites.

Patients allergic to pollen allergens often present with a history of deterioration during and after walks or at certain times of the year.

- A dog may be rinsed or hosed with water after walks. In colder climates or seasons, this can be limited to just the distal limbs.
- In patients with seasonal pruritus worst outdoors, indoor confinement with only short walks during that time may significantly decrease the clinical signs.

Symptomatic therapy

Most dogs and cats will receive glucocorticoids, antihistamines, fatty acid supplementations or a combination thereof. In refractory patients, newer and/or more expensive drugs may be considered.

Systemic therapy

Glucocorticoids: At anti-inflammatory doses, glucocorticoids are the most effective drugs for atopic dermatitis; the dose used in cats is usually higher than that in dogs (Figure 18.16). Prednisone and prednisolone are most commonly used. Some animals may not respond well to these or show excessive adverse effects such as PU/PD or polyphagia and may benefit from alternative drugs. Starting doses of various glucocorticoids are listed in Figure 18.16.

Drug	Dose	
	Dogs	Cats
Prednisone	0.5–1 mg/kg every 24–48 hours	1–2 mg/kg every 24–48 hours
Prednisolone	0.5–1 mg/kg every 24–48 hours	1–2 mg/kg every 24–48 hours
Methylprednisolone	0.4–0.8 mg/kg every 24–48 hours orally 2–40 mg/dog every 2–8 weeks for injectable depot preparation	0.5–1.5 mg/kg orally 10–20 mg/cat for injectable depot preparation
Dexamethasone	0.05–0.1 mg/kg every 48–72 hours orally	0.05–0.1 mg/kg every 48–72 hours orally
Triamcinolone	0.05–0.1 mg/kg every 48–72 hours orally 0.1–0.2 mg/kg i.m. or s.c.	0.05–0.1 mg/kg every 48–72 hours orally 0.1–0.2 mg/kg i.m. or s.c.

18.16 Glucocorticoids commonly used in veterinary dermatology and their doses.

Alternate-day to every third day therapy is preferred to daily administration; however, some dogs are controlled better on a very small dose of daily glucocorticoid rather than a fairly high dose of alternate-day administration. Atopic patients on glucocorticoid therapy may initially respond well to low doses, but may become increasingly refractory with time. Adverse effects of glucocorticoid therapy are listed in Figure18.17. Severe calcinosis cutis has been seen in dogs on 0.2 mg/kg of prednisone every other day for a few weeks to months. Although this is not common, it emphasizes that there is no 'safe' dose of glucocorticoids. Oral administration is preferred as dose adjustments are achieved more easily and quickly.

Polyphagia
Polydipsia
Polyuria
Lethargy
Exercise intolerance
Muscle wasting
Panting
Secondary infections
Delayed wound healing
Calcinosis cutis

18.17 Adverse effects seen with glucocorticoid therapy.

A sparing effect of antihistamines and fatty acid supplementations has been reported in various studies, even in patients where these antihistamines and fatty acids had not improved the condition at all on their own. Tapering a glucocorticoid to the lowest possible dose to maintain the pruritus at a very low level and then adding antihistamines or fatty acids will often result in a significantly reduced glucocorticoid requirement and should always be encouraged. The authors routinely treat atopic dogs with fixed doses of antihistamines and fatty acid supplementations at the same time and add just as much of the glucocorticoids as is needed at that particular time. If the patient shows no sign of pruritus, the dose of the glucocorticoid is decreased until mild pruritus is present. This allows tailoring of the dose to the minimum required by that particular patient at any given time as these requirements may vary from week to week and season to season.

Antihistamines: Antihistamines are used more and more commonly in the treatment of atopic dermatitis because of their safety. Their success rate in dogs is relatively low, with only an estimated 30% of atopic patients responding completely. Cats respond much better: the success rate is up to 70%. An antihistamine trial is recommended for any cat to which owners are able to administer tablets on a daily basis. As the lack of response to one antihistamine does not rule out a good response to another, patients will routinely undergo an antihistamine trial where several different antihistamines are administered one at a time for about 10–14 days. Typically, low-priced antihistamines are used first. Although sedation is seen commonly in humans, this adverse effect is not as common in small animals. Even if there is a mild sedation during the first 3–4 days, this often resolves within the first week of treatment. Commonly used antihistamines, their adverse effects and doses are listed in Figure 18.18. Two antihistamines given concurrently at their normal doses may be more effective in decreasing a patient's pruritus and a variety of combinations are used in veterinary dermatology. Giving two antihistamines concurrently does not seem to result in a significantly higher incidence of adverse effects. Only antihistamines of different classes should be administered concurrently. Antihistamines are also commonly combined with essential fatty acid supplementation. Due to their glucocorticoid-sparing activity, antihistamines are commonly used in dogs as adjunctive therapy, even if their efficacy as a sole treatment is not satisfactory.

Essential fatty acid supplementation: EFA supplementation causes an alteration of the composition and function of the epidermal lipid barrier and attempts to switch the production of inflammatory mediators such as prostaglandin E2 or leukotriene B4 to less inflammatory or non-inflammatory prostaglandins and leukotrienes. The success of this competitive inhibition varies. Complete resolution of pruritus is seen in a minority of atopic dogs only. In atopic cats, the success rate with fatty acid therapy is higher and may approach 50–70%. Dry and scaly skin in atopic patients is more likely than pruritus to respond to fatty acid supplementation.

Essential fatty acids are also known for their glucocorticoid-sparing activity and are used frequently as adjunctive therapy in combination with these and/or antihistamines and allergen-specific immunotherapy. Various products are available. They are based either on omega-3 fatty acids (such as eicosapentaenoic acid in marine fish oil), omega-6 fatty acids (such as linoleic acid in sunflower or safflower oil or γ-linolenic acid in evening primrose oil) or a combination thereof. A number of studies have evaluated the success rate of various fatty acid supplementations at various doses. At present, no clear guidelines can be given as to which type or ratio of omega-3:omega-6 fatty acid supplementation is most suited for the treatment of atopic dermatitis, although the authors prefer omega-3 fatty acids or a combination of omega-3 and omega-6 fatty acids for

Drug (Class)	Formulation	Comments	Dog Dose (D) Cat Dose (C)
Diphenhydramine (Ethanolamine)	25 mg, 50 mg tablet	Inexpensive, potentially sedating	2 mg/kg q 8–12h (D, C)
Dexchlorpheniramine (Alkylamine)	2-mg tablets, 6-mg tablets	Inexpensive, potentially sedating	2–6 mg/D q 12 h (D), 2 mg/C q 12 h (C)
Chlorpheniramine (Alkylamine)	4 mg tablets	Inexpensive, potentially sedating	2–12 mg q 12 h/D 2–4 mg q 12 h/C
Azatidine (Piperidine)	1 mg tablets		
Cyproheptadine (Piperidine)	4 mg tablets	Inexpensive, potentially sedating	2–8 mg q 12 h/D 2–4 mg q 12 h/C
Promethazine (Phenothiazine)	10 mg, 25 mg, 50 mg coated tablets	Sedating	1–2 mg/kg q 12 h (D, C)
Hydroxyzine (Piperazine)	25 mg, 50 mg capsules	Also inhibits mast cell degranulation, and is tricyclic antidepressant and teratogenic!!	2 mg/kg q 8–12 h (D, C)
Loratidine (Piperidine)	10 mg tablet, 1 mg/ml syrup		5–20 mg/D q 12–24 h 5 mg/C q 12–24 h
Cetirizine (Piperazine)	10 mg coated tablets, 1 mg/ml syrup	Inhibits exocytosis of eosinophils in humans	5–20 mg/kg q 12 h/D 5 mg q 12–24 h/C
Clemastine (Ethanolamine)	1.34 mg tablets, 0.05 mg/ml syrup	Enhances cholinergic activity of other antihistamines as these drugs are metabolized by same enzyme system in liver and concurrent administration may increase serum levels significantly	0.5–1 mg q 12 h/D
Trimeprazine (Phenothiazine)	2.5 mg, 5 mg tablets		1.25–10 mg/D, C q 8–12 h
Terfenadine (Miscellaneous)	60 mg, 120 mg tablets, 6 mg/ml suspension	Do not give concurrently with ketoconazole, cyclosporin, or erythromycin as these drugs are metabolized by same enzyme system in liver and concurrent administration may increase serum levels significantly	30–60 mg q 12 h/D
Astemizol (Miscellaneous)	10 mg tablets, 2 mg/ml suspension	Do not administer with ketoconazole, itraconazole, erythromycin, or terfenadine. Long half life!	0.25-mg/kg q 24 h

18.18 Antihistamines used for the treatment of atopic dermatitis and their doses and most common side effects. (Adapted from Mueller, 2000, with permission)

the treatment of pruritus. Products based on omega-6 fatty acids may be more suitable for the treatment of dry skin and secondary seborrhoea sicca associated with atopic dermatitis.

Approximately 50 mg/kg daily or more of eicosapentaenoic acid or linoleic acid are administered. The required dose may vary depending on the fatty acid content of the atopic patient's diet. In general, higher doses will give better response rates but also increase the risk of diarrhoea, the most common adverse effect of fatty acid therapy. Occasionally, pancreatitis and (with fish oil-based omega-3 fatty acids) bad breath are noted. The caloric density of these supplements necessitates a reduction in food intake to keep the body weight constant, particularly at higher doses.

If administering capsules to the patient is a problem, capsules can be pierced and the fatty acids mixed in with a small amount of food. Omega-3 fatty acids typically smell and taste very fishy and pets disliking fish will not eat this mixture, while animals favouring fish will be more inclined to eat it. Omega-6 fatty acids have a less intense odour and taste and may be given in food more easily. Although some controversy exists about the time period of fatty acid supplementation before effects can be evaluated, they should be administered for a minimum of 8–10 weeks, based on fatty acid concentration changes in serum and skin with supplementation.

Ciclosporin: Another drug receiving attention in human and veterinary medicine is ciclosporin. It is an inhibitor of IL-2 production, and thus T-cell activation, and is very effective in many patients with atopic dermatitis. Ciclosporin is given at 5 mg/kg daily. It is metabolized in the liver. Drugs metabolized by the same enzyme system, such as ketoconazole, prolong its half-life and have been used to decrease the dose requirement of ciclosporin for financial reasons in some countries. The ciclosporin dose may be decreased by 40–90% with concurrent ketoconazole administration at 5–10 mg/kg twice daily. Adverse effects seen include vomiting and diarrhoea. As yet, hypertension and kidney failure seen in humans have not been a problem in dogs. At doses of 15 mg/kg daily and higher given to transplant patients or patients with immune-mediated skin disease, gingival hyperplasia, weight loss, lameness, increased hair and claw growth have been reported. The long-term side effects of this form of therapy in the dog are not known. In atopic patients successfully controlled with ciclosporin, decreasing the dose below 5 mg/kg frequently leads to recurrence of clinical signs. However, the frequency of administration may be decreased to alternate days or twice weekly in some patients. This is a topic of ongoing investigation.

Pentoxifylline: Pentoxifylline has also been administered to dogs with atopic dermatitis at 10–15 mg/kg bid or tid. Although improvement of some clinical parameters has occurred in clinical studies, pruritus did not improve significantly compared with the placebo group, which is in agreement with the authors' experience. Pentoxifylline may have a place as an adjunctive therapy in dogs with mild to moderate disease.

Misoprostol: Misoprostol, a prostaglandin E2 analogue has also been evaluated as a potential treatment for canine atopic dermatitis at a dose of 6 micrograms/kg tid. As a sole antipruritic agent it does not perform well but it is effective in some individuals in combination with antihistamines and/or topical therapy.

Psychotropic agents: In animals refractory to treatment with the above outlined treatments, psychotropic agents such as amitriptyline at a dose of 1–2 mg/kg bid or fluoxetine at a dose of 1 mg/kg sid may be used. Adverse effects include all those seen with antihistamines but psychotropic agents may also result in abnormal and strange behaviour, lower the seizure threshold and induce cardiac arrhythmias.

Topical therapy

Topical therapy may also be of benefit to many patients with atopic dermatitis. A number of antipruritic shampoos are available.

Demulcents and moisturizers: These are common ingredients of shampoos. A demulcent is a high-molecular-weight compound in aqueous solution which coats the skin surface, thus protecting the underlying cells and alleviating irritation. Urea promotes hydration and is antibacterial. Glycerine is a popular vehicle and a hygroscopic agent which is absorbed into the skin. Linoleic acid is very important for the barrier function of the stratum corneum, particularly affecting transepidermal water loss. Topical application of fatty acids has been shown to affect epidermal fatty acid concentrations and may hydrate the stratum corneum by reducing transepidermal water loss. Colloidal oatmeal hydrates the stratum corneum hygroscopically by attracting and binding water passing through the epidermis.

Anti-inflammatory ingredients: Hydrocortisone, antihistamines and *Aloe vera* extracts have been incorporated into shampoos. Antihistamines and hydrocortisone presumably penetrate the epidermis and exert antihistaminic and anti-inflammatory effects in the upper dermis. The systemic absorption of hydrocortisone in shampoo form has been shown to be clinically insignificant after prolonged use. Anti-inflammatory properties of aloe vera have been reported in rats based on inhibition of cyclo-oxygenase activity and neutrophil migration. In some patients, topical therapy alleviates pruritus for several days and owners may choose to continue weekly or twice weekly shampoo therapy. Other patients do not benefit from topical therapy enough to consider this form of treatment for long-term management.

Anti-infective ingredients: Frequent use of shampoos containing antibacterial and antifungal agents such as chlorhexidine, benzoyl peroxide and miconazole is often beneficial in the management of those dogs with a particular predisposition to bacterial and yeast infections.

Summary

In summary, there is no single uniformly effective therapeutic agent or management approach for canine or feline atopic dermatitis, and the succesful remedy is usually a combination of topical treatments, systemic therapeutics and environmental changes. The management of atopic patients is frequently a challenge requiring a dedicated and educated client willing to put in significant personal, emotional and financial effort, and a veterinary surgeon willing to invest a significant amount of time to guide and advise the client long term in the search for the best therapeutic approach for that particular patient. However, this is an area of intense research in both the human and veterinary field, and it is likely that newer and more effective therapies will become available within the next decade.

References and further reading

Mueller RS (2000) *Dermatology for the Small Animal Practitioner.* Teton New Media, Jackson Hole, WY

Prelaud P and Gilbert S (2000) Atopic dermatitis. *A Practical Guide to Feline Dermatology*, ed. E Guaguere and P Prelaud, pp.10.1–10.7. Mérial, Lyon

Reedy LM, Miller WH and Willemse T (1997) *Allergic Skin Disease of Dogs and Cats, 2nd edn.* WB Saunders, Philadelphia

Scott DW, Miller WH and Griffin CE (2001) *Muller & Kirk's Small Animal Dermatology, 6th edn.* WB Saunders, Philadelphia

Willemse T (1986) Atopic skin disease: a review and a reconsideration of diagnostic criteria. *Journal of Small Animal Practice* **27**, 771–778

Willemse T, Van den Brom WE, Rynberg A *et al.* (1984) Effect of hyposensitization on atopic dermatitis in dogs. *Journal of the American Veterinary Medical Association* **184**, 1277–1280

19

Flea allergy and flea control

Gail Kunkle and Richard Halliwell

Flea allergy dermatitis (FAD) is the most common skin disease of dogs and cats throughout the world. Although fleas can serve as vectors for other diseases affecting both animals and humans (e.g. transmission of cat scratch fever due to *Bartonella henselae*) and may cause skin disease in people, the most important problem with this insect is the hypersensitivity and resulting dermatological signs that some pets develop. Until recently, recommendations for management and treatment of FAD have required a major time and financial commitment from owners to treat the pets and the indoor and outdoor environment. For many years, dermatologists have 'preached' the one fleabite theory and that for optimum clinical response the flea-allergic pet should receive NO bites. With the development of new highly effective on-animal flea adulticides and compounds that act on various stages of the flea's development, this goal has become attainable, with markedly improved clinical outcomes for pets.

Flea biology

The cat flea *Ctenocephalides felis felis* is the primary flea causing clinical disease in dogs and cats in most parts of the world. Regionally there may be areas in which *C. canis* (Ireland), *Pulex* spp., and *Echidnophaga gallinacea* are clinically important. Species of fleas that predominantly parasitize wildlife may, on occasion, infest dogs and cats. However, such infestations are usually transitory and readily controlled. Adult cat fleas are obligate ectoparasites of the animal host, and can survive for only short periods off the host once they have fed. Unlike many other flea species, *C. felis* is not a nest or den flea but one that lives, feeds and lays eggs on the host. It is the adult flea feeding on the host pet that causes the clinical signs noted in flea allergy. However, the major proportions of the parasite life cycle develop off the host in the host's environment.

In the environment, the newly emerged flea is stimulated to erupt from its pupa when there is vibration, warmth or carbon dioxide from a nearby mammal. Once settled on the pet, these fleas do not jump on and off under normal circumstances, and do not ordinarily move freely between hosts. Most adult flea mortality on dogs and especially cats is from grooming. Flea-allergic animals develop highly effective grooming skills to remove the parasites that cause them misery. This explains why flea-allergic pets often have 'no fleas'.

Optimum environmental conditions for flea propagation and survival include temperatures between 20 and 30°C with a relative humidity greater than 70% (Rust and Dryden, 1997). The eggs and adult flea faecal pellets, which are the major food source for the larvae, are often concentrated in or near pet sleeping areas. Although larvae burrow down into carpets, they do not burrow into soil. However, they can move horizontally over smooth surfaces quite rapidly to avoid light and heat, as they are susceptible to desiccation. Outdoors, larvae can easily be washed away by significant rainfall. The pupae can survive for up to several months and are the most difficult stage of the life cycle to eliminate.

It is important to recognize that in some geographical areas a wide range of non-domesticated hosts, particulary the fox, raccoon, skunk and Virginia opossum, may harbour *C. felis*. When plotting control measures the veterinary surgeon always needs to consider the life cycle and biology of the flea as well as each pet's home conditions.

The development of hypersensitivity

It seems likely that the majority of cats and dogs exposed to fleas on a long-term basis will develop hypersensitivity. Thus, when cats are maintained in colonies for the purpose of rearing fleas, most develop allergic reactions in time and this usually necessitates their removal from the colony. Nonetheless, under natural conditions, both dogs and cats are often observed to have varying, but relatively constant, flea burdens over long periods of time, and yet no obvious clinical signs. These pets may be, at least partially, immunologically tolerant. Knowledge of the factors that determine the development of hypersensitivity is thus of importance.

Flea allergen(s)

It has long been assumed that the flea allergen(s) were present in flea saliva. Indeed, close observation of flea feeding on flea-allergic dogs often reveals a papule or urticarial wheal at the site of flea feeding. This concept has received support from workers who have shown that extracts prepared from carefully dissected salivary glands are highly allergenic, as revealed by elicitation of strongly positive skin tests at high dilutions in allergic animals. As would be expected, such extracts are far more potent than are crude extracts prepared from whole fleas. However, it is important to note that the whole flea extract is the common allergen used worldwide for skin testing most suspect patients. It is commercially available, inexpensive and widely accepted.

It has been shown that a number of protein allergens are present in flea saliva and recently a major salivary allergen, termed Cte f 1, has been cloned and expressed. The allergen is recognized by sera from 80% of flea-allergic dogs (McDermott *et al*, 2000). It can be predicted that additional recombinant allergens will become available in time and may offer potential for immunotherapy.

Factors affecting the development of hypersensitivity

Dogs can be sensitized experimentally by only 15 minutes of weekly exposure to fleas (Halliwell, 1990). After 40 weeks of exposure, 77% of laboratory Beagles had an immediate intradermal test (IDT) reaction to flea salivary antigen, 44% showed a late phase reaction and 98% a delayed type hypersensitivity (DTH) reaction (McCall *et al.*, 1998) (Figure 19.1). These dogs developed clinical signs of flea allergy when challenged with flea infestations. In research, it has been shown that both dogs and cats with continuous or intermittent exposure to fleas can develop sensitization. In dogs, however, continual exposure has been shown both to delay the onset and to reduce the extent of the hypersensitivity response (Halliwell, 1990). Most animals, once allergic, remain so for life; in a minority of cases the degree of hypersensitivity may decline, or even disappear (Halliwell *et al.*, 1987). A number of studies have shown that atopic dogs are predisposed to the development of clinical FAD. Thus flea control in such animals is of the greatest importance.

Type of hypersensitivity reaction	Time of onset after allergen challenge	Details
Immediate	15 minutes	IgE-mediated. Some 15—30% of FAD dogs show no immediate hypersensitivity
Late phase	4–6 hours	Probably IgE-mediated and accompanied by an influx of basophils
Delayed-type (DTH)	24–48 hours	Cell-mediated

19.1 Flea hypersensitivity reactions. Allergic animals may have one or any combination of these.

Types of hypersensitivity involved

As noted above, when dogs suffering from FAD are exposed to the bites of fleas, there is in most cases an immediate papular eruption presumed to be mediated by IgE antibody. Biopsy findings are consistent with such a reaction. If the site of the flea bite is observed over time, a varying pattern is seen. A late phase (associated with an influx of basophils), or a DTH (cell-mediated) hypersensitivity, or both, can be noted. In other cases, the immediate and delayed phases merge imperceptibly. Which reaction patterns are the more significant in the induction of pruritus is not known. Considering the duration of persistence of the reaction, it seems that the delayed component is probably of the greater significance. However, some 15–30% of dogs suffer from DTH only. This is important, as such animals will have negative intradermal (IDT) tests at 15 minutes, reacting only at 24–48 hours. They also will have false-negative reactions to *in vitro* tests for allergen-specific IgE. Our knowledge of the situation in cats is less clear.

Clinical approach

Because FAD is the most common pruritic disease of the dog, all itchy dogs in geographical areas where fleas exist should have this diagnosis in the differential list (Figure 19.2). Sarcoptic mange and adverse food reaction are also highly pruritic. Differential diagnosis of atopy, food allergy and sarcoptic mange are discussed in Chapters 18 and 20.

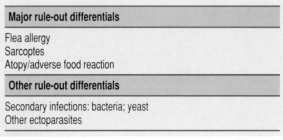

Major rule-out differentials
Flea allergy
Sarcoptes
Atopy/adverse food reaction

Other rule-out differentials
Secondary infections: bacteria; yeast
Other ectoparasites

19.2 Clinical approach to severe pruritus: differential diagnoses.

Once flea allergy is considered, a thorough history is mandatory. This should include inquiring about the environment, other pets, the lifestyle of all pets, and whether fleas, flea faeces or tapeworm segments have been noted. It is critical for the veterinary surgeon first to eliminate fleas if they are present or suspected in a pruritic pet, unless other major differentials such as sarcoptic mange take a higher priority.

The importance of the role of flea allergy in dermatology has become more apparent to veterinary surgeons as they have noted total clearing of a wide range of symptoms in both dogs and cats with the newer, highly effective flea products. Although dogs may have concurrent atopic dermatitis or adverse food reaction, it is critical to evaluate the degree of pruritus that flea allergy is contributing to the clinical signs. There are conflicting reports regarding the importance of FAD in facial and pedal pruritus as well as in otitis. Since flea eradication can be accomplished so much more easily than in the past, it is wise to investigate the flea's role early in the clinical assessment.

Diagnosis

The diagnosis of flea allergy is a clinical one, made by observation of the clinical signs and supported by a favourable response to flea control. The condition can occur in pets of any age, but classically the signs are first noted in young adulthood. In many regions of the world the signs are seasonal because of the necessary environmental conditions for insect survival.

Clinical signs

Dog

In the dog, the classical clinical signs are severe pruritus with a papular eruption, frequently involving the caudal half of the pet, especially the lumbosacral area and tail base (Figure 19.3). Most of the lesions are the result of self-trauma by the allergic dog and may include pyotraumatic dermatitis and more generalized superficial pyoderma. Many flea-allergic dogs exhibit a behaviour of jumping up suddenly and biting themselves although, because of the dog's efficient grooming, the owners often fail to observe fleas, even on careful examination. Indeed, failure to observe fleas, especially if other pets in the household have fleas, is a common feature of the flea-allergic dog or cat. With chronicity, flea-allergic dogs may develop alopecia, hyperpigmentation, lichenification and fibropruritic nodules (Figures 19.4 and 19.5).

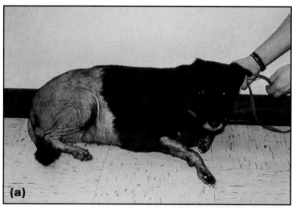

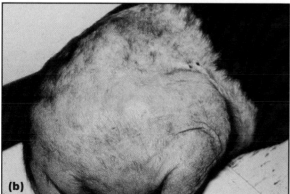

19.3 Flea allergy in an adult Labrador Retriever. Most lesions are found in the posterior half of the body. The close-up view shows self-inflicted hypotrichosis, erythema, early lichenification and excoriation.

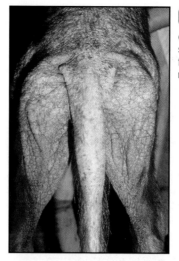

19.4 Chronic flea allergy dermatitis and secondary bacterial folliculitis in an adult mixed breed dog.

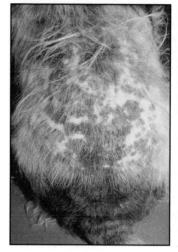

19.5 Severe canine chronic flea allergy dermatitis with alopecia, severe lichenification and fibropruritic nodules in an adult of mixed breed.

Cat

The cat with flea allergy (Figure 19.6) can present with a variety of clinical signs, including localized or generalized miliary dermatitis, focal, symmetrical or non-symmetrical, non-inflammatory or inflammatory alopecia, or eosinophilic plaque. As with the dog, self-trauma plays a major role in visible symptoms; however, the owner may not be aware of the cat's grooming. A primary papular dermatitis and/or plaques may be among the earliest of feline lesions in some cats and may necessitate clipping in order for the veterinary surgeon to see them.

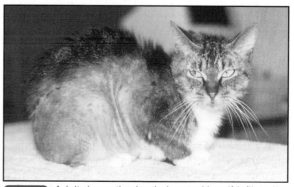

19.6 Adult domestic shorthair cat with self-inflicted symmetrical alopecia and miliary dermatitis.

Diagnostic techniques

Demonstration of fleas and/or flea faeces
Failure to demonstrate the presence of fleas and/or flea faeces, does not preclude a diagnosis of FAD. However, owners are more readily convinced of the diagnosis if a positive demonstration is made, and a number of techniques are available to assist in this:

- Flea comb
- Quick knockdown flea spray
- The patient can be placed on a sheet of white paper and its coat brushed vigorously to dislodge any fleas and flea dirt. The debris is then carefully examined, moistening the paper if necessary to aid in the demonstration of flea faeces, which will impart a red/brown tinge to the paper
- Examination of faeces for the presence of tapeworm segments should be undertaken, or, particularly in the case of cats, faecal flotation in a search for flea exoskeletons.

Intradermal tests
Many references report the usefulness of a positive IDT with flea antigen (both whole body extract and salivary allergens) to confirm the presence of flea allergy in dogs and cats. These antigens are also used in *in vitro* testing for the presence of allergen-specific IgE. Flea-allergic pets may have immediate (15 minute), late phase (6 hour) or delayed (24–48 hour) reactions or a combination (see above). There are varying reports on the percentage of animals with FAD that show immediate and delayed IDT reactions, but it has been shown that some 15–30% of patients with flea allergy will have delayed reactions only. The latter does not have a clearly observable urticarial wheal and may be demonstrable only by careful palpation or observation of localized erythema.

In vitro testing
As for IDT, the correlation of *in vitro* test results with a positive clinical response to flea control varies, depending on the study, the laboratory and the reagents used. The sensitivity and specificity of the test may be improved by the use of recombinant allergens. The test measures only antigen-specific IgE and does not document a DTH. Thus, as in the case of the immediate skin test reaction, the *in vitro* test will be negative in some 15–30% of patients with FAD.

Unfortunately, not all dogs or cats with immediate reactivity to flea antigen or positive *in vitro* reactivity to flea antigen, or both, will consistently show signs of flea allergy when bitten by or infested with fleas. Therefore, neither a positive immediate skin test, nor a positive *in vitro* test, nor both, is sufficient for definitive proof that the clinical signs noted are due to this reactivity. Regardless of *in vitro* or *in vivo* test results, fleas, when present or suspected of being present, should be eliminated first as a part of the initial therapy to determine their contribution to the clinical signs.

Response to therapy
Response to flea control alone is the best method of diagnosis. In order to make a conclusive diagnosis, the veterinary surgeon generally finds it quickest to use a rapid-acting and long-lasting flea adulticide and observe the patient for improvement of signs.

Therapeutics and management

Elimination of the flea
The veterinary surgeon needs to manage cases of flea allergy dermatitis quite differently from that of simple flea infestation (Figure 19.7). In general, successful treatment of FAD will only occur if the veterinary surgeon takes an aggressive approach to eliminating the on-pet flea population as quickly as possible. This is usually accomplished with a product that kills biting fleas quickly on the flea-allergic pet. All susceptible pets in the household of the flea-allergic pet should be treated. It is important not only to treat the allergic animal and other pets, but also to develop an individualized strategy based upon consideration of the indoor and outdoor environment, the lifestyle of the pets, and the physical and financial capabilities of the owners.

1 Assess situation
- FAD pets
- Other pets
- Environment
- Owner's abilities

2 Custom design best plan
- Rapid flea eradication
- Long-term control

3 Reassess FAD pet(s)
- Assess clinical response
- If incomplete response, consider:
  - Poor compliance
  - Inappropriate control programme
  - Concomitant skin disease
  - Wrong diagnosis

19.7 Flea control plan.

For longer-term success, most recent recommendations suggest using a flea adulticide together with an insect growth regulator (IGR) or insect development inhibitor (IDI), resulting in long-term effects on the flea life cycle, an approach known as 'integrated flea control'. This is an important attempt to minimize the development of flea resistance.

Delivery methods of antiparasitic agents
There are a wide variety of methods used to get the insecticidal compound to the flea. For on-pet use there are shampoos, rinses, collars, conditioners or lotions, powders, aerosols, foams, pump-sprays, tablets and spot-on formulations. Insecticides in some of these delivery methods may be encapsulated

in a variety of ways for slower release and entrapment in the hair coat of the animal. Among the spot-on products, there are numerous conflicting reports as to their residue and the ease of their removal by water or shampoo. Topical IGRs are usually not easily washed off.

Systemic agents may be given by mouth, by spot-on or by injection. In general, with the exception of the new product nitenpyram, these are not ideal for immediate results in flea-allergic animals. They are preferred for long-term management once the flea problem is controlled. In areas in which fleas are seasonal and all the household pets live in a contained environment, systemic or on-animal IGRs or IDIs may be sufficient if they are started well before the time of suspected flea emergence.

Environmental treatment needs have decreased but, when needed, the IGRs or IDIs do an excellent job.

Flea adulticides

A number of insecticidal compounds are available for killing the adult flea. This is important for the flea-allergic pet because the fewer fleas that bite the pet, the quicker the improvement and resolution of clinical signs. It is critical that in-contact animals, living conditions and the degree of environmental infestation be considered when dealing with a flea-allergic pet. Advantages and disadvantages of modern insecticidal compounds useful in flea control are given in Figure 19.8.

Some general concerns: Several issues arise when advantages and disadvantages of the newer flea products are discussed:

* Products applied topically may give owners with small children concerns regarding the close contact of their children with the on-animal chemical

Compound	Advantages	Disadvantages
Fipronil	Rapidly acting: kills 98–100% in 24 hours Available as a spray and spot-on Excellent clinical results Reports and history show high degree of safety Effective against ticks Not labelled for mites but appears to be effective against some Wicked on to hair from pilosebaceous units: resistant to removal	Doesn't prevent all flea bites Not a repellent Expense, especially as a spray for a large dog High quantity of alcohol in spray Label indicates use only every 30 days Vehicle can (rarely) cause local irritation On-animal chemical
Imidacloprid	Rapid flea kill ability: 98–100% in 24 hours Excellent clinical results Label permits weekly use Vehicle for coverage seems to be very effective	Expense, especially if needed weekly or biweekly May wash off after repeated swimming or bathing (controversial) Doesn't prevent all flea bites Not a repellent Vehicle can cause local irritation May not last 4 weeks in certain situations Ineffective against ticks On-animal chemical
Selamectin	Works against a wide range of parasites Label safety for young and pregnant animals Safe in ivermectin-sensitive breeds Good choice for FAD and sarcoptic mange suspects Ease of application for such multi-purpose use	Expense Takes up to 72 hours to kill fleas; not ideal for FAD pet May be paying for properties not needed Effective against only some ticks Both a systemic and topical (on-animal concerns) Vehicle can cause local irritation
Nitenpyram	Low toxicity to mammals Can be given daily No side effects and no contraindications Can be given to pregnant and nursing bitches Safe for puppies and kittens from 4 weeks of age or >1 kg in weight Fast speed of flea kill (90–98% in 4–6 hours) No residual pesticide Useful for boarding situations Short-acting: quick elimination from body Designed to be used with lufenuron when there are breakthrough fleas Only two sizes makes dosing easier Oral tablet that does not need to be given with a meal Can't be washed off	Systemic (metabolized in pet: some see this as an advantage) Very short-acting Doesn't work against ticks May need to give daily Fleas get hyperactive when dying: can be uncomfortable for pet Not anticipated to be used alone
Permethrin	Rapid activity Repellent properties Readily available Not inactivated by UV radiation Sprays and spot-ons May be useful initially on FAD dog	**TOXIC** to cats at higher concentrations Cats in direct contact with recently treated dogs may be at risk Owner can easily make error Toxicity or idiosyncratic reactions: no effective antidote Literature doesn't clearly define whether this compound is systemically absorbed

19.8 Advantages and disadvantages of a range of flea adulticides.

- Application methods are not ideal for some owners. Spraying can be difficult because large volumes are necessary, requiring many pumps be applied to a potentially uncooperative pet, and the discomfort to the owner of applying it or inhaling it may be objectionable. With the spot-on products each company provides a variety of sizes for dog and cats, which can be complicated for the owner with many pets. With the small tubes used for most spot-on applications, it is important that the liquid is applied to the animal's skin and not just placed on the haircoat and allowed to run down the side of the animal. Occasionally topical irritation, hair discoloration or alopecia can occur at the site of application. For the elderly owner, it can be difficult to squeeze all the liquid out of tiny containers
- Concern about environmental contamination is an issue for some individuals. Both fipronil and imidacloprid are also used as agricultural chemicals, often to treat seeds; some serious honey bee hive deaths have occurred in areas where sunflower seeds were treated with these chemicals. Recently the leaching of fipronil into water has killed crawfish. According to Material Safety Data Sheets (MSDSs) on both fipronil and imidacloprid, neither is safe in groundwater, lakes or ponds, both are highly toxic to bees and each has potential toxicity to fish and some birds. However, the quantity applied to pets is very minute in comparison with agricultural usage, and both compounds have been shown not to move significantly from the site of application.

Fipronil: Fipronil is a phenylpyrazole compound effective against both fleas and ticks. It acts as an antagonist at the insect GABA receptor (blocking chloride passage). Its neurotoxicity is selective, as the configuration of GABA receptors in mammals is different from that in insects. Fipronil is available in a 0.25% alcohol-based spray and as a 10% spot-on product for dogs and cats. The latter is also offered in combination with the IGR *S*-methoprene.

Imidacloprid: This is a chloronicotinyl nitroguanidine that binds to nicotinyl receptors on the postsynaptic portion of insect nerve cells, preventing acetylcholine from binding. Imidacloprid has a higher affinity for insect than vertebrate receptors; it kills insects and is relatively safe for mammals. It is available as a spot-on compound for both dogs and cats.

Selamectin: This is a semi-synthetic derivative of avermectin produced by bioengineering techniques and it is considered an endectocide due to activity against a wide range of internal and external parasites. It is a topical spot-on application and comes in a variety of sizes for dogs and cats. It is considered both a systemic and a topical agent because it is absorbed percutaneously and then distributed via the circulation back to the skin.

Nitenpyram: This product is a new generation of synthetic compounds derived from a family of drugs called neonicotinoids. It binds and inhibits specific nicotinic acetylcholine receptors.

Nitenpyram is not anticipated to be used alone for flea control. For the flea-allergic animal that has entered an area of heavy infestation, this drug may be very useful while treating other pets and the environment. It also can be used for pets entering and departing boarding kennels, veterinary facilities as well as other areas away from home. It is a fast-acting systemic insecticide with a short half-life and with virtually no mammalian toxicity and is administered in tablet form.

Pyrethrins/Pyrethroids: Natural pyrethrins, extracted from several species of the chrysanthemum, have immediate flea-killing effects via enzyme inhibition. They have little residual action and are quickly inactivated by ultraviolet light. They are often combined with synergistic chemicals, and may offer the advantage of safety on young animals or debilitated animals. In most countries, products containing pyrethrins are readily available over the counter for a variety of methods of application.

Synthetic pyrethroids, which are stable in ultraviolet light, act on sodium channels of insect nerve axons, resulting in insect excitement and then paralysis. There are many pyrethroid compounds (e.g. deltamethrin, fenvalerate, cypermethrin, permethrin, sumithrin). They have rapid flea adulticide activity and some offer repellant properties that make them useful for the flea-allergic pet entering an infested area. Permethrin is most readily available primarily as sprays (usually 2% and lower), and as spot-ons of concentrations 45% and higher, which are available over the counter in some countries, for use on dogs only.

Botanicals: Pyrethrins are botanical in derivation and, although synthetic, pyrethroids are also often included in discussions of 'natural' compounds. It is beyond the scope of this chapter to discuss all products that are used to kill fleas. There are other botanicals, such as rotenone from the root of the derris plant, which are occasionally used for killing fleas. There are many plant-derived products with various purported active ingredients that are used to kill fleas. Many of these are sold in health food stores or via the Internet as nutraceuticals without any testing for efficacy or safety. Great caution should be used with these products, as buyers have a false belief that if it is from a plant, it is safe. Some plant compounds do have wide ranges of safety but others are toxic at certain concentrations and beneficial at others. Malaleuca oil/tea tree oil, citrus extracts, and eucalyptus oil are examples of these types of compounds. In some countries, Neem tree extracts containing azadirachtin are being used for their 'natural pesticide capacity'. Additional information about many of these plant extracts, generally unsupported by science, can be located by searching the Internet. The extraction process and purification of many plants generally is not well standardized and may result in sudden adverse reactions to one 'batch' of product; idiosyncratic toxicities may be seen which may be attributable to the lack of regulation of these products. Even products such as garlic, given by some convinced that it is a repellent, can cause adverse effects in pets.

Organophosphates and carbamates: There still is a wide range of organophosphate and carbamate compounds available primarily for environmental application. In some countries there are still some on-animal products, some of which are systemically absorbed, containing these acetylcholinesterase inhibitors. Cats are more sensitive than dogs to the toxicity of organophosphates. The use of organophosphates is unjustified because of their toxicity to all mammals and their residual properties in the environment. Many countries have withdrawn the more potent organophosphates. It has been shown that years after indoor application there can still be airborne contamination with these chemicals. The availability of newer and safer products has almost eliminated their use, especially on animals, where their residual flea-killing properties were not that good and they were not that safe.

Insect growth regulators and insect development inhibitors

The availability of these agents represents a major breakthrough in flea control.

Insect growth regulators: Three IGRs are available on the world markets: fenoxycarb, methoprene and pyriproxifen. All are analogues of the insect juvenile hormone. A fall in juvenile hormone is what allows development of the pupal stage. IGRs thus prevent pupation. They are also ovicidal, and pyriproxifen has been shown to have some adulticide activity, which acts after contact with the flea rather than following ingestion (Meola *et al.*, 2000).

Although initially developed for environmental use, methoprene and pyriproxifen are available for on-animal use, either as collars or for systemic or topical application. In some countries, methoprene is available as an oral tablet. Fenoxycarb has limited availability and is generally used in the environment. Due to the ovicidal activity of IGRs, they can be highly effective in destroying eggs at the site where they are laid. The advantages and disadvantages of insect growth regulators are listed in Figure 19.9.

Insect development inhibitors: The compounds that affect the non-adult stages of the life cycle by other means than preventing pupation are termed IDIs. The most widely used of these is lufenuron, a benzylphenol urea compound, which is a chitin synthesis inhibitor. When fleas feed on blood containing appropriate concentrations, resulting larvae develop abnormal cuticles and are unable to moult to the next instar.

- Lufenuron (Figure 19.10) is available for oral use every 30 days in both dogs and cats, and for injectable use in cats every 6 months. Because of the lack of clinically important adulticide

Compound	Advantages	Disadvantages
Methoprene	Directly and indirectly ovicidal, embryocidal, larvicidal Does not wash off animal or floor with water Readily available over the counter in many forms Safe for cats Useful in combined products or with adulticides	Sensitive to UV radiation Can translocate or volatize and move away from application site
Pyriproxyfen	Ovicidal and larvicidal for fleas Not sensitive to UV radiation Long stability and potency, even outdoors Wide range of available products Safe in cats Not easily removed by bathing or grooming Can translocate to bedding	Concerns about long-term residual status: may affect beneficial insects?

19.9 Advantages and disadvantages of insect growth regulators.

Advantages	Systemic product, ease of administration Monthly only Works well for flea-allergic pet in CLOSED environment Can eliminate use of environmental pesticides Eliminates need for spraying, bathing, other topicals No residue on animal for in-contact people Safe for cats
Disadvantages	Can take up to 3 months to eliminate fleas when used alone Flea-allergic animals will continue to be bitten and show signs until life cycle is altered Animal can pick up fleas outside its environment Wild animals may maintain the life cycle, causing failure Must be given with food for adequate absorption

19.10 Advantages and disadvantages of lufenuron.

activity, it is generally used in combination with an agent that has such properties. It will in time eliminate the flea population from a controlled environment where further contamination is prevented. However, the rate of reduction in the population has been shown to be significantly slower than that achieved by the topical application of imidocloprid (Jacobs *et al.*, 1997)
- Cyromazine is an aminotriazine that also affects chitin development. Although it does not inhibit chitin synthesis, it does affect the physical features of the cuticular tissues, thus interfering with normal development (Bel *et al.*, 2000). Its precise mode of action is unknown. In some countries it is available as an oral systemic whose necessity for daily administration has precluded its widespread acceptance. It is available in the United Kingdom in a spray, with permethrin, for use in the home.

Strategies for environmental flea control

Properly applied environmental flea control has become less important with the advent of the newer potent adulticides and the availability of lufenuron. It is important to judge whether the inside or outside environment, or both, is likely to be a major problem. Close consideration of the environmental requirements for optimal survival and reproduction of the cat flea is required in order to determine this. In more temperate climates, although some contamination of the outside environment may occur, control strategies incorporating outside flea control are generally unnecessary. On the other hand, comfortable, modern-day indoor environments generally foster survival of all parts of the life cycle year round.

Control of the outside environment: In considering external environmental control, it is important to recall the preferred habitats of the flea. No stage of the life cycle will survive for significant periods in open areas, but sheltered shady areas, particularly those close to the house or kennels or with organic matter, are ideal sites.

Control can be achieved by a combination of a suitable adulticide with pyriproxifen (not methoprene, which is rapidly destroyed by ultraviolet light). One must be concerned, however, about the possible effects of such products on the more desirable forms of insect life. Organophosphates used to be very popular as adulticides for outdoor use but are now falling into disuse. Synthetic pyrethroids represent an alternative.

Control of the inside environment: Again, it is important to recall the preferred habitats. The various stages of the life cycle are not found on tile floors, or floors covered with linoleum, from which they are readily removed by routine cleaning. They will preferentially be found in carpets, especially thick carpets with deep pile, and in cracks of wooden floors. When in carpets, the larvae tend to burrow down to the base, making it more difficult to effect control.

- The value of effective vacuum cleaning must not be forgotten. It is necessary to remove the vacuum cleaner bag or empty the container immediately

- Another approach, equally environmentally friendly, is the use of light traps. Fleas are stimulated to jump when a light source is interrupted intermittently. They also move towards heat and light, with a green light being optimal. A number of commercial light traps are marketed in different parts of the world, some of which are very effective. These are most useful for monitoring the degree of infestation (see Symptomatic therapy, below)
- If it is decided that application of an IGR or an IDI, with or without an adulticide, is required, consideration must be given to the mode of application. Foggers are a popular approach, but it must be remembered that they will not be effective on areas underneath furniture. For this reason the use of hand-held applicators is preferred. IGRs have a long residual effect and application is required only once every 6–12 months. It must be remembered that the pupal stage of the flea is the most resistant to parasiticidal agents and that IGRs are not effective against pupae. Therefore, when a short-acting adulticide and an IGR are applied, it is not uncommon to find a significant reinfestation of adult fleas after 1–3 weeks. Further application of an adulticide may then be necessary
- Boric acid and its derivatives are effective and probably act on the larvae through desiccation. Properly applied, sodium polyborate is widely held to have indoor efficacy as an environmental control product for up to 1 year.

Symptomatic therapy

Symptomatic anti-pruritic therapy (Figure 19.11) was formerly an important part of the strategy for the management of FAD. However, the availability of the newer, potent ectoparasitic agents means that this is rarely necessary. There are those who maintain that symptomatic therapy should not be used, as a beneficial response may lead both owner and veterinary surgeon to conclude that the flea control programme has been successful and can be abandoned. If symptomatic therapy is employed, it must only be as part of an overall management programme, the cornerstone of which is individually tailored flea control.

Corticosteroids: These are highly effective in FAD, but should not be necessary for long-term use.

Non-steroidal anti-inflammatory agents: There are no published studies on the efficacy of other anti-inflammatory agents that are used for the control of canine atopic dermatitis in the therapy of FAD. One could predict that ciclosporin would be very effective but its use would rarely be justified in the control of a condition for which other options are available.

Shampoos: The value of shampoo therapy should not be overlooked and may be included as part of the therapeutic strategy. Although there may be a concern over their use following topical application of ectoparasitic agents, shampoos given 24 hours after

Type of drug	Drug	Recommended dose rate	Comments
Corticosteroids	Prednisone or prednisolone, oral	Dogs: 1 mg/kg bid for 3–5 days, then reduce Longer prescription should be alternate-day Cats: 2 mg/kg bid for 3–5 days, then reduce	
	Methylprednisolone acetate, injectable	Cats: 2–4 mg/kg every 30–60 days	
Non-steroidal	Antihistamines		Generally not effective for FAD pruritus
	Fatty acids		Very high doses required and takes too long for results
	Antibiotics	Follow recommendations for pyoderma	Helpful if secondary pyoderma
	Shampoo therapy and other topical anti-pruritics		

19.11 Symptomatic anti-inflammatory treatments.

application of fipronil do not reduce its effectiveness, as the agent is stored in the sebaceous glands and released over time. In the case of imidacloprid, this is debated and seems to be variable. The choice of shampoo is dependent upon the major properties required. If anti-pruritic activity is required, products containing colloidal oatmeal, proxamine or hydrocortisone may be employed. If there is significant secondary pyoderma, agents containing suitable antibacterial agents may be indicated. On the other hand, FAD is often accompanied by severe scaling, in which case antisebborhoeic agents such as coal tar, sulphur and salicylic acid or ammonium lactate may be indicated.

Other methods of flea control: DEET (*N*,*N*-diethyl-*m*-toluamide) and some citrus oils are used by some as flea repellents on host pets. Their efficacy *in vitro* does not warrant their use, considering idiosyncratic toxicities.

Flea combs can be useful to increase an owner's awareness of fleas, when used regularly. It is unlikely to be a sole means of flea control. Light traps can be useful, but are best for monitoring the degree of the problem rather than actually to eliminate fleas. Mechanical methods such as frequent vacuuming, especially in areas the pet frequents, help to remove the flea eggs and larvae, as does outdoor raking of debris and eliminating dark, warm, areas of humid ground where flea pupae may reside for months.

Summary

Once the diagnosis of flea allergy is made, the most effective means of treatment is to use a flea control programme that is individually tailored to provide optimum flea control for that patient. Although it would be easier to have only one product which would be consistently useful for all treatment, various environments, owners' needs, and the pet(s) themselves make it important to treat each case independently. However,

with the range of current products available, there is almost no reason for any flea-allergic pet to suffer from clinical signs.

References and further reading

Bel Y, Wiesner P and Kayser H (2000) Candidate target mechanisms of the growth inhibitor cyromazine: studies of phenylalanine hydroxylase, puparial amino acids, and dihydrofolate reductase in dipteran insects. *Archives of Insect Biochemistry and Physiology* **45,** 69–78

Carlotti DN and Jacobs DE (2000) Therapy, control and prevention of flea allergy dermatitis is dogs and cats. *Veterinary Dermatology* **11,** 83–98

Dean SR, Meola RW, Meola SM *et al.* (1998) Mode of action of lufenuron on larval cat fleas (Siphonaptera: Pulicidae). *Journal of Medical Entomology* **35,** 720–724

Dryden DW and Rust MK (1994) The cat flea: biology, ecology and control. *Veterinary Parasitology* **52,** 1–19

Halliwell REW (1990) Clinical and immunological aspects of allergic skin disease. In: *Advances in Veterinary Dermatology Vol 1,* ed. C Von Tscharner and REW Halliwell, pp. 106–111. Baillière Tindall, London

Halliwell REW, Preston JF and Nesbitt JG (1987) Aspects of the immunopathogenesis of flea allergy dermatitis in dogs. *Veterinary Immunology and Immunopathology* **17,** 483–494

Jacobs DE, Hutchinson MJ, Krieger KJ *et al.* (1996) A novel approach to flea control in cats using pyriproxifen. *Veterinary Record* **139,** 559–561

Jacobs DE, Hutchinson MJ, Fox MT *et al.* (1997) Comparison of flea control strategies using imidocloprid or lufenuron on cats in a controlled simulated home environment. *American Journal of Veterinary Research* **58,** 1260–1262

Klotz JH, Moss JI, Zhao R *et al.* (1994) Oral toxicity of boric acid and other boron compounds to immature fleas (Siphonaptera: Pulicidae). *Journal of Economic Entomology* **87,** 1534–1536

Marsella R (1999) Advances in flea control. *Veterinary Clinics of North America: Small Animal Practice* **29(6),** 1407–1424

McCall CA, Stedman KE, Orbus KR *et al.* (1998) Abstract #805 Experimental flea allergy dermatitis in laboratory beagles: a model for human atopic dermatitis. *Journal of Allergy and Clinical Immunology* **101,** S196

McDermott MJ, Weber E, Hunter S *et al.* (2000) Identification and cloning of a major cat flea salivary allergen (Cte f 1). *Molecular Immunology* **37,** 361–375

Meola R, Meier K, Dean S *et al.* (2000) Effect of pyriproxifen in the blood diet of cat fleas on adult survival, egg viability, and larval development. *Journal of Medical Entomology* **37,** 503–506

Rust MK and Dryden MW (1997) The biology, ecology, and management of the cat flea. *Annual Review of Entomology* **42,** 451–473

Scott DW, Miller WH and Griffin CE (2001*) Muller and Kirk's Small Animal Dermatology, 6th edn.* WB Saunders, Philadelphia

Willis EL (2000) Flea control as we enter the next century. *Veterinary Forum* May, 40–44

20

Sarcoptic mange, cheyletiellosis and trombiculosis

Cathy Curtis and Manon Paradis

Sarcoptic mange

Sarcoptic mange (also known as sarcoptic acariosis or scabies) is a non-seasonal, pruritic skin condition caused by infestation with the mite *Sarcoptes scabiei*. The disease affects many mammalian species and the variant *S. scabiei* var. *canis* occurs commonly in domesticated dogs. In contrast, there are relatively few reports of feline sarcoptic mange.

S. scabiei belongs to the Family Sarcoptidae and is a globose mite, 200–400 µm in length, with short legs. Studies in dogs and humans have demonstrated that mites applied to the skin can penetrate within 30 minutes and that they have a circadian rhythm of activity. Following infection the mites mate on the host's skin surface. The fertilized females burrow into the epidermis and tunnel through the outer layers at a rate of 2–3 mm per day, laying eggs at the turning points in their zig-zag course. The eggs hatch within a few days. After moulting through a six-legged larval and two eight-legged nymphal stages, they emerge on the skin surface as adults. The life cycle takes 14–21 days, depending on environmental conditions.

The mites are obligate parasites but can survive for limited periods away from the host. Females and nymphs appear more hardy than males and larvae, but all stages have been shown to be capable of surviving for 2–6 days at 20–25°C and as long as 19 days at 10°C and 97% relative humidity.

Feeding, oviposition and deposition of faeces within the skin expose the host to mite allergens which, in the majority of infested dogs, induce both humoral and cell-mediated immunological responses (Bornstein and Zakrisson, 1993; Arlian *et al.*, 1996). These defence mechanisms can lead to spontaneous resolution of the disease after a few months, but most dogs develop a moderate to intensely pruritic dermatosis that initially affects the pinnal margins, elbows, hocks and ventrum, and eventually progresses to involve the entire body surface.

Canine sarcoptic mange is highly contagious. Indirect infestation via fur or fomites has been reported, but the majority of mites are transmitted by direct contact with an infested dog or fox. *Sarcoptes scabiei* var. *canis* has been isolated from species other than domestic and wild canids and has been experimentally established on rabbits, guinea pigs, sheep, goats, calves, cats and humans. This lack of host specificity has therapeutic and public health implications. Theo-retically, all mammals in contact with an infested individual should be treated simultaneously to limit the opportunities for cross- and re-infestation, and an acaricide should also be applied to their environment (see below). Furthermore, owners should be informed that they could contract sarcoptic mange from their dog, although provided the animal is treated appropriately, the disease is usually self-limiting and only rarely establishes in human skin.

Clinical approach

The textbook account of sarcoptic mange describes an intensely pruritic, papulocrustous dermatosis affecting the periocular skin, pinnal margins, elbows and hocks, which may generalize with time (Figure 20.1). The disease can start anywhere, however; hence clinicians should be suspicious whenever they are presented with an isolated patch of pruritic, papular skin, especially if the owner comments that the affected area is gradually enlarging. Erythema, excoriations and traumatically induced alopecia are secondary phenomena. As the condition progresses heavy scaling may develop, particularly along the pinnal margins and at the points of the elbows and hocks. A positive pinnal–pedal scratch reflex may also be present and a recent study demonstrated that 82% of scabious dogs exhibit this reflex, compared with only 6.2% of dogs affected by other skin diseases (Mueller *et al.*, 2001).

Diagnosis

History

One of the most useful facets of the diagnostic approach to scabies is the history provided by the owner. Sarcoptic mange can affect dogs of any age or breed and there is no known sex predilection. The classic historical features are the sudden onset of intense pruritus in one or more localized areas that enlarge with time. Another clue lies in the distribution of the lesions which, in common with other infectious and ectoparasitic dermatoses, is frequently asymmetrical.

Microscopic examination

The definitive diagnosis of scabies relies on direct visualization of mature or immature mites and/or their eggs and faeces in skin scrapings, skin biopsy specimens or faecal samples. Of the three, skin scraping is practised most frequently, yet mite detection rates as low as 20% are quoted in some texts. To improve mite

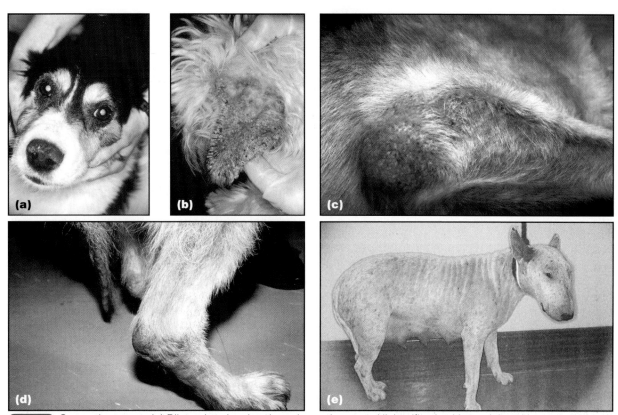

20.1 Sarcoptic mange: (a) Bilateral periocular alopecia, erythema and lichenification in an adult male crossbreed dog. (b) Left pinna of a male Lhasa Apso; note the marked degree of hyperkeratosis, particularly around the pinnal margin. (c) Elbow of an adult male German Shepherd Dog; note the hair loss and scaling. (d) Hocks of an adult male German Shepherd Dog. (e) Generalized sarcoptic mange in an English Bull Terrier bitch.

recovery, time should be taken to select the most appropriate lesions for sampling. Intact, encrusted papules at any site and/or areas of heavy scaling, particularly at the pinnal margins, elbows and hocks should be gently but firmly scraped using a size 10 scalpel blade dipped in liquid paraffin. *Sarcoptes* mites live in the epidermis and therefore the sampled area should exude a slight ooze from dermal capillaries at the end of the scraping procedure to ensure that the entire epidermis has been removed. The dislodged material is then suspended in a few drops of liquid paraffin on a microscope slide and trapped beneath a cover slip to facilitate examination and to prevent motile mites escaping from the slide. Once made, the preparation should be scanned as soon as possible at low power (X 40) and any areas of interest magnified at medium power (X 100) (Figure 20.2). Higher magnification is not usually necessary and can be counterproductive as it may distort the image of the mites.

Antibody detection

Serum samples from suspected cases can be submitted for circulating anti-*Sarcoptes* IgG detection by enzyme-linked immunosorbent assay (ELISA). This test was initially developed in Sweden in the early 1990s (Bornstein and Zakrisson, 1993) and is one of several that have since become commercially available to European veterinary surgeons as a diagnostic test for canine scabies. To the authors' knowledge, Bornstein and Zakrisson's assay is the only one which has been subjected to an independent

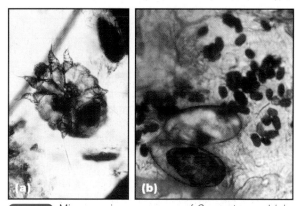

20.2 Microscopic appearance of *Sarcoptes scabiei*. (a) Adult mite in liquid paraffin (X100 original magnification). (b) Ova and faeces (scybala) in liquid paraffin (X400 original magnification).

blind controlled trial in which it performed fairly well, with sensitivity and specificity rates of 83% and 92%, respectively (Curtis, 2001). One of the controls in the study was a group of atopic dogs, all of which had negative results. Despite the fact that *Sarcoptes* and dust mites (e.g. *Dermatophagoides farinae*) share common antigens, it appears that atopic dogs sensitized to *D. farinae* do not develop circulating antibodies that interfere with the test. Conversely, dogs with scabies have been known to be sensitized temporarily to *D. farinae,* demonstrated by intradermal allergen testing (Prélaud and Guaguère, 1995), but the reason for this discrepancy is unclear.

Therapeutic trial

An alternative and commonly used diagnostic 'test' is a scabicidal therapeutic trial. Since modern acaricides are often capable of killing a range of different ectoparasite species, a favourable response to therapy is not absolute confirmation that the animal was affected by scabies. However, as the rapid alleviation of the patient's pruritus and malaise using appropriate medication is the principal aim of the attending clinician, trial acaricidal therapy is justified for any pruritic dog presenting with historical and clinical features suggestive of sarcoptic mange.

Management and therapeutics

Topical therapy

Traditionally, the most commonly used agents have been topical 'sponge-on' formulations containing monoamine oxidase inhibitors (e.g. amitraz; licensed in Europe, Canada and Australia) or organophosphates (e.g. phosmet), which need to be applied weekly or fortnightly, respectively, until clinical cure is achieved. In North America, a 2.5% lime sulphur dip is also available and is applied weekly. This has the advantage of a wider safety margin in small animals, but its foul odour and potential for staining light-coloured coats and jewellery make it unpopular with some owners. A 0.25% fipronil solution, applied by pump spray at 3 ml/kg on three occasions at 3-weekly intervals, has been used to control an outbreak of scabies in a litter of puppies (Curtis, 1996) and has also been used successfully as a sponge-on in adult dogs when applied once weekly for 2 weeks at 6 ml/kg (Bordeau and Hubert, 2000). In the authors' opinion, fipronil's main indications are early infestations or for those individuals in which the use of more potent products is contraindicated (e.g. puppies less than 12 weeks of age and pregnant or nursing bitches).

Dogs undergoing topical therapy with the products described should be treated in a well ventilated room or, ideally, outdoors. Owners of diabetic pets and those affected by diabetes mellitus themselves should be warned that amitraz can induce transient hyperglycaemia in addition to its potential sedatory and bradycardic effects. Amitraz is contraindicated in Chihuahuas. To improve acaricidal skin contact, clipping is recommended for dogs with long and/or dense coats.

Systemic therapy

Given the tedious nature of topical treatment, particularly when a number of dogs are involved, systemic therapy is an attractive alternative and several systemic macrocyclic lactones (ivermectin, milbemycin oxime, moxidectin and selamectin) have been used successfully for the control of canine sarcoptic mange. With the exception of selamectin, these drugs are not licensed for this purpose and owner consent should be obtained prior to their 'off-label' use.

Ivermectin: Ivermectin can be administered by subcutaneous injection, orally or topically as a pour-on. It should not be used in collies and sheepdogs or their crosses as it can affect the central nervous system, causing ataxia, tremors, mydriasis, salivation, depression and even coma and death. Initial experimental reports in other breeds indicated that a single dose of 200 µg/kg s.c. was effective; however, a course of treatment is preferable as this ensures that larvae emerging from the relatively resistant ova are also killed. A more reliable regimen would therefore be the administration of 200–400 µg/kg every 7 days orally, or every 14 days s.c. for 4–6 weeks (Paradis, 1998). For convenience and when large numbers of animals are involved, the pour-on formulation may be a useful and economical alternative (Paradis *et al.*, 1997).

Milbemycin oxime: Several trials involving oral milbemycin oxime as an alternative treatment for canine sarcoptic mange have recently been conducted. Using a dosing regimen of 2 mg/kg every 7 days on three to five occasions, success rates ranging from 71 to 100% have been reported (Miller *et al.*, 1996; Shipstone *et al.*, 1997; Bergvall, 1998). Another anecdotal study claims a 98% success rate with 1 mg/kg administered every 2 days on eight occasions (Christensson, 1999). Although more expensive than ivermectin, milbemycin oxime is fairly well tolerated in collies and related breeds and is therefore a safer alternative therapy in high-risk breeds; however, some collies have been found to be sensitive to higher dosages, so accurate drug dosing is essential. The drug is principally marketed as a canine heartworm prophylactic and is therefore not available worldwide.

Moxidectin: There is one anecdotal report describing the off-label use of moxidectin in canine sarcoptic mange in which 12 dogs treated with a dose of 250 µg/kg s.c. every 7 days on three occasions were cured (Wendelberger and Wagner, 1998). However, when administered orally at 400 µg/kg every 3–4 days, it may take 3–6 weeks to eradicate the mites (J. Fontaine, pers. comm.).

Selamectin: Selamectin is a novel avermectin and its spot-on formulation is the only systemic treatment licensed for the control of canine sarcoptic acariosis. Its ease of application and apparent safety in collies and related breeds make it a very appealing product . Field studies conducted by the manufacturers reported comparable efficacy rates to a reference positive-control product when the drug was applied at 6–12 mg/kg on two occasions, 30 days apart (Six *et al.*, 2000). However, the authors and other dermatologists have anecdotally reported a small number of treatment failures when using the drug according to the manufacturer's recommendations and are concerned by the potential misinterpretation of a poor response to a therapeutic trial. Consequently, many are advocating that selamectin be used primarily in confirmed cases and that it be reapplied every 2–3 weeks on at least three occasions, provided that owners are made aware of, and consent to, this extra-label use of the drug.

Contact animals and the environment

Whichever scabicidal therapeutic regimen is prescribed, all dogs known to have been in recent contact with the affected animal should be treated concurrently and grooming equipment, bedding and the domestic environment should be treated with an appropriate acaricidal spray (e.g. permethrin) to prevent possible reinfestation from these sources. Attempts should be made to limit socialization and mixing with other dogs and foxes, and persistently affected humans should consult their doctor to assess whether they themselves require scabicidal therapy. Dogs with unconfirmed scabies that fail to respond to acaricidal therapy should be reassessed and their diagnostic approach re-evaluated, as atopic dermatitis, flea bite hypersensitivity, adverse food reaction, *Malassezia* dermatitis, contact dermatitis, cheyletiellosis and otoacariosis are all major differential diagnoses.

Cheyletiellosis

Cheyletiellosis is typically a mild, albeit very contagious, dermatosis caused by mites living on the skin surface. Cheyletiellidae are relatively large (500 x 350 µm) white 'fiddle-shaped' acari with legs that protrude beyond their body margins and terminate in hair-like setae. Their most distinctive feature is a pair of crescent-shaped hooks on the accessory mouthparts (Figure 20.3). They feed on tissue fluid and lymph obtained by piercing the epidermis with a style-like chelicera and form 'pseudo-tunnels' in the scale generated in response to their activity. Following mating, adult females lay eggs which they bind to hairs with a silken thread (Figure 20.4); when shed, these hairs can also act as an environmental reservoir of infection. When the ova hatch, larvae emerge and undergo three ecdyses through two nymphal stages before emerging as adults, a process taking approximately 3–4 weeks.

The mites are obligate parasites but in addition to direct transmission, infestation may occur indirectly via fomites, such as leashes or grooming tools, or via other, larger ectoparasites such as fleas, lice and flies. *Cheyletiella yasguri* is the species most frequently isolated from dogs and *C. blakei* and

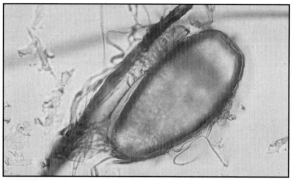

20.4 *Cheyletiella* sp. ovum in liquid paraffin (X400 original magnification). Note the thread attaching the egg to the hair.

C. parasitovorax are most commonly associated with cats and rabbits, respectively, but the Cheyletiellidae are not believed to be host-specific and may readily transfer between hosts of different species. Humans in contact with pets carrying *Cheyletiella* sp. are at risk of becoming transiently infested, producing an uncomfortable, pruritic dermatosis characterized by papular lesions which appear on the arms (Figure 20.5a), legs, trunk (Figure 20.5b), buttocks and, rarely, the face. However, as *Cheyletiella* are not capable of reproducing on humans, appropriate treatment of the pet host should prevent further infestation, making human acaricidal therapy unnecessary. Given this lack of host specificity and the fact that the mites are capable of surviving away from the host for at least 10 days in suitable environmental conditions, it is imperative that all in-contact pet mammals, their paraphernalia and the environment be included in the treatment programme.

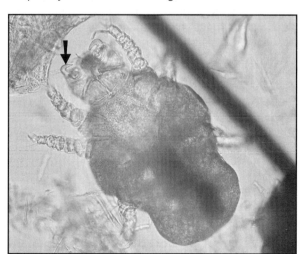

20.3 *Cheyletiella* sp. mite harvested from a canine skin scraping, suspended in liquid paraffin (X100 original magnification). Note the distinctive crescent-shaped hooks on the accessory mouthparts (arrowed).

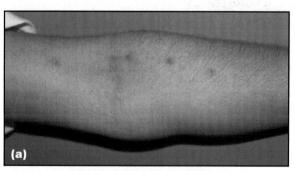

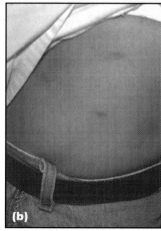

20.5 Papules on the (a) forearm and (b) trunk in a human case of cheyletiellosis.

Clinical approach

Cheyletiellosis is primarily a dorsally distributed disease characterized by mild erythema and excessive scaling (Figure 20.6). In cats, papulocrustous lesions may also develop, thus cheyletiellosis is a differential diagnosis for feline 'miliary' dermatitis. In dogs, infestation may lead to pyotraumatic dermatitis so 'hot spot' cases with concurrent dorsal or truncal dry seborrhoea should be screened for the mite. Pruritus is variable, ranging from absent to moderately severe, and young animals usually exhibit more obvious clinical signs than adults. An asymptomatic carrier status also exists and this should be borne in mind when tackling problem cases in which repeated reinfestation and zoonotic transmission is occurring.

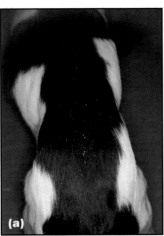

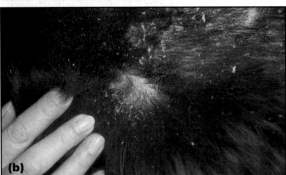

20.6 Canine cheyletiellosis. (a) Dorsal scaling in an adult Springer Spaniel. (b) Severe scaling and erythema in an adult Newfoundland.

Diagnosis

Direct observation

In cases where the history and clinical signs are suggestive of cheyletiellosis, the simplest diagnostic test is to sit or stand the animal on a dark surface and, using the hand, a brush or a flea comb, to dislodge some of the scale from the skin surface. On closer inspection, the scale may appear motile as a result of mite activity, this being the origin of the disease's alternative name: 'Walking dandruff'.

Microscopic examination

More accurate methods of diagnosis involve harvesting mites and eggs by adhesive acetate tape preparations, skin scrapings and faecal flotation. The former involves applying the sticky surface of a piece of acetate tape repeatedly along the dorsum of a scurfy animal, applying it directly to the surface of a glass slide and then examining it microscopically for evidence of mature and immature mites and their eggs. To improve detection rates, care must be taken to sample the skin surface and not just the distal ends of the hairs which may not harbour many mites/ova. Superficial skin scrapings can help to overcome this problem. Scale or, in the case of cats with miliary dermatitis, crusts should be removed using a size 10 scalpel blade and then suspended in liquid paraffin on a microscope slide beneath a cover slip. As mentioned above, the slide should then be scanned at low power and any areas of interest examined at medium power. Faecal flotation, although not performed very frequently, may be particularly useful for the detection of ingested mite and ova in cats due to their grooming habits (Figure 20.7).

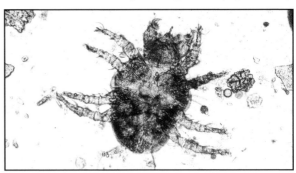

20.7 Mature *Cheyletiella* sp. mite isolated from a canine faecal specimen (x 100 original magnification).

Therapeutic trials

Despite being present in large numbers in the majority of cases, it should be remembered that *Cheyletiella* can sometimes be difficult to detect. In two separate studies investigators failed to recover mites in 15% of infested dogs and 58% of infested cats (Paradis and Villeneuve, 1988; Paradis *et al.*, 1990). Therapeutic trials with reliable acaricides are therefore indicated in suspected cases but ironically, for reasons explained above, they can only definitively rule out, as opposed to confirm, a tentative diagnosis.

Management and therapeutics

There are currently no veterinary licensed products specifically indicated for the treatment of cheyletiellosis. The infested dog or cat should be re-examined and monitored throughout the treatment period to screen for residual mites and eggs. Treatment should continue for a few weeks beyond clinical cure, until multiple tape strippings and superficial skin scrapings fail to reveal any microscopic evidence of ectoparasites.

Topical therapy

The mites are susceptible to several of the insecticidal/acaricidal formulations available. Weekly application of lime–sulphur dips, pyrethroid sprays or shampoos or amitraz solution, in conjunction with regular treatment of the environment, is effective. Care should be exercised when using pyrethroids or amitraz in cats as they are particularly sensitive to these drugs. Alternative options are two applications of a 0.25% fipronil spray, one month apart (Chadwick, 1997) and weekly bathing with a 1.0% selenium sulphide shampoo on three occasions.

Systemic therapy

Ivermectin: Animals that resent or do not tolerate topical therapy can be treated systemically with oral or injectable ivermectin at 200–300 µg/kg at 7 (orally) to 14 (s.c.) day intervals for 6–8 weeks (Paradis, 1998), provided the associated risks of adverse reaction are considered and the owner gives informed consent (see above). Another recent study reported the successful use of a 0.5% alcohol-based pour-on ivermectin formulation when applied to the withers of cats (Pagé *et al.*, 2000). The drug was well tolerated but a few animals developed a transient alopecic patch and mild scaling at the site of application and it should be remembered that kittens are more susceptible to the toxic effects of this drug compared to adult cats with rare reports of lethargy, ataxia, coma and even death occurring within 1–12 hours of administration.

Selamectin: This may provide a safer alternative to ivermectin. The results of a recent open pilot study in which it was applied to infested cats at monthly intervals on three occasions were promising (Chailleux and Paradis, in press).

Milbemycin oxime: In dogs, milbemycin oxime has been shown to be effective in the control of cheyletiellosis when given orally at weekly intervals at 2 mg/kg (White *et al.*, 2001), although the fact that some animals required up to nine treatments to control the mites may make the relatively high cost of this drug prohibitive. The use of milbemycin oxime in the control of feline cheyletiellosis has not been reported.

Contact animals and the environment
When compiling a treatment programme, the infested animal's bedding and grooming equipment should be treated with an acaricide or discarded to prevent fomite-mediated reinfestation. Washable fabrics should be cleaned at temperatures of at least 55°C and then sprayed along with the rest of the environment with a pyrethroid-containing product. As mentioned above, all in-contact mammals should be treated concurrently with a suitable acaricide.

Trombiculosis

Of the several hundred different species of Trombiculidae (chigger) mites that have been recognized, only a handful cause disease in man and animals. *Neotrombicula autumnalis* (harvest mite, berry bug) and *Eutrombicula alfreddugesi* (North American chigger) are the most familiar pathogenic mites in Europe and North America, respectively. Only the larval stages are parasitic to mammals, the remainder of the life cycle being completed in the environment, with the nymphal and adult stages feeding on vegetable matter. Canine and feline (and occasionally human) infestations are therefore seasonal, with the majority of cases occurring between June/July and November, although one British veterinary surgeon recently reported an atypical feline *Trombicula* larval infestation in January

(White, 2001). The other chiggers reported to cause skin disease in small animals are *Walchia americana*, which was isolated from a domestic cat in North America (Lowenstine *et al.*, 1979) and *Leptotrombidium subquadratum* (Heyne *et al.*, 2001), which has recently been described as an annual cause of canine and human pruritus and dermatitis in South Africa, during the southern hemisphere's summer months. Again, it is only the larval forms of these mites that are believed to be parasitic to mammals.

Clinical approach
All Trombiculidae cause papular to papulocrustous lesions at their feeding sites, which tend to be concentrated interdigitally (Figure 20.8) or along the ventral abdomen. *Eutrombicula* and *Neotrombicula* larvae, which appear as red–orange 'specks', can also affect the ears and have a particular preference for the cutaneous marginal pouch or 'Henry's pocket' (Figure 20.9). Most infestations are asymptomatic, but some parasitized animals become extremely pruritic and in extreme cases, wheals can develop at the sites of mite attachment.

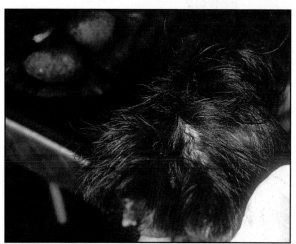

20.8 Left forefoot of a mature male Giant Schnauzer, showing the presence of multiple *Neotrombicula autumnalis* larvae in the fourth interdigital space.

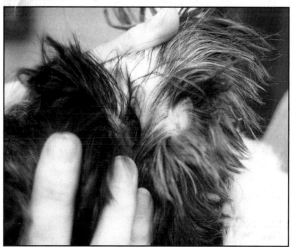

20.9 Left ear of a mature, female Shih Tzu showing the presence of an accumulation of orange-red *Neotrombicula autumnalis* larvae in the cutaneous marginal pouch ('Henry's pocket').

Diagnosis

Whenever trombiculosis is suspected, direct examination of the coat and particularly the predilection sites is warranted, as the mites are visible to the naked eye. If mites remain undetected, suspicious lesions should be scraped or even biopsied as the host's immune reaction to the mite may wall-off or 'encyst' them (Bourdeau *et al.*, 2000), making them detectable only by deep scrapings (Figure 20.10) or histopathological examination.

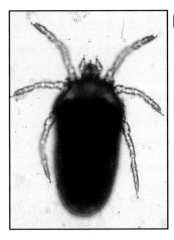

20.10

A 6-legged *Neotrombicula autumnalis* larva suspended in liquid paraffin (x 100 original magnification).

Management and therapeutics

There are currently no licensed acaricides for the treatment of trombiculosis but a variety of ectoparasiticidal dips, sprays and even otic preparations are known to be effective. Products possessing a short residual action will need to be reapplied regularly as reinfestation will occur if the dog or cat is allowed continued access to the environmental source of larval mites. A recent study demonstrated that monthly applications of a 0.25% fipronil spray controlled trombiculids in 15 of 18 dogs, with 2 of the remaining 3 dogs requiring additional, localized treatment every two weeks for repeated pedal infestations and the third dog failing to respond (Nuttall *et al.*, 1998). In the same study, three cats became reinfested within 10 days of treatment, suggesting a shorter residual action in this species. One of the authors (CC) recommends weekly spraying of the predilection sites (i.e. pinnae, ventrum and feet) with a 0.25% fipronil spray during the summer months. When the mites cause moderate to severe pruritus, intermittent, short courses of oral corticosteroids should also be prescribed to alleviate the host's discomfort.

References and further reading

Arlian LG, Morgan MS, Rapp CM *et al.* (1996) The development of protective immunity in canine scabies. *Veterinary Parasitology* **62**, 133–142

Bergvall KE (1998) Clinical efficacy of milbemycin oxime in the treatment of canine scabies: a study of 56 cases. *Veterinary Dermatology* **9**, 231–233

Bourdeau P, Degorce-Rubiales F, Breton C *et al.* (2000) Newly recognised manifestation of trombiculosis with epithelial encystment in 12 dogs. *Veterinary Dermatology* **11** (Suppl. 1), 26

Bordeau W and Hubert B (2000) Treatment of 36 cases of canine *Sarcoptes* using a 0.25% fipronil solution. *Veterinary Dermatology*, **11** (Suppl. 1), 27

Bornstein S and Zakrisson G (1993) Humoral antibody response to experimental *Sarcoptes scabiei* var. *vulpes* infection in the dog. *Veterinary Dermatology* **4**, 107–110

Chadwick AJ (1997) Use of a 0.25 per cent fipronil pump spray formulation to treat canine cheyletiellosis. *Journal of Small Animal Practice* **38**, 261–262

Chailleux N and Paradis M (in press) Efficacy of selamectin in the treatment of naturally acquired cheyletiellosis in cats. *Canadian Veterinary Journal*

Christensson DA (1999) Milbemycin oxime for treatment of infection with *Sarcoptes scabiei* in the dog. *Proceedings of the 16th annual congress of the ESVD/ECVD, Helsinki, Finland*. p. 153

Curtis CF (1996) Use of 0.25 per cent fipronil spray to treat sarcoptic mange in a litter of five-week-old puppies. *Veterinary Record* **139**, 43–44

Curtis CF (2001) Evaluation of a commercially available enzyme-linked immunosorbent assay for the diagnosis of canine sarcoptic mange. *Veterinary Record* **148**, 238–239

Heyne H, Ueckermann EA and Coetzee L (2001) First report of a parasitic mite, *Leptotrombidium subquadratum* (Acari: Trombiculidae: Trombiculinae), from dogs and children in the Bloemfontein area, South Africa. *Journal of the South African Veterinary Association* **72**, 105–106

Lowenstine LJ, Carpenter JL and O'Connor BM (1979) Trombiculosis in a cat. *Journal of the American Medical Association* **175**, 289–292

Miller WH Jr, de Jaham C, Scott DW *et al.* (1996) Treatment of canine scabies with milbemycin oxime. *Canadian Veterinary Journal* **37**, 219–221

Mueller RS, Bettenay SV and Shipstone M (2001) Value of the pinnal–pedal scratch reflex in the diagnosis of canine scabies. *Veterinary Record* **148**, 621–623

Nuttall TJ, French HC, Cheetham HC *et al.* (1998) Treatment of *Trombicula autumnalis* infestation in dogs and cats with a 0.25 per cent fipronil pump spray. *Journal of Small Animal Practice* **39**, 237–239

Pagé N, de Jaham C and Paradis M (2000) Observations on topical ivermectin in the treatment of otoacariosis, cheyletiellosis, and toxocariosis in cats. *Canadian Veterinary Journal* **41**, 773–776

Paradis M (1998) Ivermectin in small animal dermatology. Part II. Extralabel applications. *Compendium on Continuing Education for the Practicing Veterinarian* **20**, 459–469

Paradis M, de Jaham C and Pagé N (1997) Topical (pour-on) ivermectin in the treatment of canine scabies. *Canadian Veterinary Journal* **38**, 379–381

Paradis M, Scott DW and Villeneuve A (1990) Efficacy of ivermectin against *Cheyletiella blakei* infestation in cats. *Journal of the American Animal Hospital Association* **26**, 125–128

Paradis M and Villeneuve A (1988) Efficacy of ivermectin against *Cheyletiella yasguri* infestation in dogs. *Canadian Veterinary Journal* **29**, 633–635

Prélaud P and Guaguère E (1995) Sensitisation to the house dust mite *Dermatophagoides farinae*, in dogs with sarcoptic mange. *Veterinary Dermatology* **6**, 205–209

Shipstone M, Mueller R and Bettenay S (1997) Milbemycin oxime as a treatment for canine scabies. *Australian Veterinary Practice* **27**, 170–173

Six RH, Clemence RG, Thomas CA *et al.* (2000) Efficacy and safety of selamectin against *Sarcoptes scabiei* on dogs and *Otodectes cynotis* on dogs and cats presented as veterinary patients. *Veterinary Parasitology* **91**, 291–309

Wendelberger U and Wagner R (1998) Moxidectin an alternative to ivermectin? *Proceedings of the 15th annual congress of the ESVD/ECVD, Maastricht, Netherlands September 2–5*, 149–151

White W (2001) Early *Trombicula autumnalis* infection (letter to editor). *Veterinary Record* **148**, 188

White S, Rosychuck R and Fieseler K (2001) Clinicopathological findings, sensitivity to house dust mites and efficacy of milbemycin oxime treatment of dogs with *Cheyletiella* sp. infestation. *Veterinary Dermatology* **12**, 13–18

21

Demodicosis

Mark Craig

Canine demodicosis

Canine demodicosis is a skin disorder associated with higher than normal populations of demodicid mites. *Demodex canis,* a slender mite with short stubby legs and a long tapering abdomen, is host-specific and apparently a normal inhabitant of canine skin. It lives mainly within hair follicles (rarely in sebaceous glands) and feeds on cells, sebum and epidermal debris. Adult mites measure 250–300 μm x 40 μm (Figure 21.1). Both a shorter (90–148 μm long) and a longer (334–368 μm long) demodicid mite have been found in some dogs. These represent either separate species, previously unrecognized, or mutant/aberrant forms of *Demodex canis.* The short variety is believed to live only on the skin surface whereas the longer mite has been found in pilosebaceous units.

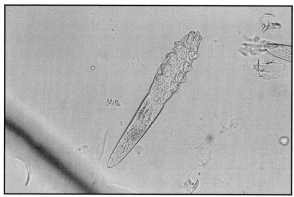

21.1 Adult *Demodex canis* from a skin scraping. (X125 original magnification.)

Predisposing factors

Pure breeds of dog appear to be more susceptible to demodicosis than crossbreeds. One North American study found a predisposition to generalized demodicosis in the following breeds: Shar Pei, West Highland White Terrier, Scottish Terrier, English Bulldog, Boston Terrier, Great Dane, Weimaraner, Airedale Terrier, and Afghan Hound. However, there may be geographical variation in breed susceptibility.

The tendency to develop demodicosis appears to be hereditary, and limited data suggest an autosomal recessive mode of transmission. Not breeding from clinical cases, or any of their siblings and parents, has been found to reduce or even eliminate the incidence of the disease in some lines.

Life cycle

The entire life cycle is spent on the skin. From lemon-shaped eggs (Figure 21.2), hatch larvae (six legs) which moult first into nymphs (eight legs) and subsequently into adults (eight legs).

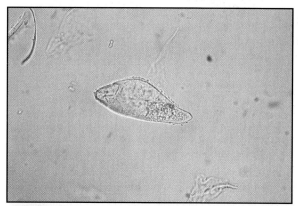

21.2 *Demodex canis* egg from a skin scraping. (X300 original magnification.)

Transmission

The only means of mite transfer appears to be from bitch to sucking puppy by direct contact during the first few days of the pup's life. Mites have been found in hair follicles from 16 hours after birth, appearing first on the muzzle. Mites are not found on stillborn puppies nor on puppies born by Caesarean section and reared away from the bitch (Scott *et al.,* 1974). There is no evidence of horizontal spread between older dogs.

Pathogenesis

It is unknown why, if the mite is a normal inhabitant of canine skin and hair follicles, it should cause skin disease in some dogs and not others. It has been suggested that virulence may vary with the strain of mite. However, within a litter of puppies exposed presumably to the same strain of mite, some individuals may have severe clinical disease whilst others remain asymptomatic.

The discovery that clinical demodicosis could be induced by giving dogs antilymphocyte serum led to the theory that the condition might be linked to immunodeficiency. Further evidence for this comes from adult dogs developing demodicosis in association with severe neoplastic or metabolic disorders, or when treated with immunosuppressive drugs. However, if puppies with generalized demodicosis were severely immunocompromised they would be expected to develop widespread systemic infections and this does not happen. Equally, most adults with debilitating diseases or given immunosuppressive drugs do not develop demodicosis.

Some studies have demonstrated immunosuppression. Initially, this was thought to be induced by the mites themselves although later studies suggested that immunosuppression was a consequence of pyoderma (a common complication of demodicosis). More recent work has shown that the immune system of dogs with demodicosis becomes more compromised with both greater populations of mites and pyoderma. However, immunological abnormalities persist following resolution of demodicosis and pyoderma, and immunosuppression is not a precondition for the development of clinical demodicosis.

A hereditary, *D. canis*-specific, T-lymphocyte defect of varying severity may be involved (Scott *et al.*, 2001). Changes in hormone levels may also encourage mite proliferation: clinical demodicosis frequently develops around 6–9 months of age, a time when many puppies are becoming sexually mature.

Clinical features

Canine demodicosis is seen mostly in pure-bred dogs under 1 year of age. It may be localized or generalized. When feet are involved, the condition is known as pododemodicosis.

Localized demodicosis

Localized demodicosis develops typically at 3–6 months of age. It is a mild disease, resolving spontaneously in 90% of cases, usually within 6–8 weeks, although lesions may wax and wane for months. Hair loss and erythema are often the presenting signs and owners may see patches of red, scaly skin (Figure 21.3), which tend not to be itchy. The face, especially around the eyes and mouth, is the most common site affected, followed by the forelegs. Hindlegs, trunk and ears are less frequently involved. Rarely, the condition may be restricted to the ear canals, producing a ceruminous, sometimes pruritic, otitis externa. It is very unusual for localized demodicosis to become generalized.

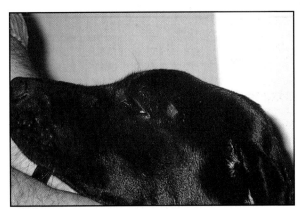

21.3 Focal alopecia above the left eye of a 5-month-old male Labrador Retriever with localized demodicosis.

Generalized demodicosis

The generalized form of the disease usually starts in the first 18 months of a puppy's life (juvenile-onset). Occasionally, it occurs *de novo* in older dogs (adult-onset). There is no universally recognized standard as to what constitutes 'generalized'. It has been suggested that fewer than six lesions indicate localized disease and 12 or more lesions indicate the generalized condition, but each patient clearly needs to be assessed individually (Scott *et al.*, 2001).

Juvenile-onset: Typical age of onset is between 3 and 18 months. Multiple poorly circumscribed areas of erythema, scaling, crusting, hair loss and hyperpigmented skin may be seen initially (Figure 21.4). Secondary pyoderma (usually associated with staphylococcal infection; less commonly *Pseudomonas* and *Proteus*) is common and leads to oedema, exudation and thick crust formation. Otitis externa may be present. Some dogs have nodules and other atypical lesions. English Bulldogs are reported to be predisposed to demodectic nodule development. Lesions are not normally itchy in the absence of pyoderma. Dogs are frequently depressed and may have peripheral lymphadenopathy. In dogs under 1-year old, generalized demodicosis resolves spontaneously in more than 50% of cases.

Adult-onset: This rare form of the disease occurs in dogs aged 4 years or more with no prior history of demodicosis. It follows a reduction in the dog's resistance to the mites, which have previously been tolerated and kept in check by a healthy immune system. The condition is often associated with systemic disease (e.g. neoplasia (Figure 21.5), Cushing's disease, hypothyroidism) or treatment with immunosuppressive drugs. Where associated with an internal disorder, demodicosis may be diagnosed before signs of that disorder are detectable. Atopic dogs with a long history of steroid therapy may sometimes develop adult-onset demodicosis.

Clinical signs are similar to those of juvenile-onset demodicosis. Severity is variable and the prognosis poor, particularly in cases where the underlying disorder cannot be corrected.

In a recent retrospective study (Renvier and Guillot, 2000) involving 28 dogs with adult-onset demodicosis, 18 dogs (64%) had pustular skin lesions and 10 (36%) had scaling lesions. Chronic glucocorticoid therapy was the most commonly identified predisposing factor (16 dogs) followed by hypothyroidism (4), neoplasia (3) and autoimmune disease (2). Pododemodicosis was seen in 5 dogs (18%).

Pododemodicosis

A dog's paws may form part of a generalized presentation or they may be the only region affected (Figure 21.6). Pedal lesions are particularly susceptible to secondary pyoderma and can be so painful as to cause severe lameness. Pododemodicosis can be very resistant to therapy, especially if lesions are infected with *Pseudomonas*. Old English Sheepdogs seem to be more prone than other breeds.

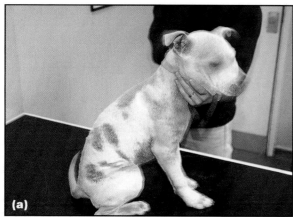

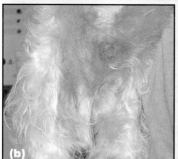
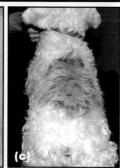

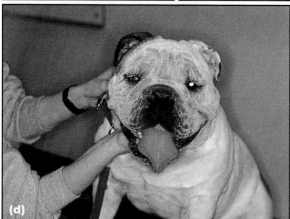

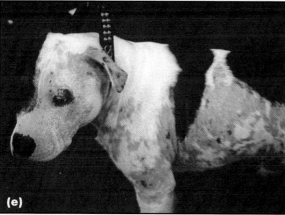

21.4 Generalized demodicosis of juvenile onset. (a) An 8-week-old female Pit Bull Terrier. (b) Ventral erythema in a 9-month-old neutered male Sealyham Terrier. (c) Dorsal alopecia and hyperpigmentation in a 17-month-old entire male Sealyham Terrier. (d) A 9-month-old entire male English Bulldog. (e) Erythema and diffuse alopecia in a one-year-old entire male Staffordshire Bull Terrier.

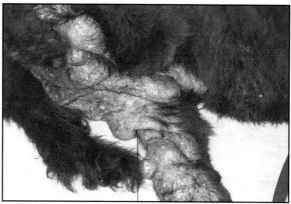

21.5 Generalized demodicosis of adult onset in an 11-year-old neutered male Newfoundland with neoplasia.

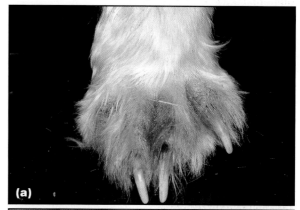

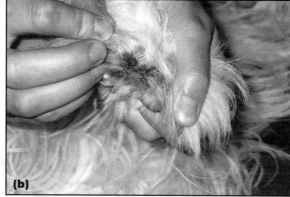

21.6 Pododemodicosis. (a) Erythema, crusting, alopecia and hyperpigmentation in a 17-month-old entire male Sealyham Terrier. (b) Interdigital erythema, exudation, crusting and hyperpigmentation in a Bearded Collie cross with pododemodicosis and *Pseudomonas* infection.

Diagnosis

A consideration of the history and clinical signs is important but to confirm the diagnosis, mites must be found. The most useful procedure for demonstrating demodicid mites is the deep skin scraping (see Chapter 3). Affected skin should be squeezed firmly to extrude mites from hair follicles. Hair plucks are also very useful, especially from areas that are difficult to scrape such as feet and face. Finding one adult mite may not be significant but if many adults or immature stages (eggs, larvae or nymphs) are found, the disease is confirmed. If in doubt, more scrapings from several parts of the body should be taken. In some cases, particularly with pedal lesions, skin biopsy specimens should be submitted for histopathology before the condition can be ruled out.

Differential diagnosis includes dermatophytosis, bacterial folliculitis and pemphigus foliaceus.

In adult-onset demodicosis, an underlying condition should always be sought through:

- Full haematology and biochemical profiles
- Thyroid evaluation (e.g. T4, TSH)
- Adrenal evaluation (e.g. dexamethasone suppression test)
- Chest and abdominal radiographs
- Urinalysis
- Heartworm serology (in countries where it is prevalent).

However, an underlying disorder may sometimes only become apparent months or even years later.

Treatment

The golden rule is always to avoid steroids no matter how tempting it is to use them. They may suppress an already compromised immune system and are contraindicated in all forms of demodicosis. In adult-onset demodicosis, response to any therapy may be incomplete unless predisposing factors have been addressed.

Localized demodicosis

The condition in most young dogs does not require specific acaricidal treatment because of the likelihood of spontaneous resolution. Therapy may be completely unnecessary but washing with benzoyl peroxide, ethyl lactate or chlorhexidine shampoos can be helpful. Glucocorticoids may further suppress a compromised immune system and can lead to the condition becoming generalized. They should be avoided.

In the USA, rotenone ointment and shampoo are licensed for treatment of localized disease.

Generalized demodicosis (including pododemodicosis)

Although the condition in many young dogs may resolve spontaneously, cases of generalized demodicosis should be treated with a suitable acaricidal product. Every effort should be made to ensure that dogs with generalized demodicosis are in optimal general health. A good diet should be given and suitable worming procedures performed regularly.

Owners should be advised to have their bitches spayed. There are two reasons for this: a bitch with a history of generalized demodicosis should not be used for breeding; and intact females may relapse or the disease become refractory to treatment when the bitch is in season. Entire male dogs should be castrated to prevent breeding.

In adult-onset demodicosis, any underlying systemic condition should be corrected if possible.

All forms of glucocorticoids should be avoided to prevent further immune system suppression. Immunostimulants such as vitamin E and levamisole have not been found to improve the cure rate of generalized demodicosis.

Treatment of generalized demodicosis can be particularly troublesome in dogs with concurrent allergic skin disease for whom only glucocorticoids provide relief. Euthanasia is sometimes indicated for dogs that fail to improve with available treatments.

Amitraz: This is the only product licensed for treating canine demodicosis in the UK and is the treatment of choice. A 0.05% aqueous solution of amitraz (500 ppm) is applied, all over, at an initial frequency of once weekly. This strength of solution is obtained by diluting 50 ml amitraz into 5 litres of water.

In the USA amitraz is licensed for use as an 0.025% solution (250 ppm) to be applied every other week.

Although frequency of application can often be reduced to every 2 weeks once the condition appears to be under control clinically, therapy should be continued until at least 1 month after scrapings have repeatedly failed to show any stages of mite, dead or alive. As an aid to monitoring the effects of therapy, skin scrapings and hair plucks should be carried out every 2–4 weeks.

Dogs with medium or long coats should be clipped to allow the solution better skin contact and greater penetration into hair follicles. Before amitraz is applied, dogs should ideally be washed to aid removal of scale, crust and exudate. For this purpose, one of the shampoos recommended above for treating localized demodicosis can be used. These shampoos may also exert antibacterial and follicular flushing activity. Appropriate systemic antibiotics are always indicated when pyoderma is present.

Amitraz should not be used in dogs suffering from heat stress, in pregnant or lactating bitches, or in puppies less than 3 months old. In Chihuahuas, amitraz has been associated with a small number of deaths for which no cause could be determined, and use of amitraz in this breed is therefore contraindicated. There are no contraindications in other small or toy breeds. Some dogs show transient erythema, sedation or vomiting following amitraz application. Lethargy and vomiting are less likely to occur if dogs are prevented from licking themselves until the product has dried.

Side effects are likely to resolve spontaneously within 24–48 hours but atipamezole has been found to reverse the sedative effects of amitraz. In some countries, yohimbine (unavailable in the UK) is used to counteract amitraz toxicity.

Amitraz is a monoamine oxidase inhibitor (MAOI) and adverse reactions have been reported in dogs and people taking other MAOIs (e.g. certain antihistamines, antidepressants and antihypertensive agents) following application of amitraz to the dog. Nausea and dizziness may occur following inhalation. Amitraz can induce hyperglycaemia and should not be used in diabetic dogs nor applied in the presence of diabetic people. In order to minimize the risk of toxicity and systemic absorption, amitraz should not be used on dogs with severe deep pyoderma lesions. It should also be avoided in dogs under, or recently given, a general anaesthetic, because of the possibility of drug interaction.

Ivermectin: Ivermectin is effective in some dogs but this product is unlicensed for any use in dogs in the UK (it is licensed in the USA as a heartworm prophylactic). Idiosyncratic toxicity reactions including ataxia, behavioural changes, tremor, mydriasis, weakness, apparent blindness, hypersalivation, depression, coma and death have been reported. It should always be avoided in Rough Collies, Shetland Sheepdogs, Old English Sheepdogs, other collie-like herding dogs, and their crosses. Its use should be limited to cases where, for whatever reason, amitraz is ineffective or poorly tolerated, and the dog is in need of treatment. The dosage most commonly recommended is 400–600 µg/kg/day orally, although those who use the drug regularly often give a small 'test dose' initially (100 µg/kg/day). The dose can be increased gradually, provided there are no adverse reactions. Owners of a few dogs treated with ivermectin by the author have reported wobbliness and vagueness. Treatment in each case was stopped immediately and problems resolved within 24 hours. Treatment should otherwise be continued for about 3–6 months, or for 1–2 months after scrapings fail repeatedly to demonstrate any mites or eggs. Great care is needed when using ivermectin in dogs and it is essential to obtain informed consent from owners before starting therapy.

Milbemycin: Milbemycin is similar in its activity to ivermectin but appears to be safer, producing (when given at 1–2 mg/kg) none of the adverse reactions associated with the latter, even in ivermectin-sensitive breeds. Milbemycin is expensive, unlicensed for use in the dog in the UK, and can only be obtained in the UK by import under licence. However, for dogs that either cannot tolerate, or do not benefit from, amitraz and ivermectin, the product can be invaluable. For generalized demodicosis, a dosage of 0.5–2 mg/kg once daily, orally, is recommended. Combination products containing lufenuron are not recommended for treating demodicosis.

Moxidectin: Moxidectin was reported to be effective in one study (Wagner and Wendlberger, 2000) involving 22 dogs with generalized demodicosis. Seventy-two per cent of dogs given moxidectin at a dose of 0.4 mg/kg/day orally were cured (mean duration of therapy 2.4 months), although treatment was stopped in 14% of cases because of side effects. Good efficacy and no side effects were reported in another study (Bensignor and Carlotti, 1996) involving eight dogs with generalized demodicosis. Like ivermectin and milbemycin, moxidectin is unlicensed for use in the dog in the UK. Case selection is important and owner consent should always be obtained.

Selamectin: There are currently no data available on the efficacy of selamectin in canine demodicosis. The use of selamectin for treating canine demodicosis is not recommended.

Lufenuron: Lufenuron is a widely used flea control agent which prevents chitin synthesis. Its role as a potential therapy for generalized demodicosis has been investigated (Schwassmann *et al.*, 1997). At mean dosages ranging from 13.3–19.3 mg/kg/day, orally, no efficacy was demonstrated in 11 adult dogs with either juvenile-onset or adult-onset demodicosis, despite high levels of the drug in the skin.

Feline demodicosis

Demodicosis is much less common in cats than in dogs. It may be more common in Siamese and Burmese cats. It is caused by excessive numbers of either or both of two species of demodicid mite: *Demodex cati* and *Demodex gatoi*. *D. cati* lives in pilosebaceous units and closely resembles *D. canis*, although its eggs are slim and ovoid rather than lemon-shaped. *D. gatoi*, a shorter mite with a broad abdomen, lives only in the superficial epidermis. This mite is considered to be contagious. The life cycle and mode of transmission are not well understood for either species.

The prognosis is better for the 'juvenile form' (occurring in cats under 3 years of age) than for the 'adult form' (seen in cats over 5 years), where an underlying disease is often present.

Clinical features

Demodex cati
Localized and generalized disease have been reported. The head and neck are the main areas affected with limbs (Figure 21.7) and trunk occasionally involved. Pruritus is variable but typically absent. Erythema, papules, pustules, localized diffuse or symmetrical alopecia, scaling, crusting, erosions, ulcerations (Figure 21.8), comedones and hyperpigmentation may be seen. Otitis externa, with a dark brown waxy discharge, has been described both in cats with normal skin and also in those with generalized demodicosis. Generalized disease is usually associated with underlying disease: hyperadrenocorticism, feline immunodeficiency virus or feline leukaemia virus infection, diabetes mellitus or squamous cell carcinoma *in situ*. A particular clinical form involving a greasy facial discharge has been reported in the Persian.

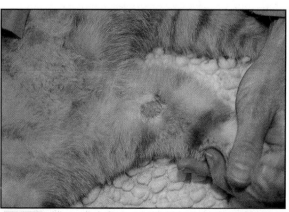

21.7 Ulcerated plaque on the hindleg of a cat with demodicosis (*D. gatoi*). (Courtesy of AP Foster.)

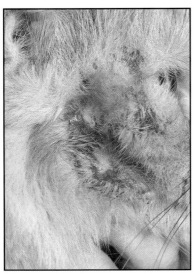

21.8

Erythema, excoriation and ulceration on the face of an aged Domestic Shorthair with demodicosis (*D. cati*). (Courtesy of AP Foster.)

Demodex gatoi

Clinical signs are similar to those described for *D. cati,* but pruritus is a more common feature. Two clinical syndromes have been described:

- Severe pruritus with lesions affecting head, neck and elbows
- Ventral pruritus, erythema and alopecia.

Symmetrical alopecia is occasionally the only presenting sign. It appears to be contagious in some reports.

Diagnosis

Diagnosis is based on history and clinical signs and confirmed by finding mites on deep skin scrapings, hair pluckings or skin biopsies. Histologically, *D. cati* is found in hair follicles whereas *D. gatoi* is found only in the stratum corneum. Differential diagnoses are listed in Figure 21.9.

Dermatophytosis
Flea allergy
Atopy
Adverse food reaction
Cheyletiellosis
Bacterial folliculitis
Pediculosis
Pemphigus foliaceus
Contact dermatitis
Feline scabies
Psychogenic alopecia

21.9 Differential diagnoses for feline demodicosis.

The possibility of underlying disease should be investigated, especially in generalized cases, through:

- Full haematology and biochemical profiles
- Tests for feline leukaemia virus and feline immunodeficiency virus
- Adrenal evaluation (e.g. dexamethasone suppression test)
- Chest and abdominal radiographs
- Urinalysis.

Treatment

Treatment of generalized demodicosis in the cat is often unrewarding. Over half the cases involving *D. cati* have serious underlying disease. Controlling the latter may be more important than killing mites. Feline demodicosis (both localized and generalized) may resolve spontaneously although this would appear to be the exception rather than the rule. There is no licensed product available for treating feline demodicosis. In the USA the treatment of choice for *D. gatoi* is lime–sulphur.

Amitraz

A 0.0125–0.025% solution of amitraz (125–250 parts per million) can be used every 5 days for 4–6 weeks. This solution is obtained by diluting 25–50 ml of amitraz in 10 litres of water (1:200–1:400 dilution); the amount of product will need to be varied in line with the formulation. At this range of concentration, amitraz is usually effective and well tolerated by cats. However, amitraz is unlicensed for use in the cat and the manufacturer does not recommend its use in this species. Possible adverse reactions include sedation, excessive salivation, anorexia, depression and diarrhoea.

Systemic endectocides

Both ivermectin (0.3 mg/kg orally) and milbemycin (dose not determined) have been recommended.

References and further reading

Bensignor E and Carlotti DN (1996) Moxidectine in the treatment of generalised demodicosis in dogs: a pilot study: 8 cases. In: *Advances in Veterinary Dermatology 3,* ed. K Kwochka *et al.,* pp. 554–555. Butterworth Heinemann, Oxford

Guaguère E (2000) Ectoparasitic skin diseases. *A Practical Guide to Feline Dermatology,* ed. E Guaguère and P Prélaud, p. 3.8, Merial, Lyon

Kwochka KW (1993) Demodicosis. *Current Veterinary Therapy,* ed. CE Griffin *et al.,* pp 72–84. Mosby Year Book, St Louis

Renvier C and Guillot J (2000) Adult-onset demodicosis in dogs: a retrospective study of 28 cases. *Veterinary Dermatology* **11,** 49

Schwassman M, Kunkle G, Hepler DI *et al.* (1997) Use of lufenuron for treatment of generalised demodicosis in dogs. *Veterinary Dermatology* **8,** 11–17

Scott DW, Farrow BRH and Schultz RD (1974) Studies on the therapeutic and immunological aspects of generalised demodectic mange in the dog. *Journal of the American Animal Hospital Association* **10,** 233–243

Scott DW, Miller MH and Griffin CE (2001) Parasitic skin diseases. In: *Muller and Kirk's Small Animal Dermatology,* 6th edn, pp. 457–476. WB Saunders, Philadelphia

Wagner R and Wendlberger U (2000) Field efficacy of moxidectin in dogs and rabbits naturally infested with *Sarcoptes* spp., *Demodex* spp. and *Psoroptes* spp. mites. *Veterinary Parasitology* **93,** 149–158

22

Staphylococcal pyoderma

Chiara Noli

Aetiology and pathogenesis

Ninety per cent of canine pyodermas are caused by *Staphylococcus intermedius*, a Gram-positive, beta-haemolytic, coagulase-producing bacterium. Other coagulase-positive and -negative staphylococci (e.g. *S. aureus*, *S. epidermidis*) and other Gram-positive and -negative bacteria (e.g. *Pseudomonas aeruginosa, Proteus* spp.*, Escherichia coli*) may be isolated occasionally. In cats *S. aureus* and *S. intermedius* are considered the main causes of pyoderma, excluding abscesses.

S. intermedius is a normal resident of canine mucous membranes and is able to colonize the skin temporarily without causing skin disease. Two bacterial populations may exist, one with pilosebaceous localization, which may occasionally colonize the skin, and a second one with mucosal localization, which may be transferred to the hair shafts by grooming and licking (Harvey and Lloyd, 1994). In a case of pyoderma these bacteria are allowed to multiply excessively on the skin surface and become pathogenic.

Pathogenic staphylococci are able to produce a variety of enzymes and toxins, whose function is not yet fully understood. Of these the best known are: toxin TSS-1 (Toxic Shock Syndrome-1 produced by *S. aureus*), responsible for the toxic shock syndrome in humans; protein A (produced by *S. aureus* and *S. intermedius*), which is able to bind the Fc portion of immunoglobulins with potent pro-inflammatory effects; the enzyme coagulase (produced by *S. aureus, S. intermedius, S. hyicus*), which allows the deposition of fibrin on the bacterial cells inhibiting their recognition by phagocytic cells; and beta-lactamase, responsible for resistance against non-protected penicillins.

No difference has been found between the array of toxins and proteolytic enzymes of *S. intermedius* isolated from healthy animals and from animals with pyoderma, but a difference in virulence has been observed. One of the most important virulence factors is adherence to host tissues. An increased adherence to extracellular matrix proteins has been observed in pathogenic staphylococci compared to those isolated from healthy dogs (McEwan, 2000).

While pyoderma is very rarely seen in cats (generally associated with systemic disease or self-inflicted lesions), in dogs it is probably the most commonly recognized skin disease. In the dog pyoderma develops each time the cutaneous balance and protective mechanisms (Figure 22.1) are disturbed. Several predisposing factors (Figure 22.2) have been recognized.

- Horny layer and its constant desquamation: eliminates surface microorganisms
- Surface hydrolipid film (from sebaceous and apocrine glands), intercellular lipids between the corneocytes and in the follicular ostia:
  - nutrients for resident microorganisms
  - inhibit pathogenic bacteria and yeasts (Ihrke *et al.*, 1978)
- Resident and transient cutaneous microflora (bacteria and yeasts):
  - inhibit multiplication of transient and pathogenic microrganisms by competing for nutritional factors and development niches

22.1 Protective mechanisms of healthy skin against penetration of pathogenic microorganisms.

Dogs

- Allergic and pruritic parasitic diseases:
  - damage to the protective epidermal barrier leads to entrance of bacteria and penetration of staphylococcal toxins, favouring the development of the infection
  - increased adhesion of bacteria to corneocytes in allergic dogs (McEwan, 2000)
  - steroidal treatment may decrease immune surveillance and favour bacterial infections
- Moisture and high temperature, especially in skin folds and dogs with a long, thick coat
- Seborrhoea, excessive skin dryness and other keratinization disorders: alterations of the horny layer or hydrolipid film, favouring bacterial skin infection
- Follicular obstructions due to demodicosis, dermatophytosis or keratinization disorders
- Hormonal imbalance: for example, hypothyroidism, hyperadrenocorticism
- Immune suppression: due to congenital, acquired or iatrogenic disease

Cats

- Severe systemic diseases: viral infections (FIV, FeLV), diabetes mellitus, hyperadrenocorticism
- Pruritus and bacterial contamination/infection of self-inflicted lesions: eosinophilic plaques, ulcerated eosinophilic granulomas, excoriations on head and neck

22.2 Factors predisposing to pyoderma.

Primary pyoderma

A pyogenic bacterial skin infection with no underlying cause is called primary pyoderma. It is not clear whether this condition is dependent on a higher bacterial virulence or on an increased host susceptibility. The dog has some anatomical characteristics that make it more susceptible than other species to pyoderma: the horny layer is very thin; the intercellular spaces are filled by lower amounts of hydrolipid film; and the follicular ostia are devoid of this protective emulsion (Mason and Lloyd, 1993). German Shepherd Dog pyoderma is a deep primary infection in which abnormalities of cell-mediated immunity have been identified. Short-haired dogs are predisposed to superficial bacterial folliculitis, with no apparent underlying cause. In these dogs staphylococcal populations have been isolated from lesional and non-lesional skin, as well as from mucous membranes (Saijonmaa-Koulumies and Lloyd, 1995).

Clinical approach

Predisposing factors
Several breeds are predisposed to different types of pyoderma or to possible underlying causes. Age is an important factor to be considered: impetigo is seen in puppies, idiopathic folliculitis of short-haired breeds in young adults, and German Shepherd Dog pyoderma in dogs older than 4–5 years. There is no gender predisposition to developing pyoderma, with the exception of vulvar skin fold pyoderma in females or where there is a gender predisposition for underlying causes (i.e. endocrinopathy due to testicular tumour).

History
Taking a proper history is essential in order to understand what underlying disease is predisposing the animal to skin infection. For example, pruritus on the extremities, muzzle and ears in a 2-year-old dog with folliculitis may suggest an underlying atopic dermatitis; polyuria, polyphagia and polydipsia in an old Poodle with a thin skin and superficial spreading pyoderma suggests an underlying hyperadrenocorticism. However, if presented with a pruritic dog with bacterial skin infection, it should be remembered that pyoderma itself is an important cause of pruritus, and that the predisposing disease may be a non-pruritic illness. In this case, it is preferable to treat with antibiotics first, in order to eliminate cutaneous signs and pruritus due to pyoderma, and re-evaluate the dog subsequently.

Clinical examination
After collecting data regarding predisposing factors and history, a thorough general and dermatological examination should be performed. The skin lesions should readily suggest a bacterial infection and its type (surface, superficial or deep; Figure 22.3). Further diagnostic investigations (cytological examination of exudates, culture and sensitivity tests etc.) confirm the diagnosis of pyoderma. Other diagnostic tools (e.g. skin scrapings, fungal cultures, antibiotic trial) are used to identify a possible underlying cause.

Surface pyodermas
Limited to the surface of the stratum corneum Skin fold infection (intertrigo) Pyotraumatic dermatitis (hot spots)

Superficial pyodermas
Infundibular portion of hair follicles and epidermis Impetigo Bacterial folliculitis Superficial spreading pyoderma Mucocutaneous pyoderma

Deep pyodermas
Whole hair follicle, dermis and occasionally subcutis Chin pyoderma (acne) Pododermatitis and interdigital granuloma Callus pyoderma Lick granuloma

22.3 Classification of pyoderma.

Erythema, superficial exudation, erosions without pustules and collarettes

Intertrigo: This is the cutaneous infection of skin folds, typically on the muzzle in brachycephalic breeds (Figure 22.4) and Shar-Peis, around the tail base in Bulldogs, around the vulva in obese females, in the interdigital skin, axillae and groin. In cats, it may be observed in the facial folds of Persians. The skin in the depth of the folds is pruritic, erythematous, humid and may harbour a whitish, greasy exudate, which, at cytological examination, contains large amounts of extracellular bacteria, corneocytes and few neutrophils.

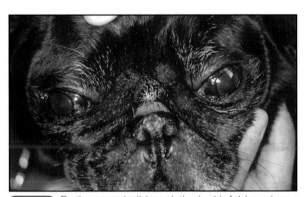

22.4 Erythema and mild exudation in skin fold pyoderma (intertrigo). (Courtesy of F. Scarampella.)

Pyotraumatic dermatitis: This is the superficial exudative and highly pruritic infection of lesions caused by chewing or scratching (Figure 22.5). These lesions are frequently associated with flea bite allergy in dogs and located on the posterior parts of the body. Other causes may be excessive skin humidity, poor ventilation and poor grooming, mostly seen in thick-coated dogs. Clinically an area of sparsely haired, humid skin and coat is observed, with mild localized cutaneous erosions. Pyotraumatic dermatitis may evolve to a superficial folliculitis, in which case satellite papules and pustules may be seen, and the lesion appears

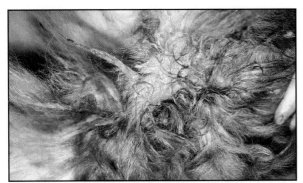

22.5 Alopecia, erosion and exudation in pyotraumatic pyoderma ('hot spot').

thicker and crusted. In cats bacterial infection may be a complication of self-inflicted lesions, such as excoriations on the face and neck, eosinophilic plaque or ulcerated eosinophilic granuloma.

Bacterial overgrowth: Recently a condition called 'bacterial overgrowth' has been recognized in dogs, characterized by an excessive number of bacteria on cytological observation of impression smear samples from glabrous skin. This condition causes pruritus, desquamation and a foul odour, and is often associated with allergic or endocrine diseases. The cutaneous signs and pruritus disappear with antibiotic therapy or with antibacterial shampoos.

Canine mucocutaneous pyoderma: This is characterized by crusts and erosions on the lips (Figure 22.6), eyelids, vulva, praeputium and anus. It has been described primarily in German Shepherd Dogs but may be seen in other breeds. Lesions usually heal completely with antibiotics, allowing a differentiation from autoimmune and metabolic diseases with mucocutaneous involvement.

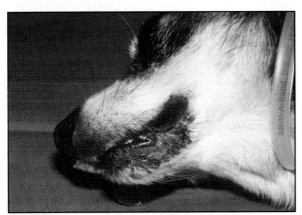

22.6 Perioral erosions, ulcerations and crusts in mucocutaneous pyoderma in a German Shepherd Dog cross.

Papules, pustules, collarettes and focal alopecia

Impetigo: Impetigo is a pustular disease that usually occurs on the abdominal skin in puppies, and rarely kittens, particularly if infested by endoparasites, badly managed or affected by viral diseases (e.g. distemper). Pustules are small and non-follicular (no hair shaft is seen in the centre of the pustule).

Bacterial folliculitis: This is the most frequent form of canine pyoderma, and is characterized by papules, follicular pustules, collarettes and patchy alopecia (Figure 22.7). This form of pyoderma is a frequent complication of allergies, ectoparasitic and endocrine diseases. An idiopathic primary bacterial folliculitis is also observed in short-haired dogs. Bacterial folliculitis has rarely been observed in cats.

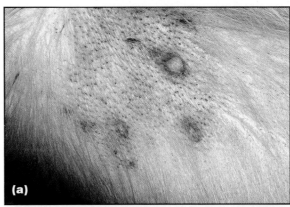
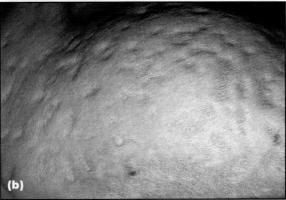

22.7 Bacterial folliculitis. (a) Pustules – the primary lesion. (b) The patchy alopecia 'moth-eaten coat' characteristic of short-haired breeds.

Superficial spreading pyoderma: This is characterized by the absence of pustules and the presence of large collarettes with an erythematous, mildly exudative leading edge of infection (Figure 22.8). This form of folliculitis is mostly seen on the trunk.

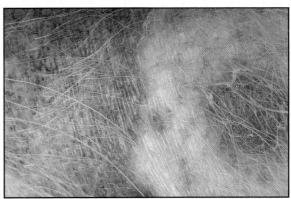

22.8 Large collarettes and an erythematous mildly exudative leading edge in superficial spreading pyoderma.

161

Deep furunculosis, haemorrhagic bullae, ulcerations, nodules and draining tracts

Deep pyoderma is characterized by ulcerative crusty lesions localized in the dermis and/or subcutis, tissue oedema and purulent to haemorrhagic exudation. Most of these infections occur in short-haired dogs and in pressure and friction areas, suggesting that mechanical trauma on hair roots may be one of the predisposing factors.

German Shepherd Dog pyoderma: This is an idiopathic deep pyoderma, with ulcerations and draining tracts on the lateral aspect of the thighs (Figure 22.9), on the trunk, on the groin and on the lips. Affected dogs are usually 5 years or older and often have a history of chronic skin disease (e.g. flea bite allergy). German Shepherd Dog pyoderma is probably a multifactorial disease associated with genetic predisposition, allergies (flea bite allergy, food allergy, atopic dermatitis), endocrinopathies (especially hypothyroidism), parasitic diseases (ehrlichiosis, leishmaniasis) and abnormalities of the cell-mediated immune system (Chabanne *et al.*, 1995; Denerolle *et al.*, 1998). However, no definitive aetiology has been determined and no definitive therapy has been identified that is able to cure this condition.

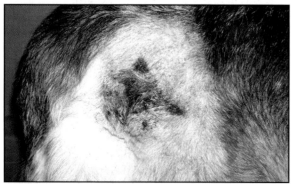

22.9 Furuncles, ulceration, draining tracts and crusts on the lateral thigh of a German Shepherd Dog.

Furunculosis: This is the result of hair follicle rupture and spillage of its content in the dermis, with surrounding pyogranulomatous or granulomatous inflammatory reaction. This can be the evolution or the complication of a bacterial folliculitis, demodicosis , dermatophytosis or follicular keratinization defect. Localized types of furunculosis are chin acne, mostly seen in short-haired breeds, interdigital pyogranulomas (Figure 22.10),

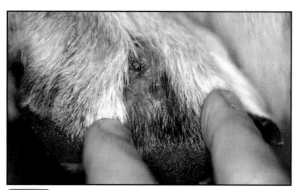

22.10 Interdigital pyogranuloma.

callus pyoderma and lick granulomas. In these conditions chronic trauma may play an important role in the development of hair follicle rupture and secondary bacterial infection.

In cats, chin acne is a keratinization disorder that leads to comedo formation. In some cases bacterial infection of abnormal hair infundibula may lead to folliculitis, furunculosis and haemorrhagic bullae.

Diagnosis

Differential diagnoses

The differential diagnoses for superficial and deep pyoderma are numerous (Figure 22.11). Furthermore, a bacterial infection secondary to these diseases is frequently seen, so that pyoderma and its differential diagnoses may coexist in the same lesions.

Condition	Differential diagnoses
Surface pyodermas	
Skin fold pyoderma (intertrigo)	None
Pyotraumatic pyoderma (hot spots)	None
Superficial pyodermas	
Bacterial folliculitis in short-haired breeds	Demodicosis Dermatophytosis
Mucocutaneous pyoderma	Autoimmune dermatoses Metabolic epidermal necrosis
Impetigo and bacterial folliculitis	Pemphigus foliaceus Sterile eosinophilic pustulosis Sterile pustular dermatitis Pustular leishmaniasis Pustular demodicosis
Superficial spreading pyoderma	Epitheliotropic lymphoma (mycosis fungoides) Dermatophytosis Adverse drug reactions (erythema multiforme or exfoliative eruptions)
Deep pyodermas	
Furunculosis	Deep fungal infections
Furunculosis on the nasal dorsum	Eosinophilic furunculosis
Abscesses and deep (nodular) pyogranulomas	Sterile nodular panniculitis Sterile pyogranulomatosis Tumoural or pseudotumoural diseases (histiocytosis)
Chin acne	Juvenile cellulitis Pyodemodicosis
Bacterial pododermatitis	Pododemodicosis Fungal pododermatitis Pemphigus foliaceus (especially in cats) Idiopathic and foreign body interdigital granulomas
Acral lick granulomas or callus pyoderma	Tumour nodules

22.11 Differential diagnoses for pyoderma.

Cytology

A sample for cytological examination may be obtained by impression smear from surface lesions, by fine needle aspiration from nodules, large pustules and bullae, or may be collected with a cotton swab, from draining tracts. Intracytoplasmic bacteria (Figure 22.12) (usually in neutrophils) confirm the diagnosis; extracellular bacteria may represent contamination. Neutrophils are degenerated and show a swollen nucleus with a low number of lobules. In superficial pyodermas large numbers of neutrophils and bacteria are seen, whereas in deep chronic infections there are variable numbers of neutrophils, macrophages, lymphocytes and plasma cells, and low numbers of bacteria.

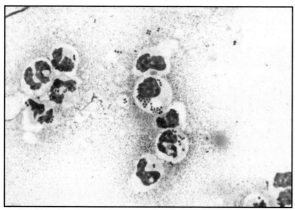

22.12 Intracellular cocci in degenerated neutrophils, diagnostic of pyoderma.

Bacterial culture and sensitivity test

A bacterial sensitivity test is advised in the following cases:

- When rods are observed on cytological examination, particularly if intracellularly in neutrophils, either alone, or in mixed infections with cocci. (The susceptibility of rods to antibiotics is unpredictable)

- When antibiotic therapy chosen empirically does not give the expected results
- When pyoderma has already been repeatedly treated and/or has frequent recurrences.

Chronically recurring cases should be thoroughly evaluated for underlying causes (Figure 22.13).

Management and therapeutics

Control of underlying causes

A satisfactory resolution of pyoderma comprises both the cure of the cutaneous signs and the prevention of recurrences. As most pyodermas are secondary infections, the identification and control of the underlying problem is mandatory for a good therapeutic success. If the underlying illness is not controlled, the pyoderma may recur after the antibiotics are interrupted. On the other hand, if the underlying cause is corrected, but the pyoderma is not treated, the bacterial infection may not heal on its own.

Systemic therapy

General principles of antibiotic therapy
While surface pyoderma may be treated with topical therapy alone, superficial and deep pyoderma require treatment with systemic antibiotics.

Choice of antibiotic: The ideal antibiotic:

- should have an antibacterial spectrum that includes *Staphylococcus intermedius*
- should reach the skin at high concentration
- should be bactericidal
- should have few or no side effects, even if used for long periods or at high dosage
- should be easy to administer, i.e orally, once or twice daily
- should not cause bacterial resistance, even if used in repeated courses of treatment
- should not be expensive, even for large breeds.

Clinical signs	Investigation	Potential underlying causes
Any superficial or deep pyoderma	Deep skin scrapings for *Demodex*	Demodicosis
Interdigital lesions	Microscopic examination of hair Fungal culture	Demodicosis Dermatophytosis
Patchy alopecia and scaling	Wood's lamp examination Collection of hair and scales for fungal cultures	Dermatophytosis
Deep lesions and draining tracts	Fungal culture Bacterial culture	Dermatophytosis Infection with 'atypical bacteria'
Pruritus	Treat the pyoderma first (and the concurrent *Malassezia* infection, if present); then re-evaluate the animal when the skin infection has cleared	Complete response and no skin lesions or pruritus left: • underlying systemic disease • idiopathic primary pyoderma Skin lesions are cured but pruritus persists: • allergic disease Skin lesions do not improve or improve only partially: • inadequate treatment • residual lesions due to underlying disease

22.13 Looking for an underlying cause for pyoderma.

Pharmacokinetics and pharmacodynamics: The drug distribution in the skin is a very important factor. Only 4% of the cardiac output reaches the subcutis and dermis, while the epidermis is not reached by any blood supply at all, and is nourished via diffusion from blood capillaries of the superficial dermis. In spite of the fact that the epidermis has no blood perfusion, in cases of superficial and deep pyoderma, systemic administration of antibiotics is always preferable to topical therapy alone, because of the strong barrier action offered by the stratum corneum.

The drug distribution within the tissues, i.e. intracellular *versus* extracellular, may also play an important role. In pyoderma the bacteria are located both extra- and intracellularly. Drugs that accumulate intracellularly include fluoroquinolones, lincosamides and macrolides. Some local factors, for example pus, necrotic debris and an acidic environment, may inhibit some drugs such as aminoglycosides, trimethoprim–sulphonamides (TMP/S), macrolides and lincosamides.

Spectrum and mode of action: In general, it is preferable to choose an antibiotic with a narrow antibacterial spectrum, as in cases requiring long-term therapy broad-spectrum antibiotics may disturb the intestinal microorganisms and cause diarrhoea. In reality this is not very common in the domestic carnivores. Narrow-spectrum antibiotics are erythromycin, lincomycin, clindamycin and beta-lactamase-resistant penicillins.

Either *bactericidal* or *bacteriostatic* antibiotics may be chosen in an animal whose immune system works normally. In animals with a compromised immune system, during immunosuppressive therapy, in deep or mixed (cocci/rods) infections, and in cases of frequent or maintenance antibiotic administration, it is important to use a bactericidal agent.

Duration and frequency of treatment: The duration of antibiotic treatment depends on the type of pyoderma and the response of the patient:

- For superficial pyoderma, the antibiotic should be administered for a minimum of 3 weeks including at least 7 days after the resolution of the clinical lesions
- In deep pyodermas, a treatment of at least 6 weeks is necessary, sometimes longer (12 weeks is not unusual), with not less than 2 weeks after clinical resolution.

The animal should be thoroughly examined by the veterinary surgeon before interruption of antibiotic therapy, particularly in cases of deep pyoderma, where the surface heals long before deeper tissues. Sometimes antibiotic therapy has to be continued until the underlying disease is controlled (e.g. atopic dermatitis or hyperadrenocorticism). This can lead to very long or repeated therapy courses, particularly in the case of hyposensitization of atopic dogs.

The frequency of administration depends on the mode of action of the antibiotic, i.e. whether it is time-dependent or concentration-dependent:

- Time-dependent agents, e.g. beta-lactamase antibiotics and all bacteriostatic drugs, work best if their concentration remains constantly above the minimum inhibitory concentration (MIC). They require administration every 8 or 12 hours
- Concentration-dependent drugs, e.g. fluoroquinolones, do not require a concentration constantly above the MIC because their efficacy is dependent on high pulse concentrations. They are better administered once daily.

Bacterial sensitivity and resistance: In the majority of cases the antibiotic may be chosen on an 'empirical' basis, i.e. without performing a bacterial culture and sensitivity test. If this test is performed, it is important to remember that the result *in vitro* does not always reflect the efficacy *in vivo*. Some drugs have low tissue distribution, or are inhibited by purulent exudates, by low pH, by organic debris, by foreign bodies (e.g. keratin in furunculosis) or by encapsulated infection foci.

Penicillin, amoxycillin and ampicillin are useless for staphylococcal pyoderma, because they are sensitive to beta-lactamase, which is produced by the majority of the isolates of *S. intermedius*.

Recently, methicillin-resistant (oxacillin-resistant) *S. aureus* (MRSA) and *S. intermedius* (MRSI) strains have been isolated (Piriz *et al.*, 1996; Gortel *et al.*, 1999). MRSA is responsible for nosocomial infections and affected dogs are usually owned by hospital employees or patients. Resistance to methicillin and oxacillin is usually associated with resistance to a wide variety of antibiotics, including those commonly used for treating canine pyoderma. Fluoroquinolones may be useful in the treatment of MRSI and vancomycin for MRSA.

Antibiotic choices for first-occurrence superficial pyoderma

Trimethoprim–sulphonamide: Trimethoprim–sulphonamide (TMP/S), at 15–30 mg/kg orally bid, is a good bactericidal drug for first-occurrence superficial pyodermas, but may not be effective in deep and strongly exudative infections, in the presence of pus and in acidic environments. Other products combined with sulphonamides are ormethoprim and baquiloprim. Resistance rates vary, depending on the country, from 1 to 50%. TMP/S is usually well tolerated by dogs and cats, though several cases of adverse reactions have been reported (Noli *et al.*, 1996), particularly in the Dobermann. The most frequent side effects in dogs are keratoconjunctivitis sicca and euthyroid sick syndrome.

Erythromycin: Erythromycin is a narrow-spectrum bacteriostatic macrolide with an excellent distribution in body tissues and cellular fluids. It is administered at 10–20 mg/kg orally every 8 hours, which may be a problem for working owners. It rapidly induces resistance in bacteria, with cross-resistance to lincomycin, thus it should be administered to animals that have never been treated with any macrolide or lincosamide, or which show bacterial sensitivity on a susceptibility test. Vomiting is the main side effect.

Lincomycin: Lincomycin is administered at 15–30 mg/kg orally bid on an empty stomach. It has the advantage of a twice-daily administration and does not cause emesis. Bacterial resistance varies between 10 and 40%, and is probably increasing (Pellerin *et al.*, 1998).

Other macrolides and lincosamides: Clindamycin (5 mg/kg orally bid or 10 mg/kg orally sid for superficial infections; 10 mg/kg orally bid for deep infections) and tylosin (10–20 mg/kg orally bid) are used with success in canine pyodermas and feline skin infections and abscesses. Azithromycin (10 mg/kg orally sid) and clarithromycin (2.5–10 mg/kg orally bid) are new bactericidal macrolides with a larger spectrum of action, a longer endurance, less development of resistance and once daily administration. Their efficacy in domestic carnivores is still to be assessed.

Antibiotics for recurrent or deep pyodermas
The following antibiotics are effective in most cases of staphylococcal pyoderma and can be chosen 'empirically' or following a susceptibility test. Bacterial resistance is usually rare, even after long or repeated treatments, and they are usually well tolerated.

Cephalosporins: First-generation cephalosporins, such as cefalexin (15–30 mg/kg orally bid) and cefadroxil (10–20 mg/kg orally bid or 20–30 mg/kg orally sid) are excellent choices for recurrent pyoderma. Side effects include anorexia, nausea and vomiting, particularly if the drug is given on an empty stomach.

Amoxicillin and clavulanic acid: This combination has a broad-spectrum bactericidal action. The recommended dosage is 12.5 mg/kg orally bid, but in some cases it may be better to use higher doses (20–25/kg orally bid or 12.5 mg/kg orally tid).

Beta-lactamase resistant penicillins: Cloxacillin, dicloxacillin, nafcillin and oxacillin (20 mg/kg orally tid) are possible alternatives but are very expensive.

Rifampin: Rifampin (5–10 mg/kg orally sid) is a bactericidal antibiotic able to concentrate inside neutrophils and macrophages and to penetrate deep, chronic, granulomatous and cicatricial lesions. It is very useful in interdigital pyoderma, callus infections and acral lick granulomas. Unfortunately, resistance develops rapidly and it should always be administered with another bactericidal antibiotic, such as cefalexin. It should not be given with enrofloxacin because enrofloxacin antagonizes rifampin's activity. Rifampin has several side effects, such as increased plasma liver enzymes, hepatitis, haemolytic anaemia, anorexia, vomiting, diarrhoea and death. It should not be administered for longer than 3 weeks. During its administration it is advised to monitor plasma liver enzymes weekly.

Fluoroquinolones: Quinolones act intracellularly and are able to kill bacteria in neutrophils and macrophages. Resistance is not frequent, although it has increased with the years. Fluoroquinolones for animal use are enrofloxacin (5 mg/kg orally sid), marbofloxacin (2 mg/kg orally sid), difloxacin (5 mg/kg orally sid) and orbifloxacin (2.5 mg/kg orally sid). The use of high dosages of enrofloxacin (10–20 mg/kg orally sid) has recently been suggested for bacteria with intermediate sensitivity. Fluoroquinolones should not be used in animals younger than one year, because they may damage bone cartilage. They should be reserved for rod infections and very difficult staphylococcal or mixed infections.

Topical therapy

Principles of topical therapy
Topical therapy is very useful, as it removes debris and crusts from the skin surface and follicular infundibula, eliminates bacteria on the horny layer, and favours drainage of exudative and deep lesions. However, with the exception of intertrigo and 'hot spots', it is rarely effective on its own in superficial and deep pyoderma, and should be associated with systemic antibiotic treatment.

Important factors for successful topical therapy are:

* Choosing the correct product, evaluating its active ingredients, vehicle, indications and contraindications, mechanism of action and residual effect
* The choice of the product formulation depends on the type, localization and extent of the lesions. Usual formulations are soaks, shampoos and creams
* Contact time should be at least 10–15 minutes, and the owner should be well instructed regarding this point
* Owner compliance is crucial. The main problems relate to cost of treatment, frequency and difficulty of application, coat type and character of the animal, odour and cosmetic appearance of the product.

Soaks
Soaks in water containing a disinfectant (chlorhexidine or iodine), better if in a whirlpool bath, are advised as an initial therapy for deep pyodermas, particularly pododermatitis. Soaks help soften crusts, decrease pruritus and pain, and promote re-epithelialization. Warm water causes peripheral vasodilation and a better antibiotic distribution to the skin. Soaks may be repeated once or twice daily for the first 3–7 days, and should not be longer than 10–15 minutes each.

Shampoos
Shampoo is the most frequently used formulation. The detergent effect helps remove debris and exudates. The active ingredients should have a contact time of at least 10–15 minutes and should then be thoroughly rinsed. Treatments are repeated initially 2–3 times weekly, then tapered to twice monthly when the disease improves. An excessively frequent use, particularly of strong agents, such as benzoyl peroxide, may lead to excessive coat dryness and skin irritation.

Benzoyl peroxide: Benzoyl peroxide 2–3% is a potent oxidant agent with an excellent broad-spectrum antibacterial effect, as well as keratolytic, antipruritic, drying, degreasing and follicular flushing properties. This product is very useful in exudative and seborrhoeic lesions and when a follicular flushing effect is needed (comedones, demodicosis). Its residual effect prevents bacterial recolonization for several hours (Kwochka et al., 1991). Disadvantages are that it may bleach dark coats, may dry the skin excessively or cause irritant contact dermatitis. A humectant rinse may be used after the shampoo in order to prevent excessive drying. This shampoo should not be used on cats.

Ethyl lactate: Ethyl lactate 10% is an excellent antibacterial agent, and is usually better tolerated than benzoyl peroxide. It penetrates rapidly in the epidermis, hair follicles and sebaceous glands, where it is hydrolysed to lactic acid and ethanol, which are both antibacterial. Ethyl lactate is less degreasing and drying than benzoyl peroxide.

Chlorhexidine: Chlorhexidine has an excellent broad-spectrum activity against bacteria, fungi and viruses. It is not irritating, sensitizing, nor inactivated by pus or exudates, and has a long residual effect. Higher concentrations (3–5%) have better effect, particularly on yeasts. It is well tolerated for repeated treatments and by cats.

Sulphur and salicylic acid: Sulphur has antibacterial, antipruritic and keratoplastic properties. Salicylic acid is keratolytic, keratoplastic, mildly antipruritic and bacteriostatic, thanks to its low pH. In combination of 2% each they have a synergistic effect. They are recommended for superficial pyodermas with dry desquamation or seborrhoea. The combination may be used in cats and is very rarely irritating. The product is contraindicated in cases of known hypersensitivity to acetylsalicylic acid or sulphonamides.

Creams

Creams and ointments are indicated for very localized bacterial skin infections, such as pododermatitis or chin acne. They should be massaged well into the skin to promote absorption and the animal should be watched for the following 10–15 minutes to prevent licking.

Mupirocin: Mupirocin is an antibiotic exclusively for topical use with an excellent bactericidal action against Gram-positive bacteria. It is not systemically absorbed but is able to penetrate well in deep, granulomatous and scarring lesions. It does not belong to any systemic antibiotic class and has no bacterial cross-resistance. A 2-week course with twice daily application is suggested.

Main causes of therapeutic failure

Pyoderma usually responds promptly to antibiotic therapy. If this is not the case or if the pyoderma recurs after therapy withdrawal, a re-evaluation of diagnosis and treatment is necessary. The main reasons for failure are:

- Wrong choice of antibiotic (inappropriate pharmacokinetics or bacterial resistance)
- Insufficient dosage or duration of treatment (immediate relapse after drug withdrawal)
- Interruption of the treatment without a clinical evaluation by the veterinary surgeon
- Incorrect administration
- Administration together with steroids or immunosuppressive drugs
- The underlying disease has not been identified or controlled
- Concurrent *Malassezia* infection that has not been identified or treated
- The diagnosis of pyoderma is wrong.

Treatment of recurrent pyoderma

If the diagnosis and treatment are correct, and no underlying cause is found, then the relapsing skin infection is considered a 'recurrent idiopathic pyoderma' and may be controlled with topical therapy, pulse or maintenance antibiotic therapy, and/or immunostimulant drugs (Figure 22.14). The relapse period is very important: if the recurrence occurs a few days after antibiotic withdrawal, the treatment period was probably too short and the antibiotic course should be repeated and prolonged. If the pyoderma recurs after several weeks or months, then a maintenance therapy should be planned.

Summary

The approach to pyoderma and its differential diagnoses is summarized in Figure 22.15.

Topical therapy

Continue regular topical therapy when the pyoderma is cleared, e.g. antibacterial shampoos every 2–4 weeks
Antibiotic creams on early localized lesions
Try application of fusidic acid to mucosal surfaces as 1% viscous eye drops twice daily: significantly reduces mucosal populations of *Staphylococcus intermedius* (Saijonmaa-Koulumies *et al.*, 1998)

Immunostimulants

Only able to stimulate a suppressed immune system; therefore, have a low success rate
Act on very specific parts of the immune system, so it is difficult to choose the correct drug
Initially given with an antibiotic; after antibiotic withdrawal, the immunostimulant is maintained, with the aim of preventing relapse

Staphage Lysate (Delmont Laboratories, Swarthmore, PA)
- Staphylococcal bacterin produced by lysis of *Staphylococcus aureus*
- Able to stimulate cell-mediated and humoral immunity
- May work as bacterial hyposensitization in dogs with staphylococcal hypersensitivity
- Give s.c. twice weekly for at least 10 weeks before evaluating its efficacy
- Maintenance therapy (every 7–14 days) may be prolonged for life
- Efficacy about 40% (DeBoer *et al.*, 1990)
- Rare side effects: vomiting, diarrhoea, hyperthermia, injection site reactions, anaphylactic shock

22.14 Treatment of recurrent pyoderma. (continues) ▶

Immunostimulants (continued)

Autogenous vaccines
- Staphylococcal vaccines are prepared with bacteria isolated from the patient's lesions
- Reportedly good results but no controlled study
- The animal is stimulated with the same bacterial strain causing its skin disease
- Vaccine has to be produced each time for each patient by a specialized laboratory

Antibiotic maintenance treatment

Antibiotics with low toxicity and low bacterial resistance: first-generation cephalosporins and potentiated penicillins
This therapeutic protocol, which may favour development of bacterial resistance, should be considered as the last resort in case of idiopathic recurrent pyoderma:
- Relapse rate >2 months; treat each relapse with a full course
- Relapse every 7–30 days: after a full course of antibiotics, full doses 3 days a week or every other week
- Relapses within 1 week: daily antibiotic therapy with 25–100% of the dose

22.14 (continued) Treatment of recurrent pyoderma.

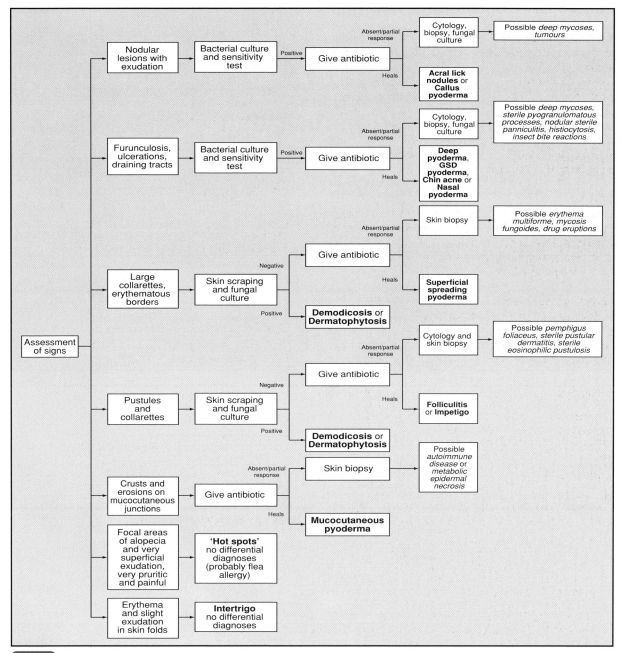

22.15 Approach to pyoderma and its differential diagnoses.

References and further reading

Chabanne L, Marchal T, Denerolle P *et al.* (1995) Lymphocyte subset abnormalities in German Shepherd Dog pyoderma. *Veterinary Immunology and Immunopathology* **49,** 189–198

DeBoer DJ, Moriello KA, Thomas CB *et al.* (1990) Evaluation of a commercial staphylococcal bacterin for management of idiopathic recurrent superficial pyoderma in dogs. *American Journal of Veterinary Research* **51(4),** 636–639

Denerolle P, Bourdoiseau G, Magnol GP *et al.* (1998) German Sherpherd Dog pyoderma: a prospective study of 23 cases. *Veterinary Dermatology* **9,** 243–248

Gortel K, Campbell KL, Kakoma I *et al.* (1999) Methicillin resistance among staphylococci isolated from dogs. *American Journal of Veterinary Research* **60,** 1526–1630

Harvey RG and Lloyd DH (1994) The distribution of *Staphylococcus intermedius* and coagulase-negative staphylococci on the hair, skin surface, within the hair follicles and on the mucous membranes of dogs. *Veterinary Dermatology* **5,** 75–81

Kwochka KW and Kowalski JJ (1991) Prophylactic efficacy of four antibacterial shampoos against Staphylococcus intermedius in dogs. *American Journal of Veterinary Research* **52(1),** 115–118

Ihrke PJ, Schwartzman RM, McGinley K *et al.* (1978) Microbiology of normal and seborrheic canine skin. *American Journal of Veterinary Research* **39,** 1487–1489

McEwan NA (2000) Adherence by *Staphylococcus intermedius* to canine keratinocytes in atopic dermatitis. *Research in Veterinary Science* **68,** 279–283

Noli C, Koeman JP and Willemse T (1996) A retrospective evaluation of adverse reactions to trimethoprim-sulphonamide combinations in dogs and cats. *The Veterinary Quarterly* **17,** 123–128

Pellerin JL, Bourdeau P, Sebbag H *et al.* (1998) Epidemiosurveillance of antimicrobial compound resistance of *Staphylococcus intermedius* clinical isolates from canine pyodermas. *Comparative Immunology, Microbiology and Infectious Diseases* **21,** 115–133

Piriz S, Valle J, de la Fuente R *et al.* (1996) In vitro activity of fifteen antimicrobial agents against methicillin-resistant and methicillin-susceptible *Staphylococcus intermedius. Journal of Veterinary Pharmacological Therapy* **19,** 118–123

Saijonmaa-Koulumies LEM and Lloyd DH (1995) Carriage of bacteria antagonistic towards *Staphylococcus intermedius* on canine skin and mucosal surfaces. *Veterinary Dermatology* **6,** 187–194

Saijonmaa-Koulumies L, Parsons E and Lloyd DH (1998) Elimination of *Staphylococcus intermedius* in healthy dogs by topical treatment with fusidic acid. *Journal of Small Animal Practice* **39,** 341–347

23

Dermatophytosis

Carol Foil

Dermatophytosis is a cutaneous infection with a keratinophilic fungus. Most cases of canine and feline dermatophytosis are caused by *Microsporum canis*, *Trichophyton mentagrophytes* or the geophilic species *M. gypseum*. In cats, 98% of cases are caused by *M. canis*. In dogs, the prevalence of infections caused by each of the three common aetiological agents varies geographically. There are numerous other species of dermatophyte that may infect domestic dogs and cats from wild animal, soil or human sources (Figure 23.1).

Species	Geographical range
Zoophilic (Normal hosts)	
Microsporum canis (cats)	Worldwide
M. equinum (horses)	Worldwide
M. nanum (pigs)	Worldwide
M. gallinae (poultry)	Worldwide
Trichophyton equinum (horses)	Worldwide
T. verrucosum (ruminants)	Worldwide
Sylvatic	
T. mentagrophytes	Worldwide
M. persicolor	Europe and Canada
Geophilic	
M. cookei	Worldwide
M. fulvum	Worldwide
M. vanbreuseghemi	Eurasia; North America
T. simii	India (primates and poultry)
M. gypseum	Worldwide
T. terrestre	Not very pathogenic
T. ajelloi	Worldwide; not very pathogenic
Anthropophilic	
Epidermophyton floccosum	Worldwide
M. audouinii	Worldwide
T. megninii	Africa; Europe
T. rubrum	Worldwide
T. schoenleinii	Africa; Asia
T. tonsurans	Worldwide; esp. South America
T. violaceum	Worldwide; rare in North America

23.1 Dermatophytes that may infect dogs or cats.

Simultaneous infection of dogs by more than one dermatophyte species may occur. Of combined infections, those caused by *M. gypseum* and *T. mentagrophytes* have been the most common.

Dogs and cats may carry many saprophytic moulds and yeasts on their haircoats and probably on dermatitic skin as well. The most common fungi isolated from the haircoats of clinically healthy dogs are *Alternaria*, *Cladosporium* and *Aspergillus* spp.

Dermatophytes may also be isolated from the haircoats of normal dogs and cats living in contaminated environments as transient flora; in cats this phenomenon has been referred to as the 'fomite carrier' state (Moriello and DeBoer, 1997). *M. canis* may cause a persistent subclinical infection of long-haired cats. *M. gypseum* may be cultured from the feet of dogs that show no clinical signs.

The prevalence of dermatophytosis in dogs is low, although this varies geographically, being higher in tropical and subtropical climates. In cats, the situation is more difficult to define. In free-roaming cats and those congregated in multi-cat facilities, the prevalence can be quite high (approaching 100% in some situations).

Dermatophytes spread between animals by direct contact or by contact with infected hair and scale in the environment or from fomites. The source of *M. canis* infections is usually an infected cat. In most *Trichophyton* infections, dogs and cats are suspected of being exposed by direct or indirect contact with rodents. *M. gypseum* and *T. terrestre* are acquired by dogs and cats from digging in contaminated areas. Infections with anthropophilic species are acquired as reverse zoonoses by direct contact with infected persons. Dermatophyte infections of pets and wild rodents involve the hair shaft and follicle (except for *T. terrestre*). Infected hair shafts are fragile and dislodged hair fragments containing infectious arthrospores are the most efficient means of transmission to other hosts. This material may remain infectious in the environment for many months.

Young animals are predisposed to acquiring symptomatic dermatophyte infections; exposure in healthy adult animals does not always lead to active infection. Excessive bathing and grooming, warm humid environments and long hair coats may predispose to infection after exposure (Moriello and DeBoer, 1997). Dermatophyte infections in healthy dogs and short-haired cats are usually self-limiting, with the infection clearing up within 8 weeks in most cases. Immunodeficient pets are at greater risk of acquiring infections and their infections may be more widespread and more prolonged. Glucocorticoid therapy is particularly likely to increase susceptibility to dermatophytosis by means of inhibiting local inflammation. Recovery from infection requires a healthy cell-mediated immune response.

Clinical features

Dermatophyte infections in both dogs and cats are highly variable in the clinical picture presented to the veterinary surgeon. Some of the clinical presentations of dermatophytosis are listed in Figure 23.2.

- Circular patch of hair loss, ± scale, ± inflammation. Singular or multiple
- Folliculitis: localized, regional or generalized
- Hair loss: Widespread to patchy
- Seborrhoea sicca with hair loss
- Miliary dermatitis in cats
- Kerion reaction – often *M. gypseum*
- Nodular dermatophytosis (Pseudomycetoma)
- Onychomycosis: nail bed inflammation and nail deformity
- Subclinical

23.2 Clinical syndromes recognized in dermatophytosis.

Dogs

Dogs may show foci of alopecia with follicular papules (Figure 23.3), scales and crusts. Dermatophytosis should be considered in any papular or pustular follicular eruption. Demodicosis and dermatophytosis may be clinically indistinguishable but can be differentiated reliably by a skin scraping. Superficial spreading folliculitis, with its spreading rings of erythema and exfoliation, is often mistaken for dermatophytosis.

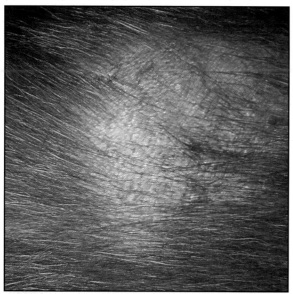

23.3 Focal patch of alopecia with follicular papules forms a classical dermatophyte lesion in a young Dobermann Pinscher. (Courtesy of V Fadok.)

Facial folliculitis and furunculosis may mimic an autoimmune skin disease (Figure 23.4). Nodular skin lesions (kerions) are a common presenting sign of *M. gypseum* (Figure 23.5). Onychomycosis causes chronic ungual fold inflammation, with or without footpad involvement, or the claw alone may be infected, which causes claw deformity and fragility.

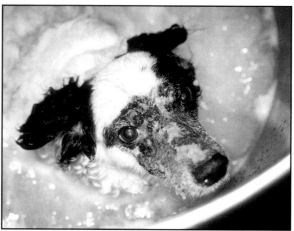

23.4 Facial *Trichophyton* dermatitis with scaling and crusting and depigmentation in a mixed breed dog. The condition can mimic autoimmune skin disease. This dog is receiving an antimicrobial whirlpool bath.

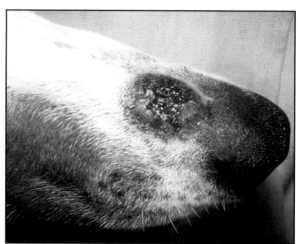

23.5 A kerion associated with focal *M. gypseum* infection, showing the boggy localized cellulitis and furunculosis, on the nose of a Whippet.

Cats

Culturing for fungi should be considered a part of the minimum database in the work-up of almost every feline skin disease because the lesions caused by dermatophytes are so variable.

Feline dermatophytosis often appears as irregular patchy alopecia with scale; this is the most common presentation in older kittens and young adult cats. In long-haired cats, this type of lesion is more difficult to detect. Other syndromes include classical circular patches of alopecia with scaling (Figure 23.6), miliary dermatitis, focal or multifocal pruritic dermatitis, onychomycosis and granulomatous dermatitis. In kittens, scaling and crusting lesions on the face and extremities are common presentations.

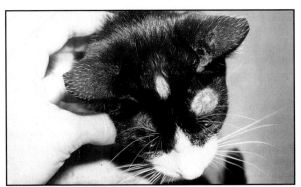

23.6 Patchy alopecia with scale on the face of a young Domestic Shorthair cat with *M. canis* infection forms a classical lesion in the older kitten or adult cat with ringworm.

Granulomatous dermatitis takes the form of a well circumscribed ulcerated nodule (Figure 23.7). The lesions occur on cats with generalized *M. canis* infection. Persistent and subclinical infections may be a problem in long-haired cats and there may be 'anatomical reservoirs' in persistently infected cats, in face folds, periocular skin or ungual folds (Moriello and DeBoer, 1997). These cases can be difficult to distinguish from fomite carriers in multiple cat households.

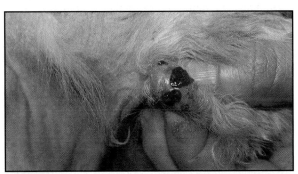

23.7 Granulomatous dermatophytosis lesion in a Persian cat with generalized *M. canis* ringworm.

Diagnosis (see also Chapter 3)

Wood's light examination

This technique can be very valuable in the hands of an experienced diagnostician, remembering that it can never be used to rule out dermatophytosis, as not all infections exhibit fluorescence. *M. canis* infections may be positive on a Wood's light examination. False-positive examinations may result from greasy scale (follicle casts) and medication. True fluorescence is quite bright, apple green, and should only be seen within the shafts of infected hairs. It is useful to pluck positive hairs for direct microscopic examination and for culture. Hairs may remain fluorescent during treatment after there are no longer any viable fungal spores in the hair. In Wood's lamp-positive infections in multiple cat households, a Wood's lamp may be used to demonstrate the extent of environmental contamination.

Direct microscopic examination

Dermatophytes form hyphae and arthroconidia within and on hair and scale, which may be seen on

examination of hairs plucked from lesions (Figures 23.8 and 23.9). Mineral oil mounts may be sufficient as a mounting medium, but visualization is facilitated by mounting in 10–20% potassium hydroxide for variable periods of time. Even in experienced hands, this technique is time-consuming and may be diagnostic in only a few cases. It may lead to misinterpretation if saprophytic fungal spores are present in the specimen. Dermatophytes never form macroconidia in tissue.

---

1. Choose hairs that appear damaged or 'dirty' from the periphery of the lesion. Scrape or pluck so as to collect the intrafollicular portion of suspect hairs.
2. Place the sample into a large drop of clearing agent (10--20% KOH) and apply a coverslip.
3. Examine with low power for fractured hair shafts with clinging debris and disrupted cuticle.
4. Examine these hairs with high power for hyphae and masses of arthrospores.

23.8 Potassium hydroxide trichogram technique. False positives result from mistaking melanin granules for spores or from the presence of saprophytic fungi on hairs. Dermatophyte elements are *never* pigmented.

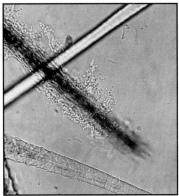

23.9 Dermatophyte hyphae and arthrospores are visible in this potassium hydroxide trichogram from an *M. canis*-infected cat. (Courtesy of P Ihrke.)

Fungal culture

Definitive diagnosis of dermatophytosis is made by culture. Several important principles should be followed to ensure accurate results.

Specimen collection

If done properly (Figure 23.10), clipping and cleaning the lesions to be cultured will reduce contaminant growth. This is most important in humid climates where saprophyte spores are common contaminants of haircoats.

---

1. Clip hair within and around lesions to 0.5 cm.
2. Pat area with alcohol-moistened gauze and allow to dry.
3. Collect hair stubble with haemostats by grasping the hair shafts close to the skin and rolling the hairs from the follicles.
- Select hairs that fluoresce in UV light or are broken and are near active inflammation, when possible
- Include scales in the sample
- Place firmly in contact with the surface of the DTM medium
- Exudates or antiseptics should not be transferred to the medium.

23.10 Culture technique for suspected dermatophytosis.

Media and incubation

Culture can readily be performed as an in-house procedure using dermatophyte test medium (DTM) (Figure 23.11). DTM consists of Sabouraud's dextrose agar, phenol red as pH indicator and antimicrobials to inhibit bacterial and saprophytic mould growth. For incubation, DTM containers should be loosely capped at room temperature and protected from UV light and desiccation. They should be inspected daily for a colour change of the medium to red and simultaneous growth of a cottony mycelium. If the colour change occurs later, which may be a result of saprophyte growth exhausting the carbohydrate in the medium, the result will be a false-positive reading.

Sabouraud's dextrose agar with:
- Antibiotic to inhibit bacterial contamination
- Cycloheximide to inhibit many saprophytic fungi
- Phenol red, a pH indicator turns red in alkaline pH. This will allow distinction between a dermatophytic type of metabolism (alkaline byproducts) and a saprophytic metabolism (acidic byproducts)

Saprophytes utilize carbohydrates preferentially. However, when these are exhausted in the medium, they will shift to metabolizing nitrogenous substances. At this point, a red colour change will occur, giving false-positive DTM results. **Dermatophytes produce the red colour change on the DTM** *simultaneously with observable growth.*

23.11 Features of dermatophyte test medium (DTM).

After 7–10 days of growth, most colonies will begin to produce spores, which will allow species identification. A suspect colony that fails to produce spores or is difficult to identify, as is often the case in *Trichophyton* spp., should be sent to a qualified diagnostic laboratory.

Zoophilic dermatophyte colonies are white to buff-coloured. Anthropophilic species may be pinkish to yellow. If blue, green, dark brown or black fungal contaminants have overgrown a colony suspected of being a dermatophyte, subculturing will be necessary.

Culturing asymptomatic animals

Brush culturing is the preferred method of obtaining specimens from asymptomatic animals. A clean toothbrush is satisfactory for this technique. The animal's haircoat is brushed thoroughly for 3 minutes. The bristles are then impressed directly into the culture medium in several sites.

Onychomycosis

When dermatophytosis is suspected as a cause of chronic paronychia, special culture techniques may be needed. In many cases the hair surrounding the ungual fold may be infected and may be cultured as for elsewhere on the body, taking special care to clip and clean to reduce contaminant growth. However, in dogs, geophilic fungi may contaminate pre-existing foot lesions, so it may be necessary to correlate cultural findings with histological demonstration of fungi in hair or claw. Otherwise, repeated isolation of fungus from the lesions may be regarded as evidence of cause. If the claws alone are affected, a scalpel blade may be used to shave fine pieces from the proximal end of clipped or surgically excised specimens for culture.

Histopathology

Examination of biopsy samples is not as sensitive as culture in the diagnosis of dermatophytosis. However, in cases where the true significance of culture results is questioned, demonstration of the organism in biopsy specimens is more definitive. Histological examination is most useful in detecting the nodular forms of dermatophytosis, i.e. kerion and granulomatous ringworm. With nodular lesions, it may be impossible to culture the organisms causing the inflammation from hair and scale.

Shaved, clipped or surgically excised specimens of claws may be submitted for histological examination in cases of paronychia, onychorrhexis or onychomadesis. If fungal organisms are present, they will be readily visible within the substance of the claw.

Therapeutics

Most animals with dermatophytosis should receive both topical and systemic therapy. In healthy animals with small individual lesions, the prognosis is good for resolution without therapy; however, resolution can be hastened by treatment, and topical treatment will reduce the likelihood of contagion. Long-haired cats and all animals with numerous lesions or widespread disease should always be given systemic therapy until culture results are negative. Cats with *M. canis* infection can remain culture-positive long after they have resolved clinically (Moriello and DeBoer, 1997). *Trichophyton* infections should always be treated systemically as well, since spreading and generalized infections are common. Kerions and granulomatous lesions do not require specific antifungal therapy unless more widespread disease is also present. The kerion should be cleansed gently to remove exudate and avoid potentiation of scarring.

Topical therapy

The goals of topical therapy are to help hasten clinical resolution in animals receiving systemic treatment and to reduce environmental contamination. When sparsely haired sites are infected and when the infection is localized, topical therapy alone may be sufficient, but care must be taken to ensure that more widespread disease is not present. Baths and rinses will remove the scale, crusts, exudate and infected hairs, reducing the potential for spread of infection to other animals and people. Agents useful in topical treatment are summarized in Figure 23.12.

The decision about whether to clip around dermatophyte lesions should be made on an individual basis. Clipping can spread infection on an animal and severely contaminate the environment in which the procedure is performed. On the other hand, careful disposal of clipped hair reduces the release of infected hair in the home environment, facilitates application of topical therapy and may stimulate new hair growth and shed of infective hairs during therapy.

Agent	Formulation	Frequency	Comments
Sodium hyposulphite (bleach)	1:10 in water	twice/week	Not on black animals!
Lime–sulphur dips (USA)	2–4% in water	twice/week	Not on white animals; preferred treatment where enilconazole not licensed
Miconazole	lotion, cream, spray, shampoo rinse	as directed twice/week	Small lesions Newest product; efficacy of shampoo unknown, but licensed as POM for use in cats in the UK as adjunct to systemic therapy
Clotrimazole	cream, lotion	as directed	Small lesions
Enilconazole	Clinafarm EC™ in USA only	twice/week	Not licensed for use on dogs or cats; 0.2% EC diluted in water at 55.6 ml per US gallon
	Imaverol™ (UK) 0.2% emulsion	twice/week	Not approved in the USA or for use on cats; licensed for dogs; very effective

23.12 Recommended topical therapy for dermatophytosis.

Drug	Dosage	Comments
Griseofulvin (microsized)	50–120 mg/kg divided bid	With a fatty meal Do not give to pregnant animals
Griseofulvin (ultramicrosized)	10–15 mg/kg divided or as a single daily dose	Do not give to pregnant animals
Itraconazole	5–10 mg/kg once daily	Give with food; check liver enzymes if anorexia develops
Itraconazole pulse therapy	5–10 mg/kg daily for one week, rest one week, repeat	Give with food
Terbinafine	30 mg/kg daily	Lower dosages are recommended by some; may not be as effective

23.13 Drugs and dosages for systemic treatment of dermatophytosis.

Systemic therapy

Drugs and dosage regimens are summarized in Figure 23.13.

Treatment with any systemic antifungal should be continued until two successive brush cultures are negative, separated by 2 weeks. The first culture can be taken after 3–6 weeks of therapy depending on the agent being used.

Griseofulvin

Treatment with griseofulvin is expensive and long term, and side effects are common. It should be used only when diagnosis is certain. Griseofulvin shows variable and incomplete absorption after oral dosing. Absorption is enhanced by administration with a fat-containing meal or by formulations containing polyethylene glycol. Particle size also greatly affects oral absorption and bioavailability.

Dosages recommended for dogs and cats are not based on modern pharmacological studies. Dosages that have proved to be effective in the largest numbers of cases are higher than manufacturers' recommendations, and significant toxicities may be encountered. The most common side effects are vomiting, diarrhoea and anorexia. These can be partially avoided by dividing the daily dosage into two administrations. Bone marrow suppression and neurological signs have occurred, probably as idiosyncratic reactions. Griseofulvin is teratogenic and must never be given during the first two-thirds of pregnancy.

Ketoconazole

Ketoconazole has been shown to be a moderately effective fungistatic drug against *M. canis* and *T. mentagrophytes*. Other imidazoles and griseofulvin are more effective, and the use of ketoconazole is reserved for those who cannot tolerate griseofulvin and for whom other drugs are not affordable. The most common side effect is anorexia. Rarely, hepatic toxicity is encountered.

Itraconazole

Itraconazole is a triazole antifungal agent that would, except for cost and the lack of veterinary licensing, be the treatment of choice for dermatophytosis in dogs and cats. It is more effective and less toxic than ketoconazole. The drug is dispensed in 100 mg capsules which can be opened and the contents divided and mixed with butter or prescription critical care diet for easy administration to cats. It should be given with food to enhance absorption. Side effects include anorexia, occasionally vomiting; rarely, it may cause liver enzyme elevation. There is no need to monitor liver enzymes routinely; these should be checked if anorexia develops.

Itraconazole can be useful in pulse therapy protocols (Columbo *et al.*, 2001) for treating long-haired cats in a heavily contaminated environment. In these settings, relapse is a common problem, and pulse treatment for several months can be used to reduce the relapse rate.

Terbinafine

This is an allylamine antifungal that is well concentrated in the skin after oral administration. It is useful for treating dermatophytosis in dogs and cats, but does not have a veterinary licence. Doses reported in the literature and anecdotally for dogs and cats have varied. Side effects include anorexia and, rarely, liver enzyme elevation.

Lufenuron

Lufenuron is a chitin synthase inhibitor used for flea control that has been reported to be useful in canine and feline dermatophytosis. The original report outlined the use of 50–60 mg/kg given once (Ben-Ziony and Arzi, 2000). Since that report, several treatment failures in challenging situations have been reported anecdotally and higher dosages and more prolonged treatment is recommended. Many dermatologists are combining monthly lufenuron at label doses with initial treatment using itraconazole or terbinafine in cats. Until controlled trials are available, use of lufenuron cannot be recommended for systemic treatment of dermatophytosis.

Vaccination

In the USA there is a licensed killed *M. canis* vaccine marketed for treatment and prevention of *M. canis* ringworm in cats. When used pre-exposure, it has been shown to lessen the severity, but not reduce the incidence, of disease in kittens subsequently exposed to virulent *M. canis*. When used after infection, it has been shown to decrease the severity and hasten the resolution of clinical lesions but does not hasten mycological cure. Most veterinary dermatologists question the value of using the vaccine in a cattery programme.

Environmental control

In each confirmed case of dermatophytosis in dogs and cats, there is an environmental clean-up problem to be handled. The veterinary surgeon must be prepared to advise the client about environmental contamination and recommend appropriate measures to prevent spread of infection. The necessity for clean-up is most serious in the case of cats infected with *M. canis*. Dermatophyte arthrospores, liberated from broken and shedding hairs of infected pets, are quite long-lived.

The most important facet of environmental clean-up is complete mechanical removal of hair by means of vacuuming. Full-strength household bleach, enilconazole preparations or chlorine dioxine disinfectants may be used to disinfect surfaces and utensils. Carpets and furnishings must be vacuumed thoroughly or removed. Clothing and bedding should be thoroughly laundered with bleach or discarded.

Public health considerations

Pet owners

Owners of cats infected with *M. canis* are at great risk of acquiring the infection. It is the most frequently reported zoonotic agent acquired from pet animals. Worldwide, the numbers of reported cases of human infection with *M. canis* is increasing. Veterinary surgeons should consider advising people adopting a new cat to have the cat evaluated for ringworm before all members of the household are exposed. Cats acquired from catteries and from animal shelters are of particular concern.

Animal health workers

The occupational risk of acquiring dermatophytosis is great. In a study of government veterinary surgeons and animal health workers conducted in Great Britain, animal ringworm was the most commonly reported zoonosis; the overall prevalence was 24%. Veterinary surgeons must be vigilant in protecting themselves and their staff from this troublesome and potentially serious zoonosis.

References and further reading

Ben-Ziony Y and Arzi B (2000) Use of lufenuron for treating fungal infections of dogs and cats: 297 cases (1997–1999). *Journal of the American Veterinary Medical Association* **217**, 1510–1513

Colombo S, Cornegliani L and Vercelli A (2001) Efficacy of itraconazole as a combined continuous/pulse therapy in feline dermatophytosis: preliminary results in nine cases. *Veterinary Dermatology* **12**, 347–350

Foil CS (1990) Dermatophytosis. In: *Infectious Diseases of the Dog and Cat, 2nd edn,* ed. CE Green, pp. 362–370. WB Saunders, Philadelphia

Moriello KA and DeBoer DJ (1997) Dermatophytosis: advances in therapy and control. In: *Consultations in Feline Internal Medicine 3,* ed. JR August, pp. 177–190. WB Saunders, Philadelphia

Scott DW, Miller WH and Griffin CE (2001) Fungal skin diseases. In: *Muller and Kirk's Small Animal Dermatology, 6th edn,* pp. 337–422. WB Saunders, Philadelphia

24

Malassezia dermatitis

Tim Nuttall

Malassezia has long been recognized as a common perpetuating factor in otitis externa (see Chapter 14). One of the most important advances in veterinary dermatology in recent years has been the realization that *Malassezia* can be associated with generalized dermatitis and that antifungal therapy can have a dramatic effect in these cases.

The *Malassezia* organism

*S*pecies and strains

Malassezia is a genus of commensal yeasts found on mammalian and avian skin. *Malassezia pachydermatis* uniquely does not require lipid supplements during culture *in vitro*. There are six lipid-dependent species: *M.furfur*, *M.sympodialis*, *M.globosa*, *M.obtusa*, *M.restricta* and *M.slooffiae*. The lipid-dependent species are most commonly isolated from humans. In contrast, *M.pachydermatis* can be recovered from a variety of animals, especially carnivores. So far only *M.pachydermatis* has been isolated from dogs, but *M.sympodialis* and *M.globosa*, as well as *M.pachydermatis*, have been isolated from cats. Seven strains of *M.pachydermatis* have been identified. None has been associated with virulence, although type Id was restricted to dogs, whilst others (e.g. type Ia) were more ubiquitous (Guillot *et al.*, 1997).

Morphology

Malassezia is a single-cell yeast with a thick cell wall (Figure 24.1). Individual cells are ovoid to globular or cylindrical. Cells in the process of budding form the characteristic 'peanut' to 'Russian doll' shape.

Ecology

Malassezia can be recovered from 3-day-old puppies, suggesting there is early maternal transfer by licking, grooming or from the vagina. *Malassezia* is commonly found in the ear canals, anal sacs, interdigital skin and mucocutaneous junctions (lips, prepuce, vagina, anus) of healthy animals. It is rarely recovered from skin elsewhere on the body. Mucosal sites in particular may be reservoirs from which yeasts are seeded onto the skin by licking and grooming. Evidence for this is seen in Basset Hounds, where successful topical treatment is associated with a reduction of both mucosal and cutaneous *Malassezia* populations.

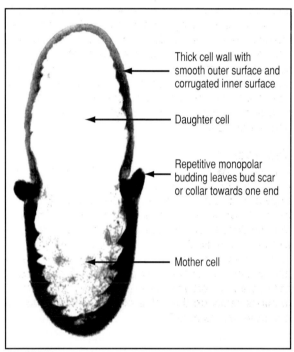

Thick cell wall with smooth outer surface and corrugated inner surface

Daughter cell

Repetitive monopolar budding leaves bud scar or collar towards one end

Mother cell

24.1 A schematic representation of a *Malassezia* yeast in the process of budding.

Malassezia yeasts colonize the superficial layers of the epidermal and infundibular stratum corneum. They appear to have a symbiotic relationship with cutaneous staphylococci, producing both mutually beneficial growth factors and a favourable microenvironment. Concurrent pyoderma frequently complicates *Malassezia* dermatitis. Furthermore, treatment regimes that also reduce bacterial numbers are superior to those with antifungal action only.

Virulence factors and host susceptibility

Precisely how a commensal organism becomes a pathogen is unclear: the balance with host defences must shift in favour of the microorganism. *Malassezia* can have a significant pathogenic role when a combination of virulence factors and microclimate allows the yeasts to overwhelm the physical, chemical and immunological host defences that normally limit colonization and proliferation (Figure 24.2).

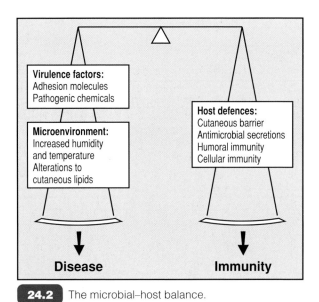

24.2 The microbial–host balance.

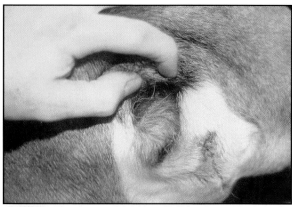

24.3 The deep tail fold in a Bulldog is an ideal site for colonization by *Malassezia*. This dog suffered recurrent bouts of *Malassezia* dermatitis, probably triggered by the warm, moist environment in the fold. Chlorhexidine scrubs and enilconazole rinses effected temporary remission, but a long-term cure required radical surgery to ablate the tail fold.

Virulence factors

M. pachydermatis expresses a variety of protein or glycoprotein adhesion molecules that bind to carbohydrate ligands on canine corneocytes. However, neither the expression of adhesion molecules nor adhesion to corneocytes *in vitro* has been associated with virulence in *Malassezia* dermatitis (Bond *et al.*, 2000). Similarly, the ability of *M.furfur* to adhere to human keratinocytes is not linked to seborrhoeic dermatitis.

Malassezia yeasts secrete various proteases, lipases, phospholipases, lipoxygenases and other enzymes, which cause proteolysis, lipolysis, alter cutaneous pH, activate complement and trigger the release of inflammatory mediators. These changes could alter the cutaneous microclimate in favour of *Malassezia* and staphylococci, as well as contributing to inflammation and pruritus. Despite this, no specific link with virulence has been demonstrated.

Host factors

The lack of an association between biological activity and virulence suggests that *Malassezia* is an opportunistic pathogen, able to establish wherever there is a permissive microenvironment.

Anatomy

Anatomical features (body folds, pendulous lips, hairy feet) (Figure 24.3), inflammation, exudates and licking can create a warm, moist microenvironment. Keratinization defects and endocrine disorders may increase humidity, and alter the quantity and quality of sebum, although the relationship between sebum production and *Malassezia* growth is unclear. Furthermore, disruption to the stratum corneum by self-trauma, keratinization or metabolic defects could also allow *Malassezia* to establish.

Breed susceptibility

Certain breeds (Figure 24.4) are predisposed to *Malassezia* dermatitis. The nature of the predilection is unclear. It could include anatomical features, specific host factors and predisposition to diseases with secondary *Malassezia* involvement. Mucosal and cutaneous *Malassezia* populations are elevated in healthy Basset Hounds, suggesting factors that facilitate *Malassezia* colonization play a role in the susceptibility of this breed.

Basset Hounds
West Highland White Terriers
Cocker Spaniels
Shih Tzus
Dachshunds
Miniature Poodles
German Shepherd Dogs
Australian Silky Terriers
English Setters

24.4 Breeds predisposed to *Malassezia* dermatitis.

Immune response

Malassezia does not invade the stratum corneum. Even so, immune responses to *Malassezia* organisms can be detected in healthy and affected dogs. At least 14 different protein antigens have been identified. Dogs with *Malassezia* dermatitis tend to recognize more antigens than healthy dogs, but no association between the pattern of antigen recognition and any particular *Malassezia* strain or virulence has been demonstrated (Bond, 2000; Chen *et al.*, 2000). Affected dogs also have elevated serum IgA and IgG titres compared to healthy dogs, but this does not appear to be protective. Basset Hounds with *Malassezia* dermatitis exhibit decreased lymphocyte responses compared to healthy dogs (Bond *et al.*, 1998) suggesting that protective immunity is associated with strong cell-mediated rather than humoral responses. Positive delayed skin test reactions, however, are seen in both healthy and affected Bassets.

A significant proportion of human patients with atopic dermatitis develop a hypersensitivity response to *Malassezia*. *Malassezia* dermatitis and otitis also frequently complicate canine atopic dermatitis. Atopic dogs have larger populations of *Malassezia* at mucosal and interdigital sites than healthy dogs. Furthermore, intradermal test reactivity to a crude *Malassezia* extract was seen in atopic, but not healthy, dogs (Morris *et al.*, 1998). In contrast, immediate skin test reactivity in non-atopic Basset Hounds with *Malassezia* dermatitis is infrequent. Recent studies have also detected higher levels of *Malassezia* specific IgG and IgE in atopic dogs than in healthy dogs (Nuttall and Halliwell, 2001). This suggests that *Malassezia* could participate in atopic dermatitis by acting as allergens or superantigens, although there is no evidence of this as yet.

Other predisposing factors
Whether *Malassezia* is a primary disease or a secondary complication is controversial. *Malassezia* has been associated with a number of primary conditions in dogs and cats (Figure 24.5), but other studies showed that dogs with atopy, keratinization defects and endocrinopathies were no more at risk of *Malassezia* dermatitis than dogs with any other dermatological problem. Treatment with glucocorticoids or antibiotics does not appear to be a factor. However, in the author's experience, primary *Malassezia* dermatitis is uncommon in most breeds, and is most frequently secondary to an underlying hypersensitivity.

Body folds
Scabies
Demodicosis
Atopic dermatitis
Adverse food reaction
Endocrinopathies
Keratinization defects
Superficial necrolytic dermatitis/necrolytic migratory
    erythema/hepatocutaneous syndrome
Zinc responsive dermatosis
Feline paraneoplastic syndrome
Feline thymoma
Feline leukaemia virus/feline immunodeficiency virus
Feline acne/facial dermatitis
Immunosuppressive therapy
Psychological stress

24.5 Possible underlying conditions in *Malassezia* dermatitis.

Zoonotic potential
Malassezia pachydermatis can transiently colonize humans. Colonization of staff members' hands from pet dogs was the likely cause of *M. pachydermatis*-associated septicaemia, meningitis, and urinary tract infections in an intensive care nursery (Chang *et al*, 1998). The yeast then persisted through patient-to-patient transmission. The elderly, AIDS sufferers or patients undergoing chemotherapy may also be at risk. This underlies the need to observe hygienic precautions when handling healthy animals, as well as those affected by *Malassezia* dermatitis.

Clinical signs

Dogs
Malassezia dermatitis can occur in any breed, although certain breeds are predisposed (see Figure 24.4). There does not appear to be any age or sex predilection.

The major clinical sign is pruritus, which can be severe, causing frenzied scratching that can be misinterpreted as a neurological problem. In the early stages there is erythema and greasy exudation, scaling and crusting (Figure 24.6). Chronic *Malassezia* dermatitis is characterized by greasy alopecia, lichenification and hyperpigmentation (Figure 24.7). Clinical signs can be focal or generalized, diffuse or well demarcated. Commonly affected sites include the ears (see chapter 14), lips, muzzle, feet, ventral neck, axillae, ventral body, medial limbs, perianal skin and tail. Affected dogs often have a rancid, musty or yeasty odour.

Less commonly dogs present with recurrent interdigital furunculosis or 'cysts'. *Malassezia* can also

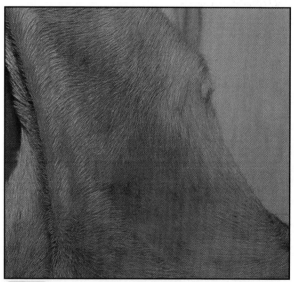

24.6 Acute, pruritic and erythematous *Malassezia* dermatitis in the axilla of a Basset Hound.

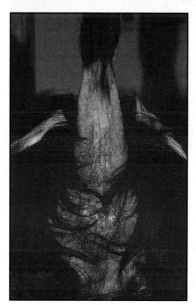

24.7 Chronic *Malassezia* dermatitis in a Cavalier King Charles Spaniel. This dog was also hypothyroid. Treatment with a 2% chlorhexidine/ 2% miconazole shampoo and thyroxine was curative, although the tail alopecia was permanent.

cause paronychia with a waxy exudate and brownish discoloration of the nails. *Malassezia* is also a rare cause of stomatitis, pharyngitis and tonsillitis.

An underlying condition (see Figure 24.5) and/or the staphylococcal pyoderma present in many cases often complicate the clinical picture.

Cats

Malassezia dermatitis is less common in cats than in dogs, but has been associated with otitis externa (see Chapter 14). Pruritus is a less constant feature than in dogs. *Malassezia* can be involved in recalcitrant feline acne and facial dermatitis characterized by erythema and comedones, with large dark tightly adherent scales and follicular casts (Figure 24.8). Other cats may present with generalized scaling and erythema. Some cats, particularly Devon Rex, present with paronychia or waxy, red-brown discoloration of the nails (Figure 24.9). Generalized erythema and greasy scaling has been associated with *Malassezia* dermatitis in cats with thymoma and paraneoplastic alopecia.

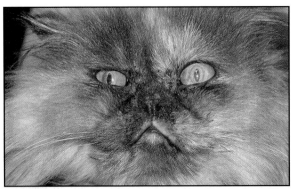

24.8 Facial dermatitis and acne in a Persian cat. The cat also had an adverse food reaction. Dietary management led to a great improvement, although weekly maintenance treatment with a 2% chlorhexidine/2% miconazole shampoo was necessary.

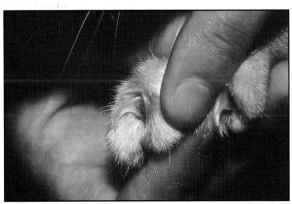

24.9 *Malassezia* paronychia and nail discoloration in a Devon Rex cat.

Diagnosis

The differential diagnosis list is extensive (Figure 24.10) and complicated by the fact that many conditions are risk factors for secondary *Malassezia* dermatitis (compare Figures 24.5 and 24.10).

Fleas
Scabies
Demodicosis
Dermatophytosis
Staphylococcal pyoderma
Atopic dermatitis
Adverse food reaction
Drug reactions
Contact dermatitis
Seborrhoea oleosa
Seborrhoeic dermatitis
Feline acne/facial dermatitis
Acanthosis nigricans
Epitheliotropic lymphoma

24.10 Differential diagnoses for *Malassezia* dermatitis.

Essentially, *Malassezia* should be considered in any *pruritic* dermatitis, particularly if associated with:

- Erythema
- Scaling
- Greasy or waxy exudate
- Hyperpigmentation, or
- Lichenification.

However, identification of *Malassezia* organisms does not preclude the possibility of an underlying condition, nor the need for further diagnostic steps. No agreed diagnostic criteria have been established. Most authors consider demonstration of elevated numbers of organisms, and a good clinical and mycological response to antifungal treatment are diagnostic.

Cytology

Cytology is quick, easy, cheap and non-invasive. Direct impression on to a glass slide is possible on accessible skin; it is helpful if the skin is very moist or waxy. Blunt scalpel blades or cotton swabs can be used to collect waxy exudate from the ears, nail folds, body folds and feet. Tape strips are effective (Figure 24.11), unless the skin is very moist or inaccessible. However, practice and proficiency, rather than technique, is most important.

Slides should be gently heat-fixed (alcohol would remove many of the organisms) and then stained in a modified Wright's stain (such as Diff-Quik®) or methylene blue. The staining solutions should be changed regularly, as yeasts can collect in them leading to false positive diagnoses. Tape strips need not be fixed before staining. Experimenting with locally available adhesive tape may be necessary to find one that resists the stain used.

Slides are initially scanned under low power (X40–X100) to check staining efficiency and to select areas with plenty of squames for closer inspection. *Malassezia* appear as small oval to peanut or snowman shapes, often forming rafts on the surface of squames (Figure 24.12). They most frequently stain blue–purple, but can appear red–pink or pale blue. Some *Malassezia* fail to stain, but their refractile cell wall can be picked out with a closed condenser. Using the oil immersion lens (X1000) is the most accurate way to find *Malassezia*, but with practice they can be easily identified using the dry lens (X400).

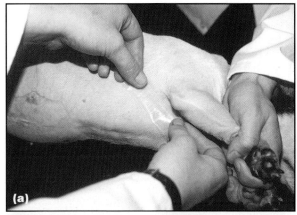

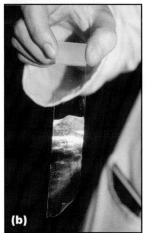

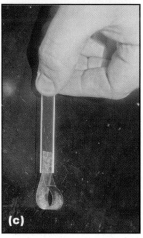

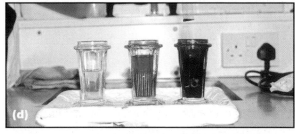

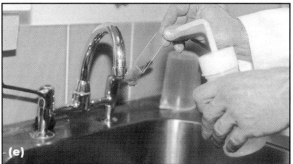

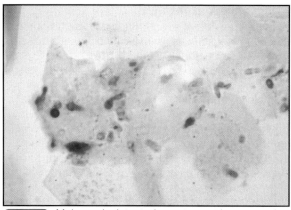

24.12 *Malassezia* detected on a tape strip preparation from the axillae of an atopic dog. The yeasts are seen as red–blue, oval to peanut shapes. The surface squames are large and angular and stain a pale blue–purple. The two small round purple objects at top right are probably staphylococci. (Diff-Quik®; X400 original magnification.)

There is no standard accepted number of organisms needed to diagnose *Malassezia* dermatitis. Estimates of *Malassezia* populations on healthy skin range from <8 yeasts/cm^2 to <1 yeast per high power field (X400). Estimates of clinically significant *Malassezia* numbers range from >2 yeasts per high power field to >10 yeasts per oil immersion field (X1000). It is likely that these figures reflect differences in technique, breed and body sites. Furthermore, *Malassezia* are often found in rafts associated with squames and may not be uniformly distributed across a slide. Hence, an individual's clinical experience and acumen is as important as relying on numbers. The author currently uses a benchmark of ≥5 yeasts per high power field. In practice, only occasional *Malassezia* yeasts are found on healthy skin.

Culture

Malassezia pachydermatis will grow on Sabouraud's medium, although the lipid-dependent species require supplemented media, such as modified Dixon's agar. Samples can be collected by swab or direct contact for quantitative and semi-quantitative culture, although this requires an incubator and supply of sterile media (Bond *et al.*, 1994). Plates should be placed in contact with the skin for 5–10 seconds, then cultured at 32–37°C for 3–7 days. Colonies are small, cream to yellow, dome shaped, smooth to slightly wrinkled, with a regular to slightly lobed edge. However, as *Malassezia* are commensal organisms, isolation is not necessarily significant. Typically, <1 colony forming unit can be isolated from healthy canine skin, but much higher populations can be isolated from the lips and interdigital skin.

Skin biopsy

Malassezia can be present in the overlying keratin crust and hair follicles, but organisms are often removed by processing. *Malassezia* can also be an incidental finding in biopsy samples from other dermatoses. The histopathology of *Malassezia* dermatitis is characterized by acanthosis, hyperkeratosis and a superficial inflammatory infiltrate.

24.11 Tape strip preparation from the axilla of an atopic Jack Russell Terrier. (a) Adhesive tape is pressed firmly against the skin several times. Squames and surface debris stick to the tape. (b) One end of the tape is attached to a glass slide. (c) The free end is attached, forming a loop. (d) If using the Diff-Quik® stain, the loop is dipped five times for 1–2 seconds in solutions 2 (red) and 3 (purple). Fixing in solution 1 is not necessary. Longer staining times may be necessary with older solutions or more material. (e) Excess stain is gently rinsed off. The free end should then be detached and the tape stuck down flat over the slide. Any excess water should be blotted and the tape examined with a microscope.

Response to treatment

Given the uncertainties surrounding the significance of the presence of *Malassezia*, a final diagnosis relies on response to treatment. A favourable response suggests the *Malassezia* were of pathogenic significance. In a study of Basset Hounds with seborrhoeic dermatitis a favourable response was correlated to the reduction in *Malassezia* populations (Bond *et al.*, 1995). However, any response must be interpreted with caution. For example, topical treatment may also eliminate staphylococcal pyoderma (e.g. miconazole/chlorhexidine) or parasites (e.g. selenium sulphide) and systemic treatment may modulate immune responses (e.g. ketoconazole). In some animals, clinical signs are not associated with elevated *Malassezia* numbers, but they do respond to antifungal agents. It is not clear if this response indicates other actions of antifungal agents or an alternative pathogenesis, such as hypersensitivity to *Malassezia*.

Treatment

Several topical and systemic treatment options are available to treat *Malassezia* dermatitis. Treatment should be tailored to the individual case.

Topical therapy

Topical therapy is generally the most cost-effective and safest treatment. However, it is also the most labour-intensive, and therefore not necessarily the most appropriate in all cases. Topical antifungal products include:

- 2% miconazole/2% chlorhexidine shampoo
- 1% selenium sulphide shampoo
- 1–4% chlorhexidine scrubs
- Enilconazole rinse.

Localized areas of *Malassezia* dermatitis (e.g. body folds) can be treated with focal application of an antifungal product, but the whole body should be treated in multifocal or generalized *Malassezia*. It is particularly important to treat the ears, mucocutaneous junctions and feet, as these are likely reservoirs of *Malassezia*. Treatment should be continued daily to three times weekly until resolution, then as necessary to maintain the improvement. Treatment with degreasing shampoos or antibacterial products may also be necessary initially. Adverse reactions are uncommon, although most of the antifungal products can be drying and irritating, and may need to be combined with emollient rinses or shampoos.

Other treatment options include imidazole-containing shampoos, lotions, ointments and creams licensed for medical use (e.g. ketoconazole, clotrimazole etc.). These are not licensed for use in animals in the UK and therefore should only be used if necessary, but the creams can be useful for treating focal lesions. Terbinafine lotion (1%) is effective in human seborrhoeic dermatitis.

Systemic therapy

Where topical therapy is impractical or ineffective, systemic triazole antifungals can be used:

- Ketoconazole   2.5–10 mg/kg orally bid
- Itraconazole   5–10 mg/kg orally sid.

However, these drugs are expensive, not licensed for animals, and can have side effects. Griseofulvin is not effective against *Malassezia*. Clinical improvement should be obvious after 7–14 days, although treatment should be continued for 7–14 days beyond clinical cure. Maintenance doses 2–3 times weekly may be necessary in some cases. Systemic or topical antibacterial therapy may also be necessary.

Side effects can include anorexia, vomiting, diarrhoea and liver damage. Ketoconazole can also be teratogenic. Haematology and serum biochemistry need to be monitored during therapy.

Prognosis

The prognosis with either systemic or topical treatment is very good in most cases. However, unless an underlying cause is diagnosed and treated, it is likely that lifelong maintenance therapy will be necessary. A greater understanding of *Malassezia* dermatitis may allow us to explore targeted treatment of the mucosal reservoir population, immunotherapy or colonization with non-pathogenic strains in the future.

Further reading

Bond, R (2000) Pathogenesis of *Malassezia* dermatitis. *Veterinary Dermatology* **11** (suppl. 1), 5–6

Bond, R, Collin, NS and Lloyd, DH (1994) Use of contact plates for the quantitive culture of *Malassezia pachydermatis* from canine skin. *Journal of Small Animal Practice* **35**, 68–72

Bond R, Elwood CM, Littler RM *et al.* (1998) Humoral and cell mediated responses to *Malassezia pachydermatis* in healthy dogs and dogs with *Malassezia* dermatitis. *Veterinary Record* **143**, 381–384

Bond R, Rose JF, Ellis JW and Lloyd DH (1995) Comparison of two shampoos for treatment of *Malassezia pachydermatis* associated seborrhoeic dermatitis in basset hounds. *Journal of Small Animal Practice* **36**, 99–104

Bond R, Wren L and Lloyd DH (2000) Adherence of *Malassezia pachydermatis* and *Malassezia sympodialis* to canine, feline and human corneocytes *in vitro*. *Veterinary Record*, 454–455

Chang HJ, Miller HL, Watkins N et al. (1998) An epidemic of *Malassezia pachydermatis* associated with colonisation of health care workers' pet dogs. *New England Journal of Medicine* **338**, 706–711

Chen TA, Halliwell REW and Hill PB (2000) IgG responses to *Malassezia pachydermatis* antigens in atopic and healthy dogs. *Veterinary Dermatology* **11** (suppl. 1), 13

Guillot J, Guého E, Chévrier G *et al.* (1997) Epidemiological analysis of *Malassezia pachydermatis* isolates by partial sequencing of the large subunit ribosomal RNA. *Research in Veterinary Science* **62**, 22–25

Morris DO, Olivier NB and Rosser EJ (1998) Type-1 hypersensitivity reactions to *Malassezia pachydermatis* extracts in atopic dogs. *American Journal of Veterinary Research* **59**, 836–841

Nuttall TJ and Halliwell REW (2001) Serum antibodies to *Malassezia* yeasts in canine atopic dermatitis. *Veterinary Dermatology* **12**, 327–332

25

Cutaneous manifestations of systemic infections

Stephen L. Lemarié

Cutaneous lesions are often the initial presenting problem of systemic infections. It is important for veterinary surgeons to recognize distribution patterns and types of cutaneous lesions associated with systemic infections. Although numerous cutaneous lesions have been described, intact and ulcerated nodules, cutaneous ulcers and draining tracts are often associated with systemic infections. When such lesions are identified, it is important to conduct a complete physical examination and diagnostic evaluation in order to establish a definitive diagnosis, an accurate prognosis and a complete therapeutic plan (see also Chapter 8).

Deep systemic mycoses

Blastomycosis

Systemic *Blastomyces dermatitidis* infection affects numerous organ systems. This dimorphic fungus grows as a saprophyte and requires sandy acid soil near water. Blastomycosis caused by *B. dermatitidis* has been identified in Africa and Central America, but is primarily a disease of North America and is endemic to the Great Lakes region and the Ohio, Mississippi and Missouri river valleys. The primary mode of infection is inhalation of spores from mycelial growth. Although an unusual presentation, solitary skin lesions in the absence of systemic disease may be the result of direct inoculation. Large breed male dogs are most commonly infected and cats are rarely infected.

Clinical signs

Cutaneous disease occurs in up to 40% of dogs with blastomycosis. Lesions may present as intact or ulcerated nodules and plaques, subcutaneous abscesses, draining tracts and large firm papules. Clinical signs in dogs can also include lameness, coughing, ocular disease, weight loss and anorexia. Multiple lesions are usually present and can occur in any distribution pattern although the face, nasal planum and digits are commonly affected. Cats can present with similar lesions to dogs, with the digits and footpads often affected.

Diagnosis

Diagnosis should be made by identification of the organism by cytological or histological evaluation.

Cytology: Exudate is collected by fine needle aspiration from intact lesions or from ulcerated or draining lesions. The cytological reaction is composed predominantly of neutrophils and macrophages, and organisms may be numerous to rare depending on the stage of the disease. Organisms are typically round to oval and yeast-like, measuring 5–20 μm in diameter. They will often demonstrate broad-based budding, with a thick refractile double-contoured cell wall.

Serology: Serological testing should be performed to help establish a diagnosis when organisms cannot be identified. The agar-gel immunodiffusion test has a sensitivity and specificity of >90% in dogs. This test is not recommended to monitor response to treatment as antibodies may persist in cured animals.

Histoplasmosis

Histoplasmosis is caused by the soil-borne dimorphic fungus *Histoplasma capsulatum*. The organism grows best in moist humid conditions and nitrogen-rich organic matter such as bat and bird excrement. The free-living mycelial stage produces microconidia, which are the source of infection in dogs and cats. Inhalation of the microconidia is the likely route of infection. Most cases occur in the central USA in the Ohio, Missouri and Mississippi river valleys although the disease is endemic throughout large areas of the temperate and subtropical regions of the world. Histoplasmosis is an uncommon disease in endemic areas.

Clinical signs

Cats are a susceptible host and most cases occur in cats less than 4 years of age. Most affected cats have disseminated disease and clinical signs can include fever, anorexia, weight loss, dyspnoea, ocular disease and depression. Skin disease is uncommon, lesions are usually multiple, can occur anywhere on the body, and can consist of draining tracts, papules, ulcers and nodules. The face, nose and pinnae may be more commonly affected.

Most affected dogs are under 4 years of age. Skin lesions similar to those in cats have been reported in dogs. Unlike cats, most dogs will present with signs of large bowel diarrhoea characterized by tenesmus, mucus and fresh blood in the stool.

Diagnosis

Diagnosis can often be made by cytological evaluation of material collected by fine needle aspiration and exfoliative cytology. Organisms are typically round yeast bodies 2–4 μm in diameter and are often contained within cells of the mononuclear phagocyte system. The inflammatory response is typically granulomatous to pyogranulomatous.

No consistently reliable immunodiagnostic test is currently available for identification of histoplasmosis in dogs and cats.

Cryptococcosis

Cryptococcosis in dogs and cats is caused by *Cryptococcus neoformans*, a saprophytic, yeast-like fungus often associated with the accumulation of pigeon droppings. *C. neoformans* is worldwide in distribution and, unlike other systemic mycoses, the prevalence of cryptococcosis in cats is equal to, or greater than, that in dogs.

Clinical signs

Cats: In cats, the nasal cavity, respiratory tract, skin, central nervous system and eyes are the most commonly affected sites. Skin (Figure 25.1) or subcutaneous lesions are present in up to 50% of feline cases. Cutaneous lesions commonly consist of multiple papules to nodules of varying sizes as well as abscesses, ulcers and draining tracts. Skin lesions can occur anywhere but are most commonly noted on the face, pinnae and paws. Nasal lesions are common in the cat and classically present as a firm to boggy swelling over the bridge of the nose or a fleshy polyplike mass in the nostril. Upper respiratory tract disease is common and may present as sneezing with a unilateral or bilateral mucopurulent, serous or haemorrhagic discharge.

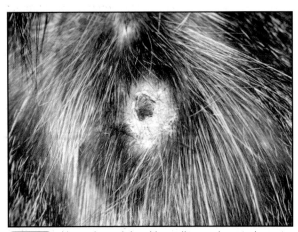

25.1 Alopecic nodule with scaling and central crust formation on the back of a cat with cryptococcosis.

Dogs: In general, cryptococcosis is an uncommon disease in the dog. Approximately 20% of cases will present with skin lesions. Skin lesions may consist of abscesses, nodules, papules, ulcers and draining tracts. Lesions of the tongue, gums and hard palate may be present. Lesions can occur anywhere but are most often found on the lips, nose and digits. The eyes and central nervous system are the other major organ systems commonly affected.

Diagnosis

Diagnosis of cryptococcosis is made by examination of direct smears of exudates or by histopathology. Inflammation is pyogranulomatous to granulomatous, and numerous round-to-elliptical yeast-like organisms, 2–20 μm in diameter, are often present. Organisms typically will display narrow-based budding and a thick clear or refractile halo.

The latex agglutination test, which detects cryptococcal capsular antigen, is a clinically useful serological test and can be used to monitor response to therapy.

Coccidioidomycosis

Coccidioidomycosis is caused by the soil-borne fungus *Coccidioides immitis*. This fungus favours sandy alkaline soil, low rainfall and elevation, and high environmental temperatures. Endemic areas for this organism include areas of Central and South America, Mexico and the southwestern USA. Infection is acquired by inhalation of arthroconidia.

Clinical signs

Abnormal respiratory signs characterized by a dry harsh cough or a moist productive cough will be present in 1–3 weeks after inhalation of the arthroconidia. In dogs, clinical signs can include intermittent fever, weight loss, lethargy, lameness and painful bony swellings, and ocular disease characterized by uveitis, keratitis and acute blindness. Generalized peripheral lymphadenopathy and gastrointestinal disease are uncommon.

Skin lesions are usually multiple and almost always occur over bony swellings. Skin lesions typically consist of nodules, papules, ulcers, draining tracts and abscesses.

Clinical signs in cats are similar to the dog, although respiratory disease is only occasionally recognized. Skin lesions in cats can consist of subcutaneous granulomas, draining tracts and abscesses. Skin lesions are the most frequent manifestation in cats and can occur with or without underlying bony involvement.

Diagnosis

Diagnosis can be made by cytological or histological identification of the organism. The organisms can be present in two forms: the spherule form (20–200 μm in diameter); and the endospore form (2–5 μm in diameter). Spherules can often be found in exudates from draining skin lesions.

Culturing the organism should be limited to laboratories with appropriate biosafety facilities.

If organisms are not identified, serology can be used to aid in confirming a diagnosis. The two most commonly utilized serological tests are the tube precipitin test, which detects primarily IgM, and the complement fixation test, which detects primarily IgG. These tests can be used in both dogs and cats.

Sporotrichosis

Sporotrichosis is caused by the dimorphic fungus *Sporothrix schenckii*. This fungus exists as a saprophyte in soil and organic matter and has a worldwide distribution. In most cases sporotrichosis is acquired via inoculation of the organism into tissues.

Clinical signs

Sporotrichosis can occur in three forms: cutaneous, cutaneolymphatic and disseminated. More than one form may be present in an individual. In dogs, the disseminated form of the disease is very rare. The cutaneous and/or cutaneolymphatic form are most common.

Skin lesions in dogs with the cutaneous form of the disease typically consist of multiple firm nodules and plaques; these lesions favour the head, pinnae and trunk but can occur anywhere. Nodules may ulcerate and form draining tracts.

The cutaneolymphatic form presents as a nodule on a distal limb with subsequent ascending infection via the lymphatics. Secondary nodules associated with regional lymph nodes may also develop. In most cases, skin lesions are not painful or pruritic and dogs are otherwise healthy.

In cats, skin lesions consist of draining puncture wounds and abscesses with cellulitis. Lesions are typically found on the head, distal limbs and tail head and are sometimes associated with cat fight wounds. Lesions may become very exudative with crusting, progressive ulceration and necrosis, which can affect underlying soft tissue. Lymphatic involvement is often not clinically apparent but is frequently present as a necropsy finding. Autoinoculation associated with grooming behaviour can result in the development of additional lesions.

Diagnosis

Diagnosis can be made by cytological or histological identification of the organism. In general, large numbers of organisms will be present in the exudates from cats, compared with very low numbers of organisms present in the exudates from canine lesions. Organisms are cigar-shaped, round or oval and measure 2–10 μm; they can be found within phagocytic cells or extracellularly.

If organisms are not evident by cytological or histological means, lesional tissue can be submitted for culture.

In canine cases, where the organism is not detected and fungal cultures are negative, fluorescent antibody detection can be helpful in establishing a diagnosis.

Because of the zoonotic potential of this organism all individuals handling suspect patients should wear gloves and properly dispose of contaminated material after use.

Zoonotic potential

Blastomycosis: There is no danger from aerosol transmission of the yeast phase. Penetrating wounds contaminated with organisms have produced infections in people. Pulmonary blastomycosis has occurred in laboratory workers exposed to the mycelial form of the fungus.

Histoplasmosis: Direct transmission from animal to human has not been reported. The mycelial form is highly infectious.

Cryptococcosis: The organism from tissues or body fluids does not spread between people or animals. The source of exposure for animals is a potential source of exposure for people.

Coccidioidomycosis: Direct spread from animals to people is very rare. The mycelial form of the fungus is highly contagious.

Sporotrichosis: Transmission of sporotrichosis to people by contact with an infected wound or exudates has been reported. Transmission is much more likely with feline sporotrichosis, presumably because of the large number of organisms found in the tissue and exudates from feline lesions.

Antifungal therapy

Antifungal therapy for deep systemic mycoses typically requires a prolonged course of therapy. Treatment should be continued for 4–6 weeks beyond clinical resolution. Patients with neurological and/or ocular disease have a poorer prognosis for cure. Despite establishing a clinical cure some patients will relapse once antifungal therapy is discontinued and may require maintenance antifungal therapy to keep their disease in remission. Guidelines for antifungal therapy in dogs and cats with deep systemic mycoses are shown in Figure 25.2.

Oomycete infections

Pythiosis

Pythiosis is caused by an aquatic pathogen, *Pythium insidiosum*; this organism is not a true fungus but a member of the protoctistid class Oomycetes. Pythiosis has a worldwide distribution but appears to be most common in wet, tropical and subtropical climates. The disease occurs in dogs but rarely in cats. Infection occurs following exposure to and/or consumption of contaminated water sources. The organism exists as a motile flagellate zoospore in water, and this stage of the organism is attracted to damaged tissue. The zoospores encyst into tissue resulting in penetration and tissue invasion.

Clinical signs

Three forms of pythiosis have been described – gastrointestinal (GI), subcutaneous and nasopharyngeal. Large-breed male dogs are most commonly affected and the GI form of the disease occurs most commonly in the dog. Any portion of the GI tract can be affected and clinical signs will be related to the region of the GI tract affected.

The subcutaneous form of the disease is most often characterized by lesions that present initially with the appearance of an abscess or lick granuloma. These lesions often first appear on the distal limbs. In some cases lesions will progress into large boggy proliferative areas with ulceration and draining tracts. Advanced lesions can be very tissue-destructive and involve underlying soft tissue (Figure 25.3). In some cases lesions will be pruritic.

Disease	Drug	Species	Dose (mg/kg)	Route	Interval	Duration
Blastomycosis	Itraconazole	dog	5	oral	24 hours	60 days
		cat	5	oral	12 hours	60 days
	Fluconazole	dog	5	oral	12 hours	60 days
	AMB lipid complex	dog	1	i.v.	3 times/week	Stop when cumulative dose reaches 12 mg/kg
	AMB	cat	0.25	i.v.	3 times/week	Stop when azotaemic or cumulative dose reaches 4 mg/kg
	AMB	dog	0.5	i.v.	3 times/week	Stop when azotaemic or cumulative dose reaches 4–6 mg/kg, then start azole; or when cumulative dose is 8–10 mg/kg when given alone
Coccidioidomycosis	Ketoconazole	dog	5–10	oral	12 hours	8–12 months
		cat	50 mg total	oral	12–24 hours	12 months
	Itraconazole	dog	5	oral	12 hours	12 months
		cat	25–50 mg total	oral	12–24 hours	12 months
	Fluconazole	dog	5	oral	12 hours	12 months
		cat	25–50 mg total	oral	12–24 hours	12 months
	AMB	dog	0.4–0.5	i.v.	48–72 hours	Until cumulative dose is 8–11 mg/kg
	Lufenuron	dog	5	oral	24 hours	4 months
Cryptococcosis	Flucytosine	cat	30	oral	6 hours	1–9 months
		cat	50	oral	8 hours	1–9 months
	and/or	cat	75	oral	12 hours	1–9 months
		dog	50–75	oral	8 hours	1–12 months
	AMB (deoxycholate)	cat	0.1–0.5	i.v.	3 times/week	Until cumulative dosage of 4–10 mg/kg is reached
		dog	0.25–0.5	i.v.	3 times/week	Until cumulative dosage of 4–10 mg/kg is reached
		cat	0.5–0.8	s.c.	3 times/week	Add each dose to 400 ml of 0.45% saline, 2.5% dextrose to a total cumulative dosage of 8–26 mg/kg
	AMB (lipid complex)	dog	1	i.v.	3 times/week	With lipid complex drug, dose per administration and cumulative dosage may be slightly increased until a cumulative dose of 8–12 mg has been reached
	Ketoconazole	cat	5–10	oral	12 hours	6–10 months
		cat	10–20	oral	24 hours	6–10 months
		dog	5–15	oral	12 hours	6–10 months
		dog	30	oral	24 hours	6–10 months
	Itraconazole	cat	5–10	oral	12 hours	6–10 months
		cat	20	oral	24 hours	6–10 months
	Fluconazole	both	5–15	oral	12–24 hours	6–10 months
Histoplasmosis	Itraconazole	both	10	oral	12–24 hours	4–6 months
	Fluconazole	both	2.5–5	oral	12–24 hours	4–6 months
	AMB	both	0.25–0.5	i.v.	48 hours	Continue until cumulative dose of 5–10 mg/kg is reached in dogs and 4–8 mg/kg in cats
Sporotrichosis	SSKI	dog	40	oral	8 hours	>2 months
		cat	20	oral	12 hours	>2 months
	Ketoconazole	dog	5–15	oral	12 hours	>2 months
		cat	5–10	oral	12 hours	>2 months
	Itraconazole	dog	5–10	oral	12–24 hours	>2 months
		cat	5–10	oral	12–24 hours	>2 months

25.2   Antifungal therapy for selected deep fungal diseases in the dog and cat. AMB = amphotericin B; SSKI = supersaturated solution of potassium iodide

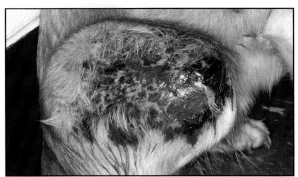

25.3 Large destructive lesion on the lateral thigh of a mixed breed dog with subcutaneous pythiosis.

The subcutaneous and nasopharyngeal forms of the disease are seen less frequently then the GI form in dogs and rarely in cats. Cats will present with similar lesions as the dog but the lesions are typically less destructive and aggressive.

Diagnosis

Cytology: A diagnosis can sometimes be made based on cytological examination: macerated tissue fixed with 10% potassium hydroxide can be evaluated microscopically for the presence of poorly septate, wide and branching hyphal elements.

Histology: Lesions are granulomatous to pyo-granulomatous with numerous eosinophils. Hyphae are typically difficult to see with routine staining and will appear as clear spaces or slightly basophilic material. Hyphae are most numerous in areas of necrosis and are often surrounded by eosinophilic material.

Culture: Tissue samples can be submitted for culture, as *Pythium* spp. will grow on blood agar and Sabouraud's dextrose agar. An indirect immunoperoxidase technique that detects *Pythium* antigen in formalin-fixed paraffin-embedded tissues is also available.

Serology: An ELISA-based serological test with high specificity and sensitivity is available at one laboratory in the USA (Louisiana State University).

Treatment

The prognosis for animals with pythiosis is poor. If possible, early and complete surgical removal of affected tissue can be curative. In general, medical therapy with antifungal agents has been unsuccessful.

Lagenidium infection

Clinical signs

Recently another organism in the class Oomycetes has been identified as a mammalian pathogen. *Lagenidium* spp. has been identified from the tissue of a small number of dogs with subcutaneous disease. These lesions were multifocal in nature, and regional lymphadenopathy was also present. Great vessel disease, pulmonary lesions, mandibular sialadenitis and a hilar mass have also been identified as necropsy findings in dogs with *Lagenidium* infections.

Diagnosis

Histologically, the lesions are characterized by severe eosinophilic granulomatous inflammation centered on poorly septate, broad hyphal organisms. The organism can be cultured on peptone-yeast-glucose medium. Molecular identification, as well as Western Blot/ELISA serology, are also available for *Pythium* and *Lagenidium* organisms.

Mycobacterial diseases

Atypical mycobacteriosis

Aetiology

Atypical mycobacteriosis in cats is most often associated with infections of Runyon group IV mycobacteria including *Mycobacterium fortuitum*, *M. phlei*, *M. smegmatis* and *M. chelonei*. These mycobacteria are non-chromogenic, rapidly growing, Gram-positive, acid-fast, aerobic, non-spore-forming bacilli. Group IV mycobacteria are ubiquitous in nature. Cats appear to be more susceptible than other animals to the development of mycobacterial skin infections, and a history of trauma is usually reported prior to the onset of clinical disease.

Cutaneous disease associated with slow-growing atypical mycobacteria is rare, and most reported cases have described disseminated disease without cutaneous involvement. *Mycobacterium avium* and *M. intracellulare* are the most common disease causing pathogens in this group. Because of similar *in vitro* growth, pigmentation and biochemical characteristics, it is recommended that *M. avium* complex be used when referring to these organisms. These acid-fast slender rods are saprophytes or facultative intracellular organisms. They are classified as Runyon group III, non-chromogens and may require weeks to months for growth in culture.

Clinical signs

Rapidly growing mycobacteria: In the cat, skin lesions associated with rapidly growing mycobacteria are most commonly found over the ventral abdomen and inguinal fat pads. Lesions are characterized by chronic or recurrent fistulous tracts and ulcers as well as purpuric macules and nodules that ulcerate (Figure 25.4). Underlying adipose tissue is thickened, firm and

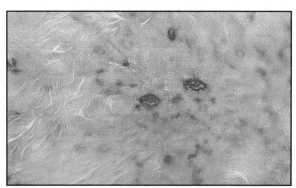

25.4 Ventral abdominal skin of an adult Domestic Long Hair cat, showing swelling, induration, purpuric macules and punctate ulcers characteristic of atypical mycobacteriosis.

nodular on palpation. In some cases large cutaneous defects, which migrate along fascial planes, are present. Most cats are systemically unaffected by their cutaneous disease and disseminated disease is rare.

Rapidly growing atypical mycobacteria infection is a rare cause of skin disease in the dog. Lesions are usually associated with trauma or dog fight wounds. Lesions are characterized by recurrent abscess, draining tracts and non-painful subcutaneous nodules which ulcerate and drain. Although few cases have been reported, the prognosis for remission with medical and surgical management appears to be better for dogs than for cats. Pulmonary and disseminated disease associated with atypical mycobacteria without cutaneous involvement can occur in the dog.

Slow-growing mycobacteria: In the cat, cutaneous involvement associated with *M. avium* complex organisms is rare. Cutaneous lesions in the cat may present as nodules or diffuse subcutaneous swellings. Anorexia, weight loss, lymphadenopathy, splenomegaly and anaemia can occur in cats with the disseminated form of the disease.

Cutaneous lesions associated with *M. avium* in the dog are rare; disseminated disease associated with *M. avium* in the dog has been reported. In general, dogs and cats are relatively resistant to infection by *M. avium* complex organisms.

Diagnosis

Culture: Diagnosis of atypical mycobacterial infections is straightforward if appropriate samples are submitted for culture and sensitivity. *Mycobacterium fortuitum* is most commonly isolated, followed by *M. smegmatis*, *M. phlei* and *M. chelonei*. Exudate from draining lesions will typically result in negative cultures, and organisms are rarely seen on exudate cytology. Lesional tissue samples that include adipose tissue should be submitted for culture and sensitivity testing as well as for histopathology.

Cytology and histology: Cytology of exudate from lesions is typically characterized as pyogranulomatous inflammation. Histopathological findings consist of varying degrees of granuloma formation, pyogranulomatous dermatitis, cellulitis and panniculitis. Acid-fast bacteria are observed in approximately 50% of cases. When organisms are present they are identified in central clear spaces of pyogranulomas. *M. avium* complex organisms are usually present in larger numbers and are more commonly identified on cytology and histopathology compared with the rapidly growing Group IV mycobacteria.

Treatment

Treatment of atypical mycobacterial infections should be based on culture and sensitivity results. The treatment period with antibiotics is typically prolonged and some patients never achieve cure or will relapse once antibiotics are discontinued. Fluoroquinolones and clarithromycin appear to be the best choice for empirical treatment while culture and sensitivity results are pending. Higher than recommended doses have been suggested for fluoroquinolones, although caution should be exercised when administering enrofloxacin to cats as doses above 5 mg/kg have been associated with blindness. Clarithromycin can be administered at 5–15 mg/kg twice daily while culture and sensitivity results are pending. Wide surgical excision of lesions can be helpful although wound dehiscence is common if all affected tissue is not removed.

Feline leprosy

Feline leprosy is a cutaneous granulomatous mycobacterial disease. The prevalence of the disease is higher in colder wet areas of the world such as Canada, northwestern USA, New Zealand, the UK and parts of Australia. Most cases appear to present during the winter months and the majority of cases reported have been in young cats between 1 and 3 years of age. Recently polymerase chain reaction (PCR) techniques have been utilized to identify *Mycobacterium lepraemurium*, the causative agent for rat leprosy, as the cause of feline leprosy. Transmission is thought to occur through the bite of infected rats.

Clinical signs

Lesions are typically single or multiple, firm to soft nodules in the skin and subcutis, most frequently on the limbs, head and trunk. Lesions may be intact or ulcerated. Regional lymphadenopathy is common; however, disseminated disease is rare.

Diagnosis

Diagnosis is made on the basis of clinical findings in conjunction with the presence of large numbers of acid-fast bacilli on histology or cytology and the absence of growth in routine cultures for *Mycobacterium* spp. The organism is very difficult to grow *in vitro*; 1% Ogawa egg-yolk medium at 35°C is recommended if culture is attempted. Cultures should be held for 3 months before being considered negative. Inoculation of infected tissue into rats and mice results in local or disseminated disease and may be helpful in establishing a diagnosis.

Treatment

If possible, excisional surgery is the treatment of choice for feline leprosy. Systemic therapy for feline leprosy has mainly been limited to clofazimine 2–8 mg/kg per day or dapsone 1 mg/kg per day. Neither of these drugs is approved for use in cats. Clofazimine appears to be well tolerated in cats, with reddish-orange skin and adipose tissue discoloration the only major side effects. Dapsone, however, has potential serious side effects in cats, which include blood dyscrasias, hepatic toxicity and neurotoxicities. Cats treated with dapsone should be monitored closely for side effects. Spontaneous remission of this disease is possible.

Canine leproid granuloma syndrome

Canine leproid granuloma syndrome is a poorly characterized mycobacterial syndrome of dogs in which nodular mycobacterial granulomas are present in the skin and subcutis. The pathogenesis of this syndrome is unknown; however, it has been speculated that biting flies may be responsible for inoculating mycobacteria into the skin of susceptible dogs. The syndrome appears to be most common in the New South Wales region of Australia although worldwide distribution is likely.

Clinical signs

The syndrome presents as single or multiple firm nodules which may ulcerate. The nodules appear to be non-painful and are most often found on the head and dorsal surface of the pinnae. Nodules may also occur on the distal limbs and trunk. Affected dogs are not systemically ill and internal organ or lymph node involvement is not a feature of the syndrome.

Diagnosis

Diagnosis of the syndrome is made by submitting nodules for histopathology. Organisms are infrequently identified on cytological examination of material collected by fine needle aspiration of the nodules. Lesions contain variable numbers of acid-fast bacilli surrounded by granulomatous inflammation. Culture and sensitivity of affected tissue should be attempted; however, in all cases cultured in this case series no mycobacterial organisms were isolated. In the case series reported by Malik *et al.* (1998), the majority of cases were from New South Wales, cases were also identified from Western Australia, Queensland, Tasmania and New Zealand. Over 90% of the dogs in this case series were short-coated breeds and approximately half the dogs were Boxers or Boxer-cross dogs.

Treatment

Favourable response to treatment with doxycycline or amoxicillin–clavulanate has been reported; however, some dogs have demonstrated spontaneous resolution of the nodules. A small number of dogs suffered with chronic lesions despite treatment.

Cutaneous tuberculosis

Tuberculosis in dogs and cats has a worldwide distribution; however, the incidence of the disease has decreased with the decline of the disease in humans and cattle. The causative agent is either *Mycobacterium bovis* or *M. tuberculosis*. In the case of *M. bovis*, dogs and cats contract the disease by consuming unprocessed meat or milk. In the case of *M. tuberculosis*, the disease is contracted via airborne transmission from an infected human. Dogs and cats are susceptible to both organisms although a higher incidence of *M. bovis* has been reported in cats.

Clinical signs

The respiratory and digestive systems are primarily affected. Cutaneous involvement is unusual but has been reported. Cutaneous lesions may present as draining tracts, nodules, plaques, abscesses or ulcers. Lesions may be single or multiple and are most common on the head, neck and limbs. Patients are usually systemically ill with fever, weight loss and anorexia.

Diagnosis

Diagnosis is made by history, physical examination, biopsy and culture results. Biopsy specimens show nodular to diffuse pyogranulomatous inflammation with few to many acid-fast organisms. These organisms are slow growers and growth may take up to 8 weeks.

Intradermal skin testing with bacille Calmette-Guérin (BCG) or purified protein derivative (PPD) is not helpful in cats but may be of use in dogs. Intradermal injection with 0.1–0.2 ml of BCG or PPD is best performed on the inner surface of the pinna. Injection sites should be evaluated in 48–72 hours. Resolved erythema at that time indicates a negative test. Severe persistent erythema with central necrosis progressing to ulceration at 10–14 days is significant. Because of the seriousness of the disease and the public health hazard most patients with tuberculosis are euthanased and treatment is usually not recommended.

Leishmaniasis

Leishmaniasis is a protozoal infection caused by numerous *Leishmania* spp. The disease has a worldwide distribution. Most cases in the Old World occur in, but are not limited to, the Mediterranean basin and Portugal. In the New World, the disease is endemic in South and Central America. Endemic foci have been identified in Texas, Oklahoma, Ohio, Michigan and Alabama, and recently in American and English Foxhound kennels in the eastern United States. The disease is transmitted by sandflies of the genus *Phlebotomus* in the Old World and *Lutzomyia* in the New World. Infections are more prevalent in the warmer months when the fly populations are increased. Rodents, domestic and wild, and other mammals can serve as reservoirs for the disease. In the Old World, most cases of canine leishmaniasis are caused by *Leishmania infantum*. In the New World, canine leishmaniasis is often associated with *L. chagasi*.

Clinical signs

The incubation of leishmaniasis is variable and can range from weeks to years. Numerous organ systems can be affected. Most dogs with leishmaniasis have cutaneous involvement; when cutaneous lesions are present, it is presumed that there is also visceral involvement.

Cutaneous lesions in dogs are typically characterized by exfoliative dermatitis with silvery scale. This process can be generalized but is typically most severe over the pinnae, head and extremities. Periocular alopecia is also a common finding. Additional cutaneous manifestations include: nasodigital hyperkeratosis, ulcerative dermatitis, onychogryposis, pustular dermatitis, nodular dermatitis, sterile pustular dermatitis and secondary bacterial pyoderma.

Numerous organ systems can be affected and clinical signs will be associated with the body system affected.

Diagnosis

Serology: Numerous tests, including ELISA, complement fixation and indirect fluorescent antibody tests, are available and will identify the presence of antibodies but do not confirm active disease. PCR amplification of *Leishmania* DNA is available. Peripheral blood can be submitted for PCR; however, lymph node tissue or bone marrow will enhance the detection of subclinical infections.

Cytology and histology: Definitive diagnosis can be made by cytological or histological identification of amastigotes from lymph nodes or bone marrow. Organisms may be free or in macrophages. Skin biopsy changes are variable with nine inflammatory patterns being characterized in dogs with leishmaniasis. Granulomatous perifolliculitis, superficial and deep perivascular dermatitis and interstitial dermatitis are the three most common patterns recognized. Orthokeratotic and parakeratotic hyperkeratosis are usually present, and the cellular infiltrate typically consists of macrophages with lower numbers of lymphocytes and plasma cells.

Treatment

Treatment of canine leishmaniasis may result in a clinical cure but relapses are to be expected. Because of the poor prognosis for cure and the public health hazard, euthanasia is often indicated.

Meglumine antimonite is most often used for treatment of leishmaniasis in dogs. Dosages range from 20–50 mg/kg s.c. twice daily to 200–300 mg/kg i.v. every other day. Clinical cure may be achieved with allopurinol at dosages of 11–15 mg/kg once daily. Combination therapy with allopurinol and meglumine antimonite appears to improve clinical response rates. Immunotherapy with an antigen derived from *L. infantum*, LiF2, in combination with meglumine antimonite has resulted in parasitological cure in some cases.

References and further reading

Greene GE (1998) Mycobacterial infections. pp. 313–325., Fungal infections. pp. 371–402., Miscellaneous fungal infections. pp. 420–423., Protozoal diseases. pp. 450–458. In: *Infectious Diseases of the Dog and Cat, 2nd edn.* WB Saunders, Philadelphia
Grooters AM (2002) New developments in oomycosis and zygomycosis. *Proceedings of 17th AAVD/ACVD Meeting, 2002, New Orleans,* 63–71
Malik R, Love D, Wigney D *et al.* (1998) Mycobacterial nodular granulomas affecting the subcutis and skin of dogs (canine leproid granuloma syndrome). *Australian Veterinary Journal* **76,** 403
Scott DW, Miller WH and Griffin CE (2001) Bacterial skin disease. pp. 312–321., Fungal skin disease. pp. 381–403., Viral, rickettsial, and protozoal skin diseases. pp. 534–538. In: *Small Animal Dermatology, 6th edn.* WB Saunders, Philadelphia

26

Pemphigus

Sandra Merchant

Pemphigus is an autoimmune dermatosis. It is characterized by the formation of anti-keratinocyte membrane autoantibodies that cause loss of adhesion between keratinocytes, leading to intra-epidermal pustule or vesicle formation. In animals, six different forms are distinguished:

- Pemphigus foliaceus
- Pemphigus erythematosus
- Pemphigus vulgaris
- Pemphigus vegetans (panepidermal pustular pemphigus)
- Canine benign familial chronic pemphigus (Hailey–Hailey disease)
- Paraneoplastic pemphigus.

Pemphigus foliaceus is the most common disease of the pemphigus complex in the cat and the dog. However, pemphigus foliaceus is much less common in the cat than in the dog.

Pathogenesis

Our understanding of the pathogenesis of pemphigus has changed dramatically in the last few years with the identification of the classic pemphigus target antigen(s) and their location in the skin and mucosa (Figure 26.1). Several questions raised from clinical observation in pemphigus (e.g. mucosal involvement in pemphigus vulgaris, lack of mucosal involvement in pemphigus foliaceus) have been answered by this target antigen identification. In addition, the entity of paraneoplastic pemphigus has been recognized and its target antigen(s) have also been identified.

Benign familial chronic pemphigus (Hailey–Hailey disease) has been documented in the dog and may have a genetic predisposition. It is an autosomal dominant genodermatosis in humans. The exact pathogenesis has not been determined for the dog. In humans the abnormality is in the desmosomal adhesion complex. Direct immunofluorescent testing is negative but electron microscopic changes include decreased numbers of desmosomes, perinuclear tonofilament aggregation and bizarre cell surface projections resembling microvilli.

Pemphigus vegetans (a deep panepidermal pustular form of pemphigus) has been observed in the dog. Clinically, it resembles pemphigus foliaceus but the course of the disease seems to be more severe and it has different histological features. This cannot be explained on the basis of the epithelial antigens involved as they are identical to those for pemphigus foliaceus.

Paraneoplastic pemphigus has been reported in the dog. In addition to possible cross-reacting antibodies attacking epithelial plakins, it may be that induction of autoimmunity is due to a dysregulated cytokine production by tumour cells. However, plakin-specific autoantibodies are not restricted to canine paraneoplastic pemphigus but can also be seen in pemphigus vulgaris (Olivry et al., 2000).

A multiple-hit hypothesis proposes that signs of pemphigus disease result from the synergistic and cumulative effects of autoantibodies targeting both acetylcholine receptors and desmoglein antigens (Grando, 2000). It can be speculated that this is why nicotinamide may work in treating canine pemphigus foliaceus. Nicotinamide binds to the acetylcholine receptors and could in theory protect the epidermis from the autoantibodies.

Disease	Antigen	Location	Clinical Significance
Pemphigus foliaceus	Desmoglein 1-A desmosomal transmembrane molecule	Superficial keratinocytes	Most intensely expressed in muzzle and ear
Pemphigus vulgaris	Desmoglein 3-A desmosomal transmembrane molecule	Oral, other stratified squamous epithelia	Highest expression in oral cavity, oesophagus, anus
Pemphigus vegetans (panepidermal pustular pemphigus)	Desmoglein 1	?	?
Paraneoplastic pemphigus	Envoplakin and Periplakin: intracellular desmosomal plaque proteins	Intracellular epithelial antigen	Cross-reaction between epithelial and tumour plakin antibodies

26.1 Pathogenesis of pemphigus in dogs and cats.

Both endogenous and exogenous factors have been implicated in the pathogenesis of pemphigus in humans (Marsella, 2000). Endogenous factors recognized include:

- Genetics
- Hormone
- Neoplasms.

Possible exogenous factors are:

- Drugs
- Nutrition (thiol-containing foods)
- Viral infections
- Physical agents (burns, ultra-violet radiation)
- Environmental factors
- Emotional stress
- Contact dermatitis.

Clinical approach

Pemphigus foliaceus

For pemphigus foliaceus in the dog, there is no age or sex predilection. There may be a breed predilection, with Akitas, Chow Chows, Dachshunds, Bearded Collies, Newfoundlands, Dobermanns and Schipperkes predisposed. For pemphigus foliaceus in the cat, there is no apparent age, sex or breed predilection. There are no seasonal or environmental risk factors for either the cat or the dog.

Cats

Cats affected with pemphigus foliaceus usually have lesions that begin on the face or digits (Figure 26.2) The disease may remain confined to the initial sites or it may spread to other locations either rapidly or very slowly over several months. Pruritus is variable. Early lesions consist of erythematous macules that progress through a pustular phase to dry, honey-coloured crusts. The pustules are very often grouped, giving the appearance of large crusted plaques. The lesions may occur in a polycyclic or arciform pattern. Alopecia and increased epilation are frequently found in more chronically affected areas.

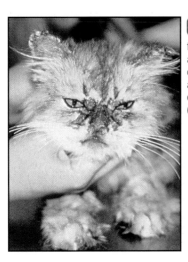

26.2 Feline pemphigus foliaceus: erythema, alopecia and crusting on the pinnae and in a butterfly pattern over the muzzle. (Courtesy of C. Foil)

Lesions can remain localized or can generalize. Localized lesions are commonly seen on the bridge of the nose, the muzzle, the nasal planum, periocular region, the pinnae, area around the nipples, the foot-pads and the nail beds. Systemic manifestations of lymphadenopathy, lameness, pyrexia and depression may be seen, especially with generalized disease. With nail fold disease, the skin may be erythematous, swollen, eroded or crusted. Nail fold lesions may occur alone or in combination with pad disease. Pad lesions include pustules, crusting, scaling and pitting.

Dogs

Three forms of pemphigus foliaceus appear to exist in the dog (Figure 26.3). Pemphigus foliaceus has been seen in dogs from 6 months to 12 years of age. Most dogs develop spontaneous disease between 4 and 5 years of age and require life-long therapy. In drug-induced pemphigus, once the offending agent is discontinued, remission is often lifelong. Chronic disease-associated pemphigus usually develops in older animals, is lifelong and may be more difficult to control.

Type of PF	Clinical associations
Spontaneous	Akitas, Chow Chows predisposed
Drug-induced	Labrador Retrievers and Dobermann Pinschers predisposed?
Chronic disease related?	Long history of chronic skin inflammatory skin disease

26.3 Three putative forms of pemphigus foliaceus in the dog.

The primary lesion in canine pemphigus is a pustule. Early lesions can be erythematous macules that rapidly progress to a pustular stage. The follicular or non-follicular pustules are very fragile and after rupture are replaced by yellow to brown crusts (Figure 26.4). Lesions may begin around the nasal planum and eyes, dorsal muzzle, lip margins and pinnae (Figure 26.5a). The distribution of pustules may be non-truncal which would be just opposite of the truncal pustule distribution seen with staphylococcal folliculitis (Figure 26.5b). The pustules may be seen forming a circular shape on an erythematous base (Figure 26.5c). Nasal depigmentation can be seen.

Slightly over one-third of cases are generalized at the onset; if left untreated, approximately 60% of cases will generalize within 6 months.

Pruritus and pain are variable.

Mucosal and oral lesions are rare. Paronychia is uncommon but hyperkeratotic and fissured foot pads can be seen (Figure 26.6). In some cases, foot pad disease may be the only clinical sign. Severe cases may develop bacterial cellulitis. Alopecia and seborrhoea may be seen in more chronic cases. Lethargy, anorexia, fever and limb oedema may occur.

The disease commonly has a waxing/waning course and waves of pustules can be very acute and dramatic followed by days to weeks of crusting and little activity.

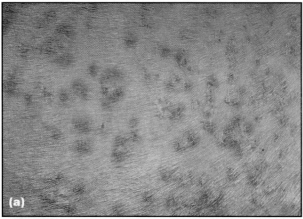
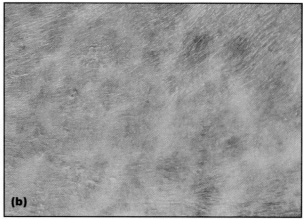

26.4 Canine pemphigus foliaceus. (a) Ruptured pustules with honey coloured crust. (b) Ruptured pustules with honey coloured crusts on an erythematous base.

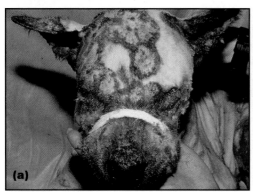
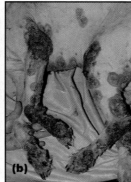
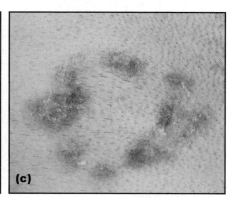

26.5 Pemphigus foliaceus in a Chow Chow. (a) Circular erythematous rings of pustules concentrated on the head. (b) The lesions have a non-truncal distribution. (c) Lesions in a circular configuration that is not seen with staphylococcal folliculitis.

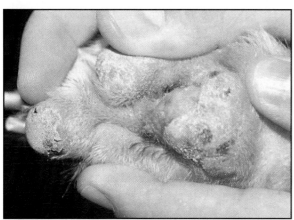

26.6 Canine pemphigus foliaceus: cracked and fissured footpads on a Golden Retriever cross.

Pemphigus erythematosus

Pemphigus erythematosus has been reported in the dog and cat and is classified as a variant of pemphigus foliaceus that is restricted to the head. No age or sex predilection has been noted. Rough Collies and German Shepherd Dogs appear to be predisposed. Dogs with pemphigus erythematosus may have a positive antinuclear antibody titre and positive immunofluorescence at the basement membrane zone.

The clinical signs are characterized by an erythematous pustular dermatitis of the face and ears. As the pustules are fragile, a typical presentation would include crusts, scales, alopecia and erosions (Figures 26.7 and 26.8) Pruritus and pain are variable. The nose frequently becomes depigmented (Figure 26.8b). Depigmentation can be an early sign with pemphigus erythematosus whereas it is a later sign in pemphigus foliaceus. Occasionally skin lesions will be seen on the paws or genitalia.

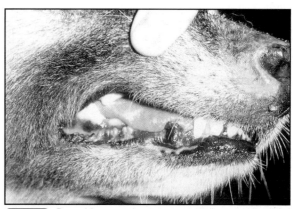

26.7 Pemphigus erythematosus: mild depigmentation around the mouth of a mixed breed dog. (Courtesy of K. Beale)

191

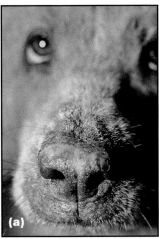

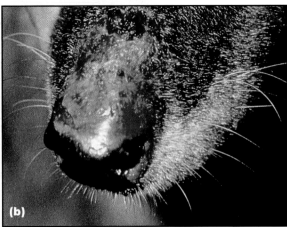

26.8 Pemphigus erythematosus. (a) Crusting and alopecia on the muzzle of a mixed breed dog. (Courtesy of M. Brignac) (b) Nasal and dorsal muzzle depigmentation.

vegetans and pemphigus erythematosus) has been proposed as the name for this extremely rare variant of the pemphigus complex (Wurm *et al.*, 1994). This may be a deep form of pemphigus foliaceus or pemphigus erythematosus.

Paraneoplastic pemphigus

Paraneoplastic pemphigus has been rarely documented in dogs (Walder and Werner, 1996; Lemmens *et al.*, 1998; Carlotti *et al.*, 1999). Clinical signs varied from severe ulcerations and erosions of the oral cavity and skin around orifices and ungual folds, to milder depigmenting and erosive disease of the face, to a pemphigus foliaceus-like syndrome.

Diagnosis

Diagnosis is based on clinical history, physical examination findings, cytology and histopathology. Possible differential diagnoses are shown in Figure 26.9. Adjunctive tests include direct and indirect immunofluorescence testing as well as immunoperoxidase staining. Appropriate diagnostic tests should be run prior to initiation of any anti-inflammatory or immunosuppressive therapy.

Pemphigus vulgaris

Pemphigus vulgaris has been reported in the cat and dog with no age, breed or sex predilection noted. It is a more serious disease than pemphigus foliaceus, as the lesions develop deeper in the epidermis and leave erosions and ulcerations.

It is a vesicular/bullous, erosive to ulcerative disease that may affect the oral cavity, mucocutaneous junctions, skin or any combination. At the time of involvement, 75–90% of animals will have oral cavity lesions and about 50% will have oral cavity involvement as the first clinical sign. Cutaneous lesions occur most commonly in the axillae and groin but pemphigus vulgaris limited to the skin is rare. Ulcerative paronychia and onychomadesis may be the only presenting sign. Pruritus and pain are variable. Systemic signs include anorexia, depression and fever.

Pemphigus vegetans

Pemphigus vegetans has been documented only in the dog. No age, sex or breed predilection has been reported. It is a vesicular/pustular disorder that evolves into verrucous vegetations and papillomatous proliferation.

The most common area affected is the face but other sites can be involved. Oral lesions are not seen. Pruritus and pain are variable. Panepidermal pemphigus (as a pemphigus variant combining pemphigus

---

Pemphigus foliaceus

Pyoderma, dermatophytosis, demodicosis, cutaneous adverse drug reaction, discoid lupus erythematosus, dermatomyositis, other diseases of pemphigus complex, keratinization disorders, sterile eosinophilic pustulosis, linear IgA pustular dermatosis, erythema multiforme, necrolytic migratory erythema, cutaneous T-cell lymphoma, leishmaniasis and zinc-responsive dermatosis

Pemphigus vulgaris

Bullous pemphigoid, epidermolysis bullosa acquisita, linear IgA bullous dermatosis, systemic lupus erythematosus, erythema multiforme, toxic epidermal necrolysis, cutaneous adverse drug reaction, candidiasis, idiopathic ulcerative dermatitis, necrolytic migratory erythema, T-cell lymphoma

Pemphigus erythematosus

Bacterial pyoderma, dermatophytosis, demodicosis, facial pemphigus foliaceus, discoid and systemic lupus erythematosus, dermatomyositis, cutaneous adverse drug reaction, leishmaniasis, zinc-responsive dermatosis.

A differential diagnosis list for nasal depigmentation would include: discoid and systemic lupus erythematosus, cutaneous T cell lymphoma, contact dermatitis, vitiligo, uveodermatological syndrome

Pemphigus vegetans

Bacterial and fungal granulomas, benign familial chronic pemphigus, cutaneous neoplasia

Paraneoplastic pemphigus

Pemphigus vulgaris, bullous pemphigoid, systemic lupus erythematosus, erythema multiforme, toxic epidermal necrolysis, cutaneous T cell lymphoma, adverse cutaneous drug reaction

26.9 Differential diagnoses for the various types of pemphigus.

Cytology

Cytology of an intact pustule (Tzanck preparation) is obtained by puncturing the pustule, expressing its contents on to a glass slide and staining the sample. Cytology reveals non-degenerative neutrophils in a case without a secondary bacterial infection, eosinophils, and few to many acantholytic keratinocytes (epithelial cells from the stratum spinosum or stratum granulosum) (Figure 26.10). Bacteria and degenerating neutrophils indicate a secondary bacterial infection. A few acantholytic keratinocytes can been seen in other diseases, including bacterial folliculitis and dermatophytosis. (Parker and Yager, 1997). Large numbers, rafts or clusters of acantholytic keratinocytes are very suggestive of pemphigus.

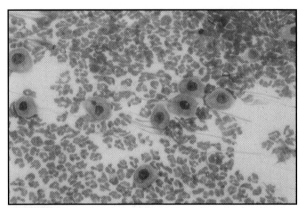

26.10 Acantholytic keratinocytes with a background of non-degenerating neutrophils (Diff-Quik®; X1000 original magnification).

Biopsy

The most important diagnostic tool is the skin biopsy. It is important to obtain several active primary lesions; submission of three or four intact pustules/vesicles is ideal. The biopsy must be performed carefully to avoid rupture. Less ideal is submission of a newly developed crust where acantholytic cells may be seen. A 4 mm punch may be used for very small primary lesions but a 6 mm size is preferred to obtain an intact lesion without rupture. The samples should be placed in formalin for histopathology and sent to a pathologist with an interest in dermatopathology.

Tissue immunohistochemistry can be performed on the skin biopsy sample. Direct immunofluorescence and immunoperoxidase staining are used to differentiate pemphigus foliaceus from pemphigus erythematosus. With improved testing methods, indirect immunofluorescence testing results have become more accurate. In one study, 64.3% of canine pemphigus foliaceus serum samples were positive when bovine oesophagus substrate was used (Iwasaki *et al.*, 1996).

Histopathology

Pemphigus foliaceus: Subcorneal to intragranular pustules can bridge several hair follicles. These pustules are composed of acantholytic epidermal cells, non-degenerating neutrophils and eosinophils (Figure 26.11). The follicular outer root sheath may be included in the acantholytic and pustular process.

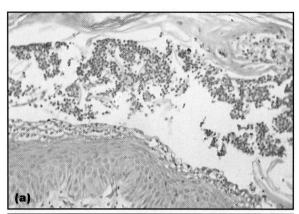

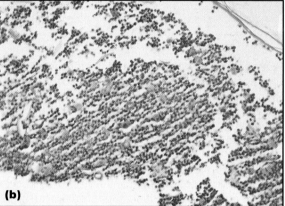

26.11 Pemphigus foliaceus. (a) Subcorneal to intragranular pustule with acantholytic keratinocytes and non-degenerating neutrophils (X400 original magnification). (b) Scattered large pink acantholytic keratinocytes with non-degenerating neutrophils comprising a subcorneal pustule (Haematoxylin and eosin; X1000 original magnification).

Immunohistochemical staining demonstrates intercellular antibody deposition within the upper epidermal layers.

Pemphigus erythematosus: The histopathology in pemphigus erythematosus is identical to that in pemphigus foliaceus except that it can have a lichenoid cellular infiltrate of mononuclear cells, plasma cells and neutrophils or eosinophils or both. Scattered hydropic basal cells and apoptotic epidermal cells can also be seen. Pigmentary incontinence may be a feature.

Immunopathologically, these cases may have a low positive antinuclear antibody titre and basement membrane immunoglobulin deposition as well as intercellular antibody deposition within the upper epidermal layers.

Pemphigus vulgaris: This condition is characterized by suprabasilar acantholysis with resultant cleft and vesicle formation. Basal epidermal cells remain attached to the basement membrane zone, resembling a row of tombstones (Figure 26.12). The dermal inflammatory reaction may be scant and perivascular or prominent and interstitial to lichenoid. Immunohistochemical staining is similar to that for pemphigus foliaceus.

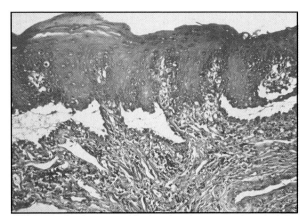

26.12 Canine pemphigus vulgaris: a suprabasal cleft with basal cells at the bottom of the cleft in a 'row of tombstones' (Haematoxylin and eosin; X400 original magnification).

Pemphigus vegetans: This is characterized by papillated epidermal hyperplasia, papillomatosis and intraepidermal microabscesses which predominantly contain eosinophils and acantholytic keratinocytes. Immunohistochemical staining is similar to that for pemphigus foliaceus.

Paraneoplastic pemphigus: This form has suprabasilar intraepithelial acantholysis, keratinocyte necrosis and hydropic degeneration of basal and sometimes suprabasal cells.

Indirect immunofluorescence reveals an anti-keratinocyte membrane staining pattern at all suprabasal layers. Direct immunofluorescence testing has not been performed. In humans, immunofluorescence is positive in the intercellular spaces, with some cases showing granular linear complement deposition along the epidermal basement membrane zone.

Management and therapeutics

Therapy for pemphigus includes the use of glucocorticoids in combination with other immunosuppressive agents. Such combination therapy may yield better results than glucocorticoids alone.

Glucocorticoids

Glucocorticoids may control the signs of pemphigus in approximately 20% of cases at doses that do not cause unacceptable side effects.

An induction dose of 2.2–4.4 mg/kg/day of oral prednisone or prednisolone is used in the dog. Induction doses of prednisone or prednisolone in the cat range from 4.4–6.6 mg/kg/day. Induction doses should be continued until disease remission is obtained. Time to disease remission varies from 2 to 4 weeks in most cases. The steroid dose is then slowly tapered over 8–12 weeks until a maintenance target dose of 1.1 mg/kg every other day in the dog and 2.2 mg/kg every other day in the cat is achieved.

Glucocorticoid pulse therapy in the dog is reserved for the severe case or the patient that has been on intermittent glucocorticoids at lower doses without achieving disease remission. Intravenous methylprednisolone sodium succinate is administered at 11 mg/kg in 250 mg of 5% dextrose in water over a 1–3 hour time period daily for 1–3 days. When remission is obtained, oral glucocorticoid therapy is initiated at immunosuppressive doses and tapered more quickly to the maintenance target dose listed above.

If oral prednisone or prednisolone is not effective alone or in combination, dexamethasone at 0.1–0.2 mg/kg orally bid, tapered to 0.05–0.1 mg/kg every 48–72 hours, or triamcinolone at 0.2–0.3 mg/kg bid, tapered to 0.1–0.2 mg/kg every 48–72 hours, can be used. Triamcinolone may be more effective in the cat in controlling signs of pemphigus but causes significant signs of iatrogenic hyperadrenocorticism in the dog.

Very mild focal lesions may be controlled initially with topical glucocorticoids. Potent topical glucocorticoids such as betamethasone or fluocinolone acetonide should be used until the lesions have resolved and then a less potent topical glucocorticoid, hydrocortisone, should be chosen for long-term maintenance. Problems associated with topical glucocorticoids are usually limited to cutaneous atrophy causing skin that is easily traumatized.

Combination therapy may prolong remission and reduce side effects associated with higher dose glucocorticoid therapy. Drugs commonly used as steroid sparing agents include azathioprine and chlorambucil.

Azathioprine

Azathioprine is used in the dog at a dose of 2–4 mg/kg orally every 24–48 hours. It should be used with caution or not at all in the cat due to the risk of severe bone marrow suppression. The dose of azathioprine is usually not tapered unless bone marrow suppression occurs or when an animal in remission is tapered from daily to every-other-day dosing.

Adverse effects of azathioprine include myelosuppression, pancreatitis and hepatotoxicity. A complete blood count and platelet count should be initially monitored every 2 weeks for 1–2 months and then every 2–3 months. Azathioprine has a slow onset of action, taking 3–6 weeks to produce clinical effects. During the initial portion of the lag phase, induction doses of glucocorticoids should be used. If bone marrow suppression occurs, azathioprine is discontinued until the cellular count returns to normal. Azathioprine can usually be reinstituted at half the original dose.

Chlorambucil

Chlorambucil at 0.1–0.2 mg/kg orally every 48 hours may be used as a steroid sparing agent in the dog and cat. It is most often used in dogs that cannot tolerate azathioprine and is a commonly used steroid sparing agent in the cat. Adverse effects include hepatotoxicity and bone marrow suppression and thus monitoring is similar to that used for azathioprine.

Cyclophosphamide

Cyclophosphamide is another alkylating agent that can be used in the dog and cat in combination with glucocorticoids. The dose is 1.5–2.5 mg/kg orally every 48 hours. Side effects of cyclophosphamide therapy include bone marrow suppression and haemorrhagic cystitis, which tend to limit its use in pemphigus.

Gold salts

Gold salts (chrysotherapy) can be used in the dog and cat as steroid sparing agents or alone to maintain pemphigus in remission after steroids have been tapered and discontinued. They are probably more effective given intramuscularly (aurothiomalate or aurothioglucose) but are also available in an oral formulation (auranofin).

In dogs, aurothioglucose is given at 1 mg/kg weekly i.m. until remission occurs, then once every 2 weeks for several months, and then once every 1–2 months. In cats, aurothioglucose is given at 1–2 mg/kg weekly i.m. or aurothiomalate at 1 mg/kg weekly i.m. until remission occurs, then decreased as for dogs. The lag phase for gold salt therapy may be 2–3 months or more. An increased dose of 2 mg/kg may be needed in some cases. The oral dose is 0.1–0.2 mg/kg sid.

Adverse side effects include hepatotoxicity, bone marrow suppression, thrombocytopenia, cutaneous drug eruption, stomatitis, proteinuria and sterile abscesses. Eosinophilia may precede the occurrence of a cutaneous drug eruption. A complete blood count and urinalysis should be performed every 2 weeks during the first few months of therapy then every few months thereafter. Liver enzymes should be checked monthly initially, then every few months thereafter.

Ciclosporin

Ciclosporin has had limited success in treating pemphigus foliaceus in the dog and cat. The initial induction dose is 20 mg/kg sid. It is tapered to 10 mg/kg every 48 hours once remission is obtained. It is often used in conjunction with glucocorticoids. Side effects include gastrointestinal disturbances, pyoderma, bacteruria, nephrotoxicity, gingival hyperplasia and a papillomatous dermatitis.

Tetracycline and nicotinamide

Tetracycline and nicotinamide (niacinamide in USA) has been used in the dog with variable success. The dose is 500 mg of tetracycline and nicotinamide given orally tid for dogs weighing more than 10 kg and 250 mg of both given orally tid for dogs up to 10 kg. After remission has occurred, the dose may gradually be tapered to once daily.

Adverse side effects in dogs include vomiting, diarrhoea, lethargy, anorexia and increased liver enzyme activity. These side effects are usually attributed to the nicotinamide.

Doxycycline may act as an immunomodulatory drug in the cat and may be tried at 100 mg per 5 kg with or without nicotinamide.

Dapsone and sulfasalazine

Dapsone and sulfasalazine are occasionally used to treat pemphigus.

The dosage of dapsone is 1 mg/kg every 8–12 hours and dosage of sulfasalazine is 22–44 mg/kg tid.

A clinical response should be seen in 4–6 weeks. A limited number of cases have been treated with this drug regimen and minimal responses have been seen.

Potential side effects of dapsone include anaemia, neutropenia, thrombocytopenia, hepatotoxicity, gastrointestinal signs and skin reactions. Sulfasalazine can cause keratoconjunctivitis sicca and tear production should be checked. Complete blood counts and chemistry panels should be performed every 2 weeks for the first 6 weeks and reduced in frequency after the dosage has been decreased.

Mycophenolate mofetil

Mycophenolate mofetil (CellCept®) has been used to treat pemphigus in humans and pemphigus foliaceus in the dog. In the few dogs given mycophenolate mofetil at 22–39 mg/kg/day divided every 8 hours, approximately 50% responded to treatment. No serious side effects were seen. However, all dogs needed concurrent glucocorticoids to control their pemphigus foliaceus (Byrne and Morris, 2001).

In humans, treatment of paraneoplastic pemphigus with normal immunosuppressive agents is routinely unrewarding unless the primary tumour is successfully managed medically, or surgically removed.

References and further reading

Aoki M, Nishifuji K, Amagai M et al. (2000) Distribution and expression of desmosomal proteins, desmoglein 1 and 3 in canine skin and mucous membrane. Veterinary Dermatology 11 (suppl 1), 2

Byrne KP and Morris DO (2001) Study to determine the usefulness of mycophenolate mofetil (MMF) for the treatment of pemphigus foliaceus in the dog. Proceedings of the Annual Members Meeting of the American College of Veterinary Dermatology and the American Academy of Veterinary Dermatology 16, 72

Bystryn JC and Steinman NM (1996) The adjuvant therapy of pemphigus. Archives of Dermatology 132, 203–212

Carlotti DN, Pin D and Buyse S (1999) Concurrent superficial pemphigus and multifocal cutaneous metastatic mammary carcinoma in a dog: a paraneoplastic disease? Proceedings of the Annual Members' Meeting of the American College of Veterinary Dermatology and the American Academy of Veterinary Dermatology 15, 75

Grando SA (2000) Autoimmunity to keratinocyte acetylcholine receptors in pemphigus. Dermatology 201, 290–295

Hertl M (2000) Humoral and cellular autoimmunity in autoimmune bullous skin disorders. International Archives of Allergy and Immunology 122, 91–100

Iwasaki T, Shimizu M, Obata H et al. (1996) Effects of substrate on indirect immunofluorescence test for canine pemphigus foliaceus. Veterinary Pathology 33, 332–336

Lemmens P, deBruin A, deMeulemeester J et al.(1998) Paraneoplastic pemphigus in a dog. Veterinary Dermatology 9(2), 127–134

Marsella R (2000) Canine pemphigus complex: pathogenesis and clinical presentation. Compendium of Continuing Education for the Practicing Veterinarian 22(6), 568–572

Olivry T, Alhaidari Z and Ghohestani RF (2000) Anti-plakin and desmoglein autoantibodies in a dog with pemphigus vulgaris. Veterinary Pathology 37, 496–499

Parker WM and Yager JA (1997) Trichophyton dermatophytosis – a disease easily confused with pemphigus erythematosus. Canadian Veterinary Journal 38(8), 502–505

Robinson ND, Hashimoto T, Amagai M et al. (1999) The new pemphigus variants. Journal of the American Academy of Dermatology 40(5), 649–671

Shanley KJ, Goldschmidt MH, Sueki H et al. (1993) Canine benign familial chronic pemphigus. Advances in Veterinary Dermatology 2, ed. PJ Ihrke et al., pp. 353–365. Pergamon Press, Oxford

Suter MM, Crameri FM, Olivry T et al. (1997) Keratinocyte biology and pathology. Veterinary Dermatology 8(2), 67–100

Suter MM, Ziegra CJ, Cayatte SM et al. (1993) Identification of canine pemphigus antigens. In: Advances in Veterinary Dermatology 2, ed. PJ Ihrke et al., pp. 367–380. Pergamon Press, Oxford

Walder EJ and Werner A (1996) A possible paraneoplastic skin disease with features of erythema multiforme and pemphigus foliaceus in a dog. *Proceedings of the 12th Annual Members Meeting of the American College of Veterinary Dermatology and the American Academy of Veterinary Dermatology* **12**, 70

White SD, Carlotti DN, Pin D *et al.* (2002) Putative drug-related pemphigus foliaceus in four dogs. *Veterinary Dermatology* **13**, 195–202

Wurm S, Mattise AW and Dunstan RW (1994) Comparative pathology of pemphigus in dogs and humans. *Clinics in Dermatology* **12**, 515–524

27

Blistering and erosive immune-mediated skin disease

Aiden P. Foster

The aim of this chapter is to review some of the skin conditions associated with blistering and ulceration that usually involve an aberrant immune response to the basement membrane, blood vessels and (directly or indirectly) the hair follicles. These include, most notably, lupus erythematosus and vasculitis. These conditions are uncommon and can provide a profound diagnostic challenge to the clinician in terms of establishing an underlying cause. The prognosis may vary: some cases resolve spontaneously, while others require life-long immunosuppressive therapy, and some conditions may be fatal. A detailed consideration of the pathogenesis of such diseases is beyond the scope of this chapter and the reader is referred to the textbook by Scott *et al.* (2001) and to the references cited.

Discoid (cutaneous) lupus erythematosus

Human discoid lupus erythematosus

Human DLE is a chronic and relatively benign form of cutaneous lupus, with coin-shaped, indurated, erythematous, scaly, alopecic skin lesions with follicular plugging, most frequently involving the face. The term 'wolf' is associated with the reddened, gnawed appearance of the circumscribed or discoid lesions. The lesions vary in size and appearance but are usually well defined patches and plaques. Marked hyperkeratosis may be associated with wart-like lesions. Some lesions have peripheral hyperpigmentation with central hypopigmentation and central atrophy. There may be tumid lesions associated with reticulate telangiectasia, chillblains, nail changes and intraoral lesions (Rowell and Goodfield, 1998).

The histological findings usually include: hyperkeratosis with follicular plugging; epidermal atrophy or acanthosis; colloid bodies (homogenous eosinophilic staining of individual keratinocytes undergoing apoptosis); vacuolar alteration at the dermoepidermal junction; and an infiltrate composed primarily of lymphocytes, which is dense at the epidermal–dermal interface and also present in the superficial and deep dermis and adjacent to the periadnexal structures. Additionally, DLE is associated with basement membrane thickening and increased mucin in the dermis (David-Bajar and Davis, 1997; Sontheimer, 1997).

Sontheimer (1997) reviewed the far from settled debate about the classification of human lupus erythematosus (LE), particularly the cutaneous manifestations. These manifestations may be LE-specific or non-specific. The former are subdivided into acute, subacute and chronic cutaneous lupus erythematosus (A/S/CCLE). Cutaneous disease may or may not be present with systemic LE (SLE). Human DLE is a form of CCLE.

Canine discoid lupus erythematosus

There has been discussion about the appropriateness of using the human-derived DLE disease terminology in dogs with an apparently photosensitive dermatosis that usually involves the nasal planum, with histological changes of a lymphoplasmacytic interface dermatitis, in a lichenoid and/or hydropic pattern. The histological changes are not specific for lupus (they may also be seen with gingival inflammation, mucocutaneous pyoderma, pemphigus foliaceus and pemphigus vulgaris). The changes may also include pigmentary incontinence, hydropic degeneration of basal keratinocytes, apoptotic keratinocytes, thickening of the basement membrane and a dermal infiltrate of mononuclear and plasma cells around the blood vessels and adnexal structures. These differences in histological findings and clinical signs have led to the proposal that the term cutaneous lupus erythematosus (CLE) should be used instead of DLE where there are signs typical of (photosensitive) cutaneous lupus with a predominantly nasal location in the dog.

Other forms of CLE may include German Shorthaired Pointer lupoid dermatosis, also termed exfoliative CLE (ECLE), and ulcerative disease of Shetland Sheepdog and Rough Collie (UDSSC), a vesicular variant of CLE, formerly considered a severe form of dermatomyositis (Vroom *et al.*, 1995; Jackson and Olivry, 2001). It remains unclear where idiopathic symmetrical lupoid onychodystrophy fits into this classification system (see Chapter 16).

The pathogenesis of cutaneous lupus erythematosus is thought to involve autoreactive T cells that stimulate B cells to produce antibodies to a variety of nuclear proteins. Ultraviolet light may initiate the process of expression on keratinocytes of autoantigens through apoptosis and the secretion of chemoattractants for lymphocytes. Antibodies are deposited at the basement membrane, and epidermal basal cells are damaged, leading to subepidermal vesicle formation and immune complex deposition at the basement membrane zone (BMZ) (Casciola-Rosen and Rosen, 1997).

DLE is considered to be one of the most common autoimmune skin conditions in the dog and particularly seems to affect long-nosed breeds including Rough Collies and the German Shepherd Dog. The clinical lesions of canine DLE may include, initially, erythema, depigmentation and scaling with the loss of the cobble-stone appearance of the nasal planum. The black nasal planum may change to a grey/white colour. The lesions usually occur on the junction between the nasal planum and haired skin, the alar folds, and may spread to involve the dorsal aspect of the muzzle. Lesions may also be seen in the mouth, and on the pinnae and genitalia. As the lesions evolve, erosions, ulceration and crusting develop (Figure 27.1). In severe cases nasal bleeding may develop.

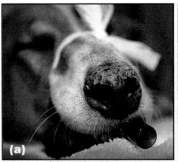
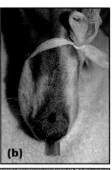
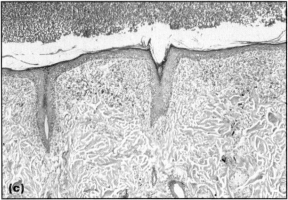

27.1 CLE (DLE) in a 5-year-old Rough Collie bitch. (a) Typical crusting, ulceration and depigmentation of the nasal planum. (b) Alopecia and scaling of the muzzle. (c) Histology shows typical intense lymphoplasmacytic interface dermatitis. (H&E; x40 original magnification).

Diagnosis
Differential diagnoses for DLE include:

- Cutaneous lupus erythematosus
- Pemphigus foliaceus/erythematosus
- Infectious folliculitis: staphylococci, dermatophytosis/furunculosis including demodicosis/sterile eosinophilic furunculosis
- Epidermotropic lymphoma, also called cutaneous T cell lymphoma
- Drug reaction
- Trauma
- Contact dermatitis
- Uveodermatitis
- Dermatomyositis.

Diagnosis is usually achieved after ruling out infectious and parasitic causes with deep skin scrapes and hair plucks looking for *Demodex* mites, hair plucks for dermatophyte culture and skin cytology looking for secondary bacterial involvement. A general anaesthetic is preferable to sedation for the potentially bloody task of collecting a variety of biopsy samples for histological evaluation. Skin tissue could also be submitted for fungal and bacterial culture. Serological tests such as anti-nuclear antibody (ANA) are usually negative.

Treatment
Please refer to Chapter 26 for detailed information about immunosuppressive drug therapy for immune-mediated skin disease. Current therapy includes:

- Topical glucocorticoids bid
- Topical ciclosporin (1% or 2% ointment or solution, applied sparingly, bid or tid, for 1–2 months)
- Topical tacrolimus (under investigation)
- Topical sunblockers (see Chapter 29)
- Vitamin E 400–800 mg/day (400–800 IU/day); side effects may include anorexia, so should be administered 2 hours before or after feeding
- Essential fatty acids
- Niacinamide and tetracycline.

Topical therapies are often difficult to apply effectively because the dog will lick its nose and remove the treatment. Vitamin E and essential fatty acids seem to work in some cases and should be administered for 6–8 weeks to take full effect. There is the potential for the condition to wax and wane slightly, giving the impression that there has been a response to therapy. In severe cases, especially where there is nasal bleeding, one should consider immunosuppressive therapy. Niacinamide (nicotinamide) is difficult to obtain as a 500 mg tablet in the UK so it may be worth contacting a referral dermatologist for sources of such medication. The attraction of all of the above therapies is the low potential for adverse side effects. For details on oral glucocorticoids, azathioprine and chlorambucil see Chapter 26.

Nasal flap plastic surgery is an option for extreme cases.

Feline cutaneous (discoid) lupus erythematosus
While DLE is well recognized as a dermatological entity in dogs, it is rarely reported in cats. There is no apparent age, sex or breed predisposition.

Clinical signs consist of periocular crusts, erythema, vesicles and papules on the pinnae, and scaling and crusting of the footpads with focal depigmentation. The nasal planum may be affected by depigmentation, ulceration and crusting. There may be plaque-like erythematous excoriations involving the pinnae, neck, abdomen and groin; or generalized crusting and scaling.

Skin biopsies may show histological changes of an interface dermatitis with hydropic degeneration of basal cells, a mononuclear infiltrate with positive immunofluorescence for IgM and complement. ANA titres are low.

Treatment may consist of oral prednisolone or dexamethasone or injectable methylprednisolone. One case has been reported which developed signs consistent with systemic lupus erythematosus (SLE) (Willemse and Koeman, 1989).

German Short-haired Pointer lupoid dermatosis

This is a rare condition limited to the breed. Cases have been identified in the UK, Europe and USA. Clinical signs are recognized early in the first year of life. An inherited predisposition is suspected.

Clinical signs may wax and wane, and include a generalized exfoliative dermatosis that may also include a bacterial folliculitis (Figure 27.2). There is no sex predisposition.

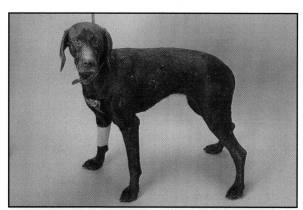
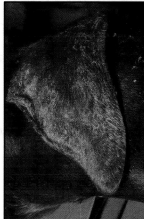
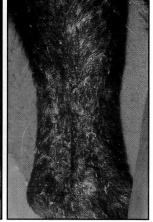

27.2 Exfoliative CLE (ECLE) or German Short-haired Pointer lupoid dermatosis in a 2-year-old bitch with generalized marked fine scaling on the trunk, muzzle, pinna and medial hock.

ANA tests are negative. Histological findings include a lymphocyte-rich interface dermatitis indicative of a lupoid condition and leading to the term exfoliative CLE (ECLE). Therapeutic options are limited but may include essential fatty acids and bathing with anti-seborrhoeic agents.

Ulcerative disease of Shetland Sheepdog and Rough Collie (UDSSC)

This is a rare condition limited to these two breeds and formerly considered a variant of dermatomyositis (see Chapter 11). The underlying pathogenesis is poorly understood. It is considered to be a vesicular variant of CLE (Jackson and Olivry, 2001). Young to middle-aged dogs of either sex develop an ulcerative dermatosis involving the ventral abdomen, axillae, groin and medial thighs. The condition can wax and wane. The ulcerations may be influenced by ultraviolet light and can be serpigenous, annular and polycyclic.

There are no distinct clinicopathological findings; ANA titres are negative. Histological findings are distinctive with a lymphocyte-rich interface dermatitis and folliculitis, and vesiculation of the dermo-epidermal junction.

Therapy options may include glucocorticoids, azathioprine, niacinamide and tetracyclines, vitamin E and pentoxifylline (Figure 27.3) but the condition is difficult to manage.

- Methylxanthine derivative and phosphodiesterase inhibitor
- Rheological and immunological properties, minimal cardiac effects
- Has immunomodulatory properties, including the inhibition of the pro-inflammatory cytokines TNF-α, IL-1, IL-12 and IFN-γ and upregulation of anti-inflammatory IL-10
- Stimulates wound healing: improved via stimulation of collagenase production
- Interferes with adhesion of inflammatory cells to endothelial cells and keratinocytes. This decreases the infiltration of inflammatory cells, especially neutrophils, into inflamed skin
- Decreases blood viscosity by inhibition of platelet aggregation
- In small animal skin diseases it has been used in vasculitis syndromes, contact allergic dermatitis, erythema multiforme, dermatomyositis and ulcerative dermatitis syndrome of the Rough Collie. It has been used anecdotally in a number of other canine skin diseases
- The optimal dose is unknown but may be of the order of 10–15 mg/kg bid or tid in dogs (supplied as a 400 mg tablet); with food if necessary
- Side effects are not commonly reported

27.3 Properties and uses of pentoxifylline (see Marsella *et al.*, 2000).

Systemic lupus erythematosus (SLE)

Canine systemic lupus erythematosus

SLE is a rare disease in the dog and has been the subject of numerous investigations since it was first documented in 1965 (Lewis *et al.*, 1965; Chabanne *et al.*, 1999a,b; Scott *et al.*, 2001).

Clinical signs

Canine SLE is a rare multisystemic autoimmune disorder which most frequently involves the musculoskeletal, haematopoietic, cutaneous and urinary systems. The following list of criteria is based on that proposed by Scott *et al.* (2001), which is adapted from the criteria of the American Rheumatism Association and Chabanne *et al.* (1999b). Four of these criteria must be met in order to establish a diagnosis of SLE:

- Polyarthritis: non-erosive
- Renal nephropathy: proteinuria

- Dermatopathy including one of:
  - erythema
  - discoid rash
  - photosensitivity
  - oral or nasopharyngeal ulceration
- ANA serology positive
- Haematological abnormalities: anaemia, thrombocytopenia, leucopenia
- Immunological disorders including, for example, changes in numbers of CD4+ and CD8+ T cells
- Neurological disorders: seizures/psychosis
- Serositis: pericarditis and/or pleuritis.

Other signs that may be present include polymyositis, fever, pneumonitis, generalized peripheral lymphadenopathy and lymphoedema. Cutaneous findings may be variable, generalized or localized, including seborrhoea, alopecia, erythema, vesicles and bullae, footpad ulcers and hyperkeratosis, refractory secondary bacterial pyodermas, panniculitis and nasal dermatitis.

Diagnosis

In view of these numerous signs, SLE presents a major challenge in terms of establishing a diagnosis. Samples for haematology, serum biochemistry, urinalysis, serum ANA, Coombs' antibody test, bone marrow aspirate, lymph node biopsy, joint aspirate, radiography, bacterial and fungal cultures, skin biopsy and skin scrapes may be required to rule out the numerous differential diagnoses potentially associated with the cutaneous and other signs.

The classical cutaneous histological features include a lymphocyte-rich lichenoid and/or hydropic interface dermatitis which may involve the hair follicles. There may also be vasculitis, panniculitis, subepidermal clefting, thickening of the basement membrane and intrabasal to subepidermal vesicle formation. Canine SLE may be associated with LE non-specific diseases including bullous SLE (subepidermal vesicles and blisters) and pemphigus foliaceus. Immunohistochemical (IHC) staining methods may reveal deposition of immunoglobulin and/or complement at the basement membrane zone. Such IHC staining, however, is like ANA serology in that positive results are not specific and do not allow a definitive diagnosis to be made.

Treatment

If there is no evidence for an underlying disease cause in the SLE complex, immunosuppressive therapy must be relied upon to control the disease. Glucocorticoids, azathioprine, gold salts, cyclophosphamide, chlorambucil, niacinamide and tetracyclines could be considered (Chabanne et al., 1999b; Scott et al., 2001). See Chapter 26 for details of dosages for treatment of immune-mediated skin disease.

Feline systemic lupus erythematosus

SLE is a rare disease in the cat with similar systemic signs to canine SLE. Cutaneous manifestations of feline SLE are exceptionally rare and may include generalized seborrhoea, exfoliative erythroderma, alopecia, scaling and crusting involving the face, pinnae, neck (Figure 27.4), ventrum and limbs, and crusting of all digital pads.

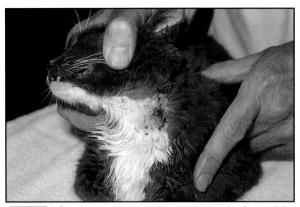

27.4 Crusting and ulceration on the neck of an adult Domestic Shorthair diagnosed with systemic lupus erythematosus on the basis of a positive antinucleur antibody test, thrombocytopenia and Coombs' test-positive non-regenerative anaemia. (Courtesy of C Foil.)

The histological features may include interface dermatitis, and interface folliculitis, epidermal basal cell and follicular basal cell vacuolation with necrosis. Evidence of the immunological basis for the latter changes is lacking in the cat. In addition, there is often immunohistochemical evidence of immune complex deposition at the basement membrane zone (BMZ).

Glucocorticoid therapy with 4 mg/kg per day for 1 month initially was effective in establishing control of one case with a positive ANA titre, oral ulceration, thrombocytopenia and typical cutaneous changes (Vitale et al., 1997).

Vasculitis

Vasculitis is inflammation of a blood vessel wall. It may be primary, or secondary to inflammation, infection, neoplasia, drugs or, especially, vaccination (see Box 27.1). There is accumulation of cells within the vessel wall, injury with necrosis and degeneration of endothelial and smooth muscle cells, and fibrin deposition. The cells that predominate may include macrophages, neutrophils and lymphocytes. Eosinophils may be seen, with necrosis of collagen and smooth muscle. Some vasculitides are cell-poor and some are granulomatous. Neutrophilic forms may be leucocytoclastic where neutrophil nuclei undergo pyknosis and karyorrhexis leading to nuclear dust. Fibrinoid necrosis may be present: an association of complement, fibrin, immunoglobulins and platelets, within the vessel wall and lumen, appearing as an eosinophilic mush. Such histological findings are frequently transient and are followed by signs of a vasculopathy where tissue changes suggest vascular compromise. There may be dermal oedema, collagen smudging, hair follicle atrophy, degeneration of vessel walls, perivascular cuffing with mononuclear cells. However, the term vasculopathy may also be applied to thromboembolic accidents and to occlusion of vessels with fibrin thrombi associated with sepsis and vascular toxins.

In human medicine there has been considerable debate about the definition of systemic vasculitides, particularly primary systemic vasculitis syndromes. The classification of such syndromes is based on size and location of vessels and the results of immuno-histochemical studies, which implicate a variety of immune mechanisms including allergic (IgE type 1 hypersensitivity), antibody-mediated including anti-neutrophil cytoplasmic antibodies (ANCA), immune complex formation and granulomas (Gross *et al.*, 2000).

In veterinary medicine few primary systemic vasculitides are recognized. One example is a multisystemic necrotizing vasculitis of small vessels in Beagles, called juvenile polyarteritis syndrome (JPS). Secondary vasculitides have been associated with the causes shown in Figure 27.5 (not intended to be a complete list).

Infections
Bacterial, including endocarditis (e.g. *Staphylococcus intermedius*) Mycobacterial Fungal Viral (e.g. FIP, FeLV, FIV, parvovirus) Protozoal (e.g. *Leishmania*) Rickettsial (e.g. Rocky Mountain Spotted Fever, *Ehrlichia*, *Borrelia*) Sarcocystosis
Vaccination
Rabies Allergen immunotherapy Sera
Drugs
Anti-infectious (e.g. Fenbendazole, Itraconazole, Ivermectin, Metronidazole) Enalapril Furosemide Imodium Metoclopramide Phenobarbital Phenylbutazone
Allergies
Food Insects and other arthropods Eosinophilic granuloma Severe scabies Flea hypersensitivity
Immune-mediated
SLE DLE Rheumatoid arthritis
Other
Plasma cell pododermatitis Malignancies Ulcerative colitis JPS of Beagles
Idiopathic
50% of all cases are idiopathic

27.5 Some causes of secondary vasculitis.

Cutaneous vasculopathies are usually secondary to an underlying process in which the small vessels, especially the post-capillary venules, are the focus of the disease process. There are several distinct cutaneous syndromes in dogs that are considered to be forms of vasculopathy, including a proliferative thrombovascular necrosis of the pinnae, familial cutaneous vasculopathy of the German Shepherd Dog, and cutaneous and renal glomerular vasculopathy of the Greyhound. Another syndrome associated with vasculitis is neutrophilic leucocytoclastic vasculitis of Jack Russell Terriers (Parker and Foster, 1996). Alopecia and focal crusting are observed on distal extremities and bony prominences. Histological changes include dermal oedema, leucocytoclastic vasculitis and ischaemic degeneration of hair follicles (Nichols *et al.*, 2001; Affolter, 2000).

Vasculitis is rarely reported in cats. Clinical signs may include ulceration of the footpads, pinnae and the lips. Anecdotally there have been associations with feline leukaemia virus, vaccine injection-site reactions and drug reactions, including topical flea products.

Clinical signs

- Skin affected in dependent areas and extremities, especially the paws (including sloughing pads (see Chapter 15), claws, pinnae, face (Figure 27.6), lips, tail, scrotum and oral mucosa
- Purpura (Figure 27.7), macules, plaques, haemorrhagic bullae, papules, pustules, necrosis, ulcers, acrocyanosis
- Oedematous plaques, urticaria, lymphoedema, pain, erythema
- Septal vasculitis and panniculitis
- Pitting oedema of limbs, ventral trunk, head and scrotum
- Anorexia, depression, pyrexia, pain, pruritus
- Polyarthropathy, myopathy, neuropathy, hepatopathy, thrombocytopenia, anaemia, lymphadenopathy.

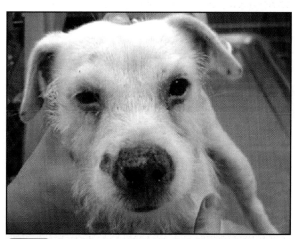

27.6 Facial lesions of erosions and alopecia associated with vasculitis in a young Jack Russell Terrier. (Courtesy of C Foil.)

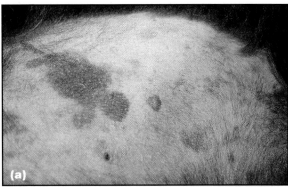

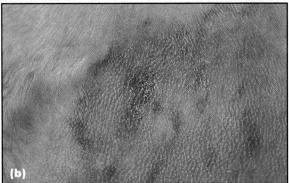

27.7 (a) Purpuric macules in a dog with idiopathic leucocytoclastic vasculitis. (b) Figurate purpuric erythema in a dog with idiopathic systemic vasculitis. (Courtesy of C Foil.)

Once the clinical examination has suggested a vasculitis process, one may consider the following classification system proposed by Outerbridge (outlined in Affolter, 2000):

- Infectious
- Non-infectious:
  - Exogenous antigens – drugs, food additives, vaccines (Box 27.1)
  - Endogenous antigen – neoplasia, connective tissue diseases (SLE)
  - Unknown – define by blood vessel size, type and location; by inflammatory infiltrate.

This may help the clinician to establish an underlying cause with appropriate diagnostic tests.

Diagnosis

Differential diagnoses for cutaneous vasculitis may include cold agglutinin disease, disseminated intravascular coagulation (DIC), coagulopathy, SLE, lymphoreticular neoplasia and frostbite.

Vasculitides in veterinary medicine are a diagnostic challenge: small blood vessel damage is a consequence of a variety of disease processes where the immune system targets blood vessel walls. True vasculitis is often a transient process followed by more chronic changes often termed vasculopathy. The diagnosis usually relies upon carefully collected skin/organ/lymph node biopsies and appropriate histological findings.

Blood samples may show lymphopenia, leucocytosis with left shift, eosinopenia, leucopenia, neutropenia, monocytosis, normochromic normocytic

Box 27.1: Canine ischaemic dermatopathy/folliculopathy

An ischaemic dermatopathy is characterized by changes in the hair follicles and dermal collagen associated with a vasculitis or vasculopathy. Histological findings may include an interface mural folliculitis, cell-poor interface dermatitis, attenuated (or faded) hair follicles and vasculopathy. The clinical signs may include alopecia, erosions or ulcerations with crusting and hyperpigmentation. The lesions may be due to a combination of immune-mediated destruction or ischaemic alteration of hair follicles secondary to a vasculopathy. Three forms are recognized.

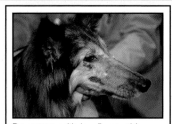

Dermatomyositis in a 5-year-old Shetland Sheepdog bitch, showing focal alopecia and erosions.

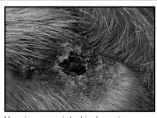

Vaccine-associated ischaemic dermatopathy. (Courtesy of C Foil.)

Dermatomyositis
This is described in Chapter 11; see Ferguson *et al.* (2000) for case reports.

Post-vaccine vasculitis
This is an uncommon but well recognized alopecic condition, primarily reported in the USA and associated with the administration of routine vaccines, especially rabies vaccines (Vitale *et al.*, 1999). Clinical signs are usually localized to the dorsal interscapular region. Histological findings usually include lymphocyte inflammation and vasculitis in the deep dermis and panniculus at the injection site. Complete surgical excision is indicated.

Post-vaccination ischaemic dermatopathy
An idiopathic ischaemic dermatopathy has been recognized with similar histological findings to dermatomyositis and post-vaccine vasculitis. The cutaneous lesions are generalized and are not limited to any particular age or breed. Lesions are particularly found on pinnal margins, bony prominences, pads, tail tip and periocular regions. In some cases lesions have developed after the administration of a rabies vaccine. This condition may respond to pentoxifylline and vitamin E.

anaemia and thrombocytopenia. Results may include increased serum liver enzymes and triglycerides, hypoalbuminaemia, hyperglobulinaemia and hyperfibrinogenaemia. Despite an exhaustive investigation for an underlying cause of the vasculitis/vasculopathy, many cases prove to be idiopathic.

Therapeutic options

If there is no evidence for drugs, neoplasia, infection or immune-mediated disease as the underlying cause, one is left with a variety of therapeutic modalities. The outcome is dependent upon the organs affected and removal of underlying factors. Glucocorticoids have been the mainstay of treatment, using immunosuppressive doses. Alternative therapies may include pentoxifylline (see Figure 27.3), sulfasalazine and dapsone.

Sulfasalazine is reduced to 5-aminosalicylic acid and sulfapyridine. It inhibits oxygen radical-mediated damage by neutrophils and polymorphonuclear leucocyte chemotaxis via downregulation of integrins. Side effects include keratoconjunctivitis sicca and hepatopathy. Dapsone has a variety of proposed effects, particularly the chemotaxis of neutrophils. It is not licensed for use in the dog, and side effects may include blood dyscrasias and thrombocytopenia.

Dapsone and prednisone have been reported to be effective in the treatment of neutrophilic leucocytoclastic vasculitis of Jack Russell Terriers.

In view of the rarity of vasculitis it should be no surprise that there is limited evidence (i.e. from clinical trials) for a beneficial response to these drugs. The mainstay of therapy has been steroids and, in some cases, sulphonamides, but these are often associated with marked side effects.

Erythema multiforme

Erythema multiforme (EM) is an uncommon disease in dogs. As the name suggests the clinical presentation can be variable. In humans it is associated with drug administration, viral diseases and neoplasia. Hinn *et al.* (1998) reviewed the human literature and a series of canine cases of EM and toxic epidermal necrolysis (TEN). In their proposed classification EM was associated with flat or raised, focal to multifocal, target or polycyclic lesions with EM minor (EMm) associated with up to one mucosal surface and EM major (EMM) associated with more than one mucosal surface. There were no distinct histopathological changes to distinguish EMm from EMM or TEN, and previous drug therapy was not associated with EM of either type.

The pathogenesis of the disease in the dog is considered to involve a variety of mechanisms including the upregulation of the expression of MHC II, CD44 and ICAM-1 adhesion molecules on keratinocytes. There are CD8+ T lymphocytes recruited to the epidermis and dermis and these are thought to be responsible for the apoptosis of epidermal and follicular keratinocytes which is a characteristic feature of EM (Affolter *et al.*, 1998).

Clinical approach

In a review by Scott and Miller (1999), the clinical signs observed in the dog included vesiculobullous and/or ulcerative lesions in most cases and maculopapular eruptions in others. The distribution involved the ventrum (especially the axilla and groin), mucocutaneous junctions, oral cavity and footpads (Figures 27.8 and 27.9). There appears to be no age or sex predilection. There may be a particular association with drugs, especially antibiotics and potentiated sulphonamides, but this is usually presumed in veterinary patients because provocative testing is rarely done. Drug-mediated disease may become apparent within 3 weeks of administration and resolve within a similar time frame. Many cases of EM are idiopathic and resistant to therapy.

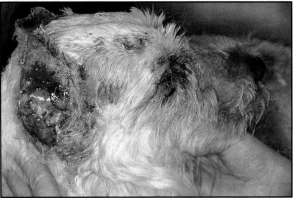

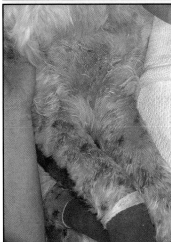

27.8 Generalized erythema multiforme, with no apparent underlying cause, in an 8-month-old female Bouvier des Flandres. The dog died from *Pseudomonas* septicaemia.

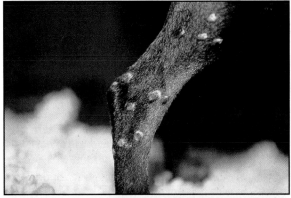

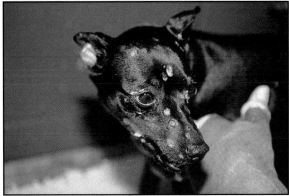

27.9 Idiopathic erythema multiforme in a one-year-old male Miniature Pinscher. There are multiple focal scaling nodules. Histological changes were consistent with EM. No apparent cause was identified and the lesions resolved spontaneously.

Erythema multiforme (EM) is a very rare disease in the cat and is usually associated with drug administration, particularly cefalexin, amoxicillin, penicillin, griseofulvin, aurothioglucose and sulfadiazine. Clinical signs observed in cats include vesiculobullous and ulcerative lesions, or maculopapular eruptions. The lesions are most likely to be found at mucocutaneous junctions and on the trunk.

Diagnosis

The diagnosis is achieved by skin biopsy: vesicular lesions should have histopathological changes of full thickness necrosis of the epidermis with subepidermal clefting. The maculopapular lesions are associated with histopathological changes of an interface dermatitis, with single cell keratinocyte necrosis, and lymphocyte and macrophage satellitosis.

Therapy

There remains considerable debate about the use of medication to treat EM. Some authors recommend glucocorticoids and azathioprine as per the treatment of other immune-mediated skin disease such as pemphigus foliaceus. Anecdotal reports suggest pentoxifylline, ciclosporin and etretinate may be beneficial, or even a change of diet as for a food intolerance (see Chapter 18).

Toxic epidermal necrolysis

Toxic epidermal necrolysis (TEN) is a rare disease involving the skin and oral mucosa. The study of Hinn *et al.* (1998) classified TEN as, distinct to EM, erythematous or purpuric macular to patchy eruptions involving >50% of the body surface with >30% epidermal detachment, and reported an association particularly with potentiated sulphonamides and beta-lactam antibacterial agents. In some cases the aetiology is unknown. The histological hallmark of TEN is full-thickness epidermal necrosis and minimal dermal inflammation. There may also be basal cell hydropic degeneration. In effect this is a cutaneous reaction pattern that warrants close investigation for underlying causes.

The clinical signs of generalized vesiculobullous disease with stomatitis, and in some cases, footpad lesions, pyrexia, pain and lethargy, are usually followed in due course by a fatal outcome. Supportive therapy to provide fluids and control of secondary infection is important. As in EM, there is debate about the value of treatment with glucocorticoids.

Bullous pemphigoid

Bullous pemphigoid disease is a rare blistering disorder reported in dogs and more recently cats, pigs and horses, which involves the formation of autoantibodies to the basement membrane type XVII collagen molecule (also termed BPAG2 bullous pemphigoid antigen 2, or BP180) which is a 180 kd transmembrane protein (see Chapter 1). Clinical signs may include vesicular, erosive and crusting dermatitis of the lips,

pinnae, hard and soft palate, abdomen, axilla and the digits. Histological findings include characteristic subepidermal vesicles, clefting with mild perivascular to moderate lichenoid inflammation which may include, notably, eosinophils and neutrophils. Treatment is as for other immune-mediated skin diseases, such as pemphigus foliaceus, but the prognosis is poor.

Mucous membrane pemphigoid (MMP)

Dogs and some cats have been described with this rare subepidermal blistering disease, seen primarily in or around the oral cavity, nasal planum, ear canal, eyes, anus and genitalia. Autoantibodies have been described directed against BPAG2 (Olivry and Chan, 2001).

Epidermolysis bullosa acquisita

Epidermolysis bullosa acquisita is another rare skin disease particularly seen in young Great Danes, with either generalized or localized lesions. Erythematous urticarial patches, vesicles and ulcers are seen on the face, groin, axilla, abdomen, footpads, oral cavity and mucocutaneous junctions. In the localized form, the pinnae and trunk may have scattered lesions. The pathogenesis is thought to involve autoantibodies targeting the anchoring fibrils containing collagen VII (see Chapter 1) leading to subepidermal blistering. Bullous pemphigoid and epidermolysis bullosa acquisita are extensively reviewed by Olivry and Chan (2001).

References and further reading

Affolter VK (2000) Cutaneous vasculitis and vasculopathy. *Clinical Program Proceedings, Fourth World Congress of Veterinary Dermatology, San Francisco,* pp. 207–211

Affolter VF, Moore PF and Sandmaier BM (1998) Immunohistochemical characterization of canine acute graft versus-host disease and erythema multiforme. *Advances in Veterinary Dermatology 3,* ed. C von Tscharner *et al.,* pp.103–115. Butterworth Heinemann, Oxford

Casciola-Rosen L and Rosen A (1997) Ultraviolet light-induced keratinocyte apoptosis: a potential mechanism for the induction of skin lesions and autoantibody production in LE. *Lupus 6,* 175–180

Chabanne L, Fournel C, Monier J *et al.* (1999a) Canine systemic lupus erythematosus. Part I Clinical and biological aspects. *Compendium on Continuing Education for the Practicing Veterinarian 21,* 135–141

Chabanne L, Fournel C, Rigal D and Monier J-C (1999b) Canine systemic lupus erythematosus. Part II Diagnosis and treatment. *Compendium on Continuing Education for the Practicing Veterinarian 21,* 402–421

David-Bajar KM and Davis BM (1997) Pathology, immunopathology and immunohistochemistry in cutaneous lupus erythematosus. *Lupus 6,* 145–157

Ferguson EA, Cerundolo R, Lloyd DH *et al.* (2000) Dermatomyositis in five Shetland Sheepdogs in the United Kingdom. *Veterinary Record 146,* 214–217

Gross WL, Trabandt A and Reinhold-Keller E (2000) Diagnosis and evaluation of vasculitis. *Rheumatology 39,* 245–252

Hinn AC, Olivry T, Luther PB *et al.* (1998) Erythema multiforme, Stevens–Johnson syndrome, and toxic epidermal necrolysis in the dog. *Journal of Veterinary Allergy and Clinical Immunology 6,* 13–20

Jackson HA and Olivry T (2001) Ulcerative dermatosis of the Shetland Sheepdog and Rough Collie may represent a novel vesicular variant of cutaneous lupus erythematosus. *Veterinary Dermatology 12,* 19–27

Lewis RM, Schwartz R and Henry WB (1965) Canine systemic lupus erythematosus. *Blood 25,* 143–160

Marsella R, Nicklin CF, Munson JW *et al.* (2000) Pharmacokinetics of pentoxifylline in dogs after oral and intravenous administration. *American Journal of Veterinary Research* **61,** 631–637

Nichols PR, Morris DO and Beale KM (2001) A retrospective study of canine and feline cutaneous vasculitis. *Veterinary Dermatology* **12,** 255–264

Olivry T and Chan LS (2001) Autoimmune blistering dermatoses in domestic animals. *Clinics in Dermatology* **19,** 750–760

Parker WM and Foster RA (1996) Cutaneous vasculitis in five Jack Russell Terriers. *Veterinary Dermatology* **7,** 109–115

Rowell NR and Goodfield MJD (1998) The 'Connective Tissue Diseases'. In: *Textbook of Dermatology, 6ᵗʰ edn,* ed. RH Champion *et al.,* pp. 2437–2575. Blackwell Science, Oxford

Scott DW and Miller WH (1999) Erythema multiforme in dogs and cats: literature review and case material from the Cornell University College of Veterinary Medicine (1988–1996) *Veterinary Dermatology* **10,** 297–309

Scott DW, Miller WH and Griffin CE (2001) Immune-mediated disorders. In: *Small Animal Dermatology, 6ᵗʰ edn,* pp. 742– 756. WB Saunders, Philadelphia

Sontheimer RD (1997) The lexicon of cutaneous lupus erythematosus – a review and personal perspective on the nomenclature and classification of the cutaneous manifestations of lupus erythematosus. *Lupus* **6,** 84–95

Vitale CB, Ihrke PJ, Gross TL *et al.* (1997) Systemic lupus erythematosus in a cat: fulfillment of the American Rheumatism Association criteria with supportive skin histopathology. *Veterinary Dermatology* **8,** 133–138

Vitale CB, Gross TL and Magro CM (1999) Vaccine-induced ischemic dermatopathy in the dog. *Veterinary Dermatology* **10,** 131–142

Vroom MW, Theaker MJ, Rest JR *et al.* (1995) Lupoid dermatosis in five German Short-Haired Pointers. *Veterinary Dermatology* **6,** 93–98

White SD (2000) Non-steroidal immunosuppressive therapy. In: *Current Veterinary Therapy XIII,* ed. RW Kirk *et al.,* pp. 536–538. WB Saunders, Philadelphia

Willemse T and Koeman JP (1989) Discoid lupus erythematosus in cats. *Veterinary Dermatology* **1,** 19–24

28

Metabolic dermatoses

Kevin P. Byrne

In veterinary dermatology, fewer skin diseases have a known association with specific underlying systemic or metabolic disease than in human dermatology. It is difficult to determine whether this is because of species differences or because of the inherent difficulty of examination of haired skin *versus* non-haired (glabrous) skin. It is easy to take for granted that a thick pelage is an obstacle that must be surmounted in order to detect less obvious skin lesions. Subtle lesions may require careful clipping of selected areas of the hair coat in order to be appreciated fully. Concerned owners of ill pets will often allow such clipping if its importance is explained to them.

The cutaneous lesions that are presented by metabolic diseases may be characteristic enough to establish the underlying disease with some certainty. Alternatively, the cutaneous lesions may be less specific and serve only as a starting point in the diagnostic work-up, such as the case with the digital crusting and hyperkeratosis of canine hepatocutaneous syndrome. Nevertheless, cutaneous lesions associated with metabolic disease are useful to the clinician.

The identification of cutaneous lesions of metabolic disease is similar to identification of cutaneous lesions of any cause and includes two major aspects:

- Lesion type: e.g. papule, plaque, macule or patch, modified by the presence or absence of hair loss
- Distribution of lesions: perhaps more important than lesion type.

In this chapter, three different metabolic dermatoses are discussed: superficial necrolytic dermatitis (metabolic epidermal necrolysis); zinc-responsive dermatosis; and vitamin A-responsive dermatosis. For each condition the cutaneous component and the correlated underlying systemic disorder are described, with emphasis on aspects that are clinically useful.

Superficial necrolytic dermatitis

The underlying disorder in superficial necrolytic dermatitis (SND) is hepatocutaneous syndrome or glucagonoma syndrome.

Gross lesions of superficial necrolytic dermatitis (necrolytic migratory erythema, metabolic epidermal necrolysis) are a combination of surface crusts (dried exudate) and hyperkeratosis (excessive stratum corneum). Crusts overlie the more severe lesions where trauma and/or secondary infection has resulted in erosion and/or ulceration of the epidermis. In all reported canine cases, lesions involve the footpads and digits (Figure 28.1) prompting the common presenting complaint of 'sore feet' by the dog's owner. Lesions are often present at mucocutaneous junctions (perioral (Figure 28.2), periocular, perianal, perivulvar, preputial and scrotal).

The pathogenesis of lesions of SND is not definitively known, as with necrolytic migratory erythema (NME), the analogous skin disease in humans. Since levels of

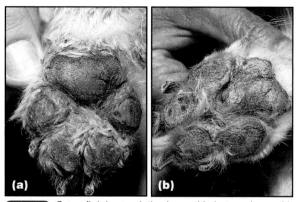

28.1 Superficial necrolytic dermatitis in two dogs with hepatocutaneous syndrome. There are gross lesions of crusting and hyperkeratosis on the digits and footpads of (a) an 8-year-old male mixed breed dog and (b) a 6-year-old Shetland Sheepdog.

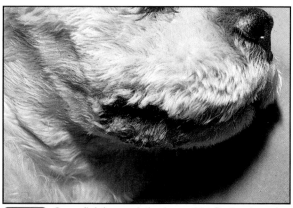

28.2 Superficial necrolytic dermatitis. Perioral crust formation in the same dog as shown in 28.1a.

plasma amino acids are decreased in both SND and NME, and since the skin requires a substantial supply of amino acids in order to function, an abnormality in protein metabolism is believed to be involved. An abnormality in glucagon metabolism may be a factor since the underlying disorder in most humans with NME is a glucagon-secreting tumour (glucagonoma syndrome) and glucagon directly affects protein metabolism. However, glucagon levels in humans with a glucagon-secreting tumour do not always correlate with the severity of their NME. Also, the vast majority of dogs with SND have a concurrent hepatopathy instead of a glucagon-secreting tumour. Other theories in the pathogenesis of SND include abnormal zinc and/or fatty acid metabolism (Byrne, 1999).

Hepatocutaneous syndrome

The most common underlying disorder for canine SND is the hepatocutaneous syndrome (HS). The initiating factors in the pathogenesis of the hepatopathy are not known. It is possible that SND is a result of liver pathology and this is supported by a small number of reported cases that developed SND after a toxic insult to the liver (Little *et al.*, 1991; Foster *et al.*, 1997). However, it is possible that the liver pathology and SND develop coincidentally due to a mechanism that is not yet known.

Clinical approach

Most reported cases of canine HS are in dogs 5 years of age or older. Either gender may be affected, although a higher incidence in males is reported in some series of cases. Common complaints from owners of dogs with HS are sores on the feet, lethargy, anorexia and weight loss. Polyuria and polydipsia may be reported where diabetes mellitus has developed. The extent of lesions at extrapodal sites is variable, although it appears that lesions develop at additional areas as the disease progresses. Since there are reported cases of canine SND due to toxic hepatopathy, it is worthwhile evaluating the history in light of exposure to hepatotoxins, including medications which are potentially hepatotoxic, such as anticonvulsants.

A summary of clinical findings is shown in Figure 28.3.

Crusts, ulcers and hyperkeratosis on feet and possibly
  mucocutaneous junctions
Liver enzymes elevated
Hypoalbuminaemia
Diabetes mellitus develops frequently
Secondary bacterial pyoderma common
Characteristic ultrasonographic findings
Characteristic histopathology

28.3 Pertinent clinical findings in superficial necrolytic dermatitis/canine hepatocutaneous syndrome.

Diagnosis

Differential diagnoses for crusting and/or hyperkeratotic lesions of the footpads include:

- Pemphigus foliaceus
- Zinc-responsive dermatosis
- Contact dermatitis
- Drug eruption.

When lesions are present on haired skin this list should include folliculitis (bacterial, dermatophyte or demodicosis).

Serum chemistry: Results of serum chemistry panels are usually supportive of hepatopathy and reveal, in descending order of frequency:

- Elevations in serum alkaline phosphatase (ALKP), alanine transferase and aspartamine transferase, with an elevation in ALKP occurring in almost all cases reported
- Elevation in fasting or postprandial serum bile acids is typical
- Hyperglycaemia, if not overt diabetes mellitus, is common
- Hypoalbuminaemia may be present
- Complete blood count may reveal non-specific findings such as a mild to moderate non-regenerative anaemia and stress leucogram.

Skin cytology: Skin cytology of lesions of SND normally reveals only inflammation and secondary bacterial pyoderma and/or yeast dermatitis.

Skin scrapings: Skin scrapings and dermatophyte culture are useful in determining the presence of demodicosis or dermatophytosis, respectively.

Skin biopsy: Examination of a skin biopsy by a qualified dermatopathologist is necessary for the diagnosis of SND. Punch or wedge biopsy techniques are adequate for specimen collection. Taking specimens from non-weight-bearing footpads or from lesions at the footpad/haired skin junction is preferable to taking specimens from the centre of weight-bearing pads, assuming that sufficient lesions of adequate quality are available. Care should be taken to keep overlying crusts intact or include them with the submission, as they may be necessary for proper diagnosis. Ulcerated areas and areas with very thick crust should be avoided. It may be advisable to collect a specimen from at least four different sites, as it is not unusual for all the dermatopathological findings needed for diagnosis of SND to be present on only one of every three or four specimens.

The prominent histopathological findings in canine SND are hyperplasia of the deep and middle layers of the epidermis and parakeratotic hyperkeratosis of the stratum corneum, with an intervening area of epidermal pallor or necrolysis in the superficial epidermis. Additionally, there may be exocytosis of inflammatory leucocytes into the epidermis with crust formation on the surface. Epidermal pallor may not be found as readily in specimens from older lesions (Gross *et al.*, 1992). It should be noted that, except for epidermal pallor/necrolysis, the histopathology of SND would be difficult to distinguish from zinc-responsive dermatosis. Secondary bacterial infection is typical and yeast organisms (*Malassezia*) are occasionally seen. Histopathological findings compatible with SND, in association with the clinical and laboratory abnormalities described above, support the diagnosis of HS and the initiation of therapy.

Investigation of liver pathology: While awaiting results of dermatopathology, further investigation of the liver abnormalities is indicated. If not already performed, fasting and post-prandial bile acid assessment may be indicated. Ultrasonography is useful in the diagnosis of HS in dogs, and the typical findings in canine SND are areas of hyper-echogenicity intermingled with areas of hypo-echogenicity in a 'Swiss cheese' pattern (Jacobson *et al.*, 1995). If feasible, hepatic biopsy is useful for confirming liver pathology compatible with hepatocutaneous syndrome: histopathology reveals parenchymal collapse with areas of nodular regeneration. Alternatively, a biopsy may determine the presence of other liver pathology. Additionally, it may be useful to consider the possibility of hyperadrenocorticism in individual cases and proceed with diagnostics accordingly, especially if results of abdominal ultrasonography are not compatible with HS.

Prognosis

In general, canine HS is a disease with a guarded to poor prognosis. Development of diabetes mellitus is not uncommon and worsens the prognosis. Even though the majority of reported cases die within a short time of diagnosis, recent information suggests that the disease in *some* dogs appears to be controlled or ameliorated with aggressive nutritional therapy. Even though HS carries a poor prognosis, owners should be made aware that some dogs regain a good quality of life that may last a year or more with continual therapy. This therapy has two major components: nutritional and dermatological.

Management and therapeutics

Nutritional therapy: The way dietary changes are carried out in dogs with HS is likely to be important. Since these dogs have evidence of aberrant protein metabolism (decreased levels of plasma amino acids), it is logical to assume that they are intolerant of inadequate calorie or protein intake during periods of anorexia. So, when attempting a diet change it is best to do so gradually, e.g. over the course of 3–4 days. If a dog refuses to eat a new diet then the food eaten previously should be resumed while an alternative diet plan is quickly formulated. If a dog stops eating after addition of a supplement to its ration, then the supplement should be administered separately from the diet, or an alternative supplement found. Care should be taken to avoid medications or treatments that cause the dog gastric upset or reduce its appetite.

Nutritional therapy includes increasing the content and quality of protein in the dog's daily ration as well as supplementing zinc and essential fatty acids. Following this, supplementation of the dog's normal diet with boiled egg yolks, three to six per day, will increase further the quality and quantity of protein intake, although some dogs dislike boiled eggs and refuse them. Another protein supplement that can be used is powdered casein; again palatability can be an obstacle with some dogs. One

protocol utilized at University of California Davis is based on a prescription diet containing high quality protein to which is added a casein-based supplement. An alternative to this is to use a critical care prescription diet.

Supplementation of the daily ration with a zinc supplement and a fatty acid supplement is recommended. Zinc supplements used include zinc sulphate (1–2 mg/kg bid) or zinc gluconate (1.5–3.5 mg/kg bid). A supplement containing essential fatty acids is also given; these supplements should contain vitamin E to reduce oxidation of fatty acids.

A nutritional therapy receiving wider use in dogs with HS is intravenous administration of amino acids. The author routinely recommends this to owners. The most commonly cited protocol uses an 8.5% or 10% crystalline amino acid solution produced for parenteral administration in humans. Approximately 25 ml/kg of body weight is administered via a jugular catheter over 6–8 hours. The treatment is repeated every 7–10 days. A possible contraindication to this treatment would be signs of hepatoencephalopathy in a patient with severe liver failure. The author recommends a trial of three treatments for dogs with HS to evaluate response. Until more information on the true efficacy of this treatment is available, amino acid therapy appears worthwhile given the poor prognosis of HS otherwise. A summary of nutritional management of dogs with SND is shown in Figure 28.4.

Balanced diet with high-quality protein (e.g. containing skeletal meat)
Additional protein supplementation (e.g. powdered casein, hard boiled eggs)
Zinc supplementation
Fatty acid supplementation
Intravenous amino acids: 8.5–10% parenteral solution via jugular vein at 25 ml/kg over 6–8 hours

---

28.4 Nutritional management of canine superficial necrolytic dermatitis.

Dermatological therapy: Management of the gross lesions includes:

- Careful clipping of hair from borders of lesions to improve drainage and facilitate topical therapy
- If lesions are moist, careful washing with a shampoo will help to remove exudate. Use of a topical therapy with a liquid or lotion base will have a similar effect. Active ingredients should be chosen based on the type of secondary infection present, e.g. chlorhexidine or benzoyl peroxide if bacterial pyoderma is present, miconazole or clotrimazole if yeast organisms are present
- Some dogs with SND develop hard projections of keratin that cause discomfort due to friction on opposing skin surfaces. Spot application of an emollient such as petroleum jelly or a keratolytic such as urea/salicylic acid cream to these projections will soften them and alleviate some discomfort

• Antibiotic therapy for controlling secondary bacterial pyoderma is usually necessary and can be started while waiting for results of dermatopathology. The antibiotic should be known to be useful in treatment of canine staphylococcal pyoderma and should be one that is unlikely to exacerbate a hepatopathy. Examples include cefalexin, cefadroxil and clavulanic acid-potentiated amoxicillin. Selection of an antibiotic, based on culture and sensitivity of material from lesions, may be necessary if cytology reveals presence of rod organisms or if bacterial pyoderma shows no evidence of resolution with appropriate empirical antibiotic therapy (see Chapter 22).

Topical therapy and especially antibiotic therapy of skin lesions of SND can be expected to relieve discomfort in the dog with HS; however, the response is likely to be inadequate without concurrent nutritional therapy.

Glucagonoma syndrome

Glucagonoma syndrome (GS) appears to be a much less common cause of canine SND than is HS. Glucagonoma is a functional malignant tumour of the alpha islet cells of the pancreas. In dogs, the tumours are relatively small and may not be detected via standard imaging techniques.

Clinical approach
Presenting complaints, physical and dermatological examination findings are indistinguishable from those of HS.

Diagnosis
Figure 28.5 shows the distinction of GS and HS after histopathological diagnosis of canine SND.

Dermatopathology: As in HS, dermatopathology of lesional skin from dogs with GS reveals SND.

Serum chemistry: Clinical laboratory findings in dogs with GS often reveal hyperglycaemia, presumably due to the excessive glucagon secretion from these tumours and, less commonly, elevations in alkaline phosphatase and alanine transferase. Fasting or postprandial serum bile acids are usually unremarkable.

When dermatopathology reveals SND in a dog with normal serum bile acids, and hepatic ultrasonography does not reveal findings characteristic of HS, the possibility of GS should be considered. In humans, serum glucagon levels are routinely performed during the workup of individuals suspected of having GS. Serum glucagon determination for veterinary species is not commercially available. Some human hospital laboratories that perform the assay may be helpful and accept a canine sample, but such laboratories are not likely to have determined normal values for dogs and results will need to be compared with values in veterinary publications.

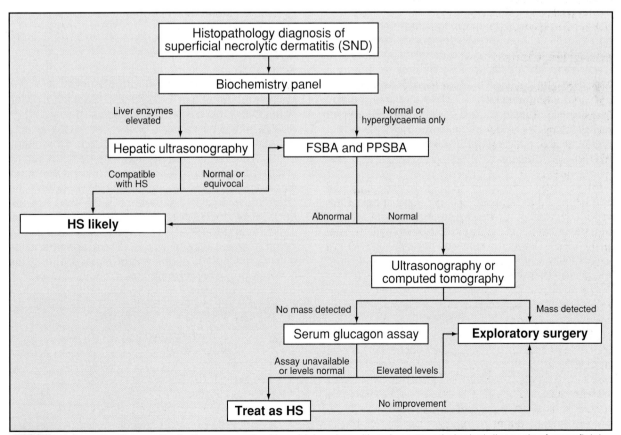

28.5 Schematic diagram illustrating one method by which a dog with a dermatopathological diagnosis of superficial necrolytic dermatitis is investigated to determine if the underlying cause is hepatocutaneous syndrome (the more common cause) or glucagonoma syndrome.

Imaging techniques: Ultrasonography of the pancreas does not detect glucagonoma reliably. In almost all reported cases of canine GS, exploratory laparotomy was required to determine the presence of a pancreatic neoplasm. In humans, standard imaging for an individual suspected of having GS would include computed tomography (CT), often with the use of contrast material to highlight these highly vascular tumours. With the increasing availability of CT for veterinary patients, abdominal CT may become useful for locating a pancreatic tumour prior to exploratory laparotomy in a dog suspected of having GS.

Exploratory laparotomy: If a pancreatic mass is not identified by imaging in a dog with a presumptive diagnosis of GS, then a decision is made whether to perform exploratory laparotomy. Elevation of serum glucagon is supportive of a decision to perform laparotomy.

Management and therapeutics

Surgery: Since metastasis of glucagonoma is common, complete excision may not be possible, although if a single tumour is present excision may be curative. Importantly, most reported cases of canine GS die post-operatively and this surgery may require an experienced surgeon and a facility with an intensive care unit for post-operative care.

Other therapy: If surgery is not feasible, or if complete resection of the tumour is not possible, therapy with octreotide, a somatostatin analogue that inhibits glucagon secretion, may provide temporary reduction in glucagon levels. This drug is expensive, and improvement, although significant, may be only temporary if tumour metastases are present (Byrne, 1999; C Foil, personal communication, 2001). Nutritional therapy and therapy of lesions used in dogs with HS can be used in dogs with GS to ameliorate the disease, but may not be effective in the face of persistent hyperglucagonaemia.

Feline SND

SND appears to be much less common in cats. One reported case of SND was determined to have a pancreatic carcinoma and a GS-like presentation (Patel *et al.*, 1996). The author has seen one case of SND-HS in a cat with skin and liver histopathology identical to the disease in dogs.

Zinc-responsive dermatosis

Zinc is found in all cells. It is a cofactor for over 60 different enzymes in mammals. It is also involved in gene transcription and membrane function, where it stabilizes lysosomal membranes and controls lipid peroxidation. As with most nutrients, not all that is ingested will be absorbed and the proportion of zinc absorbed from the intestinal tract can be affected by a variety of factors, including:

- Intestinal malabsorption
- Diarrhoea
- Certain amino acids
- Chelators
- Fibre
- Some minerals such as copper, iron, and calcium.

Any of these, or a combination, in combination with low dietary intake could cause a zinc deficiency.

Zinc deficiency results in keratinization defects in epidermis, hair, wool and horny appendages, and can result in delayed wound healing. Zinc deficiency can also lead to depressed immune responses. Topical zinc (zinc oxide) products have therapeutic uses that include facilitated healing of wounds and burns.

Cases of zinc-responsive dermatosis can usually be categorized into two separate syndromes, distinguished primarily by age, signalment and the bioavailability of zinc in the dog's diet (Figure 28.6). The dermatological signs are the same for both syndromes.

Syndrome I

This syndrome occurs more commonly in northern-breed dogs such as Siberian Husky, Alaskan Malamute, American Eskimo and Samoyed (Scott *et al.*, 2001), although other breeds can be affected. Age of onset as early as 2–9 months and as late as 10–11 years has been reported (Colombini, 1999; White *et al.*, 2001). A genetic defect resulting in decreased absorption of zinc from the intestinal tract appears to be involved in Huskies and chondrodysplastic Malamutes. There does not appear to be any gender predilection. In susceptible individuals the disease can be exacerbated by oestrus, pregnancy or stress. There appears to be a tendency for development of lesions during the late autumn or winter months.

Feature	Syndrome I	Syndrome II
Ulceration and crusting	Typically periocular or perioral, then extremities and pressure points	Typically periocular or perioral, then extremities and pressure points
Secondary skin infections	Common	Common
Breed disposition	'Northern' breeds, (Husky, Malamute); other breeds	Large breeds
Zinc	Poor assimilation/utilization, inherited in Husky and Malamute	Poor bioavailability (dietary), especially in puppies

28.6 Features of canine zinc-responsive dermatosis syndromes I and II

Clinical approach

The skin lesions of syndrome I are primarily crust lesions with variable erythema and alopecia; lesions may be symmetrical or asymmetrical. Lesions are most likely to occur in the periocular or perioral areas (Figure 28.7), followed by limbs (especially pressure points), footpads, pinnae, muzzle and the perigenital area (Colombini, 1999). Lesions may also involve the glabrous skin of the nasal planum. In 40–60% of cases, pruritus is reported and in a small number of cases this may be directed at the pinnae (White *et al.*, 2001). Secondary bacterial or yeast infections are common.

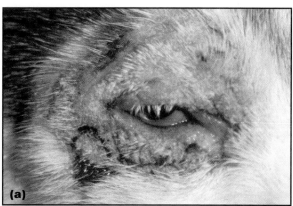

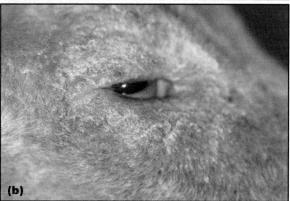

28.7 Zinc-responsive dermatosis. (a) Periocular alopecia, crusting and erythema in a 2-year-old female Malamute. The photograph was taken after skin scraping had been performed above the eye and before a skin biopsy (circle below eye). (b) Periocular alopecia and crusting in an 18-month-old male Dobermann Pinscher. There is less erythema than in (a).

Diagnosis

Differential diagnoses for these dermatological findings include:

- Bacterial folliculitis
- Dermatophytosis
- Demodicosis
- Superficial necrolytic dermatitis (SND)
- Pemphigus foliaceus
- Pemphigus erythematosus
- Discoid lupus erythematosus (for nasal planum lesions)
- Systemic lupus erythematosus.

If pruritus is present, then appropriate underlying pruritic diseases should also be considered.

Definitive diagnosis is made by skin biopsy and dermatopathology followed by response to zinc supplementation. When taking skin biopsies, care should be taken to avoid ulcerated or thickly crusted areas which may lack intact (non-ulcerated) epidermis.

The most frequent dermatopathological finding is epidermal parakeratosis. Other findings include parakeratosis of follicular epithelium, orthokeratotic hyperkeratosis, epidermal hyperplasia, crust and variable dermal inflammation. Response to an appropriate dosage of zinc supplement administered for an appropriate length of time allows a definitive diagnosis.

Management and therapeutics

Zinc supplementation: Therapy of zinc-responsive dermatosis syndrome I is by zinc supplementation. Dietary zinc is not the central issue in syndrome I as it is in syndrome II; however, dogs with syndrome I may experience recurrence of lesions if fed diets with low zinc bioavailability (Colombini, 1999). An initial dose (based on elemental zinc content) of 1 mg/kg per day may be given, with a 50% dosage increase each month until resolution of lesions. A recent study advocated a higher starting dose of 2–3 mg/kg per day of elemental zinc (White *et al.*, 2001). The daily dose should be divided and given with meals to reduce occurrence of vomiting. Lifelong therapy is usually required; relapses occur within 2–6 weeks if therapy is discontinued.

Zinc solutions for injection are available in some countries and may be used in place of oral supplementation. Intramuscular injection of a total dose of 600 mg of elemental zinc per month has been reported (White *et al.*, 2001).

Other therapy: Essential fatty acid supplementation may also be helpful in some dogs with zinc-responsive dermatosis. Since oestrus may exacerbate lesions, intact female dogs whose zinc-responsive dermatosis is difficult to control may improve after ovariohysterectomy. Secondary bacterial pyoderma, if present, is treated appropriately. Topical therapy is used to clean the skin of exudate, to soften hard keratin deposits and to aid in treatment of secondary infections.

Breeding from affected Huskies and Malamutes should be discouraged because of the apparent heritability of this condition.

Syndrome II

Syndrome II, a less common manifestation of zinc-responsive dermatosis, occurs in puppies of many breeds, often larger breeds. It has been reported in Great Danes, Dobermanns, Beagles, German Shepherd Dogs, German Short-Haired Pointers, Standard Poodles and Rhodesian Ridgebacks.

Syndrome II appears to be an issue of reduced dietary zinc bioavailability. Supplementation of the diet with excessive calcium can interfere with zinc absorption. High-cereal diets may also result in poor zinc absorption due to high dietary levels of phytate which can bind zinc in the gastrointestinal tract.

Clinical findings in syndrome II are similar to those of syndrome I. Secondary bacterial infections may be more prominent with syndrome II, sometimes resulting in regional or generalized lymphadenopathy.

Therapy for syndrome II is based on making appropriate corrections to the puppy's diet to increase zinc bioavailability, such as discontinuing calcium supplementation and changing to a balanced commercial diet containing less cereal and having more protein derived from meat sources. Zinc supplementation can be used to hasten resolution of lesions, although it should not be necessary after dietary corrections have been instituted. However, some dogs may need to continue zinc supplementation until maturity (Colombini, 1999).

Vitamin A-responsive dermatosis

Although not a vitamin A deficiency, this dermatosis is responsive to supplementation of the diet with additional vitamin A. It has been reported primarily in Cocker Spaniels. It has also been reported in Labrador Retrievers and Miniature Schnauzers and may occur in other breeds.

Clinical approach
Skin lesions are characterized by focal or multifocal hyperkeratotic plaques which, on closer examination, reveal marked follicular hyperkeratosis resulting in 'fronds' of keratosebaceous material protruding from follicular orifices and encircling of the base of hair shafts with the same material (follicular 'casts'). Lesions may be more evident on the ventrum or lateral chest and abdomen (Figure 28.8).

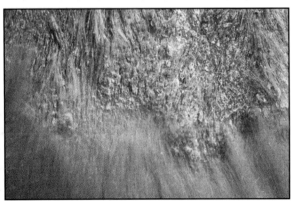

28.8 Vitamin-A responsive dermatosis in a 4-year-old female Cocker Spaniel. This severe case shows marked follicular hyperkeratosis.

Diagnosis
Differential diagnoses include:

- Idiopathic seborrhoea
- Sebaceous adenitis
- Atypical demodicosis (i.e. follicular hyperkeratosis exceeds alopecia)
- True vitamin A deficiency (rare in dogs fed commercial diets)
- Hypervitaminosis-A (history of excessive dietary vitamin A)
- Endocrinopathy, such as hyperadrenocorticism, with secondary seborrhoea
- Follicular dysplasia.

Rule-out of most differentials is possible: skin scrapings (for demodicosis), dermatopathology (for sebaceous adenitis and follicular dysplasia) and proper laboratory evaluation for hyperadrenocorticism may be performed.

Dermatopathological findings of vitamin A-responsive dermatosis include profound follicular orthokeratosis. Diagnosis is made by rule-out of differential diagnoses and response to treatment.

Management and therapeutics
Treatment of vitamin A-responsive dermatosis is via supplementation with vitamin A (retinol) at 10,000 IU per day (or 625–800 IU/kg per day). Response is usually seen in 2–3 months. Lifelong therapy is required.

References and further reading

Byrne KP (1999) Metabolic epidermal necrosis – hepatocutaneous syndrome. *Veterinary Clinics of North America: Small Animal Practice* **29**, 1337–1355

Colombini S (1999) Canine zinc-responsive dermatosis. *Veterinary Clinics of North America: Small Animal Practice* **29**, 1373–1383

Foster AP, Panciera DL and Cooley AJ (1997) Recognizing canine hepatocutaneous syndrome. *Veterinary Medicine* **92**, 1050–1055

Gross TL, Ihrke PJ and Walder EJ (1992) *Veterinary Dermatopathology: A Macroscopic and Microscopic Evaluation of Canine and Feline Skin Disease*, pp. 46–48. Mosby-Year Book, St. Louis

Jacobson LS, Kirberger RM and Nesbit JW (1995) Hepatic ultrasonography and pathological findings in dogs with hepatocutaneous syndrome: new concepts. *Journal of Veterinary Internal Medicine* **9**, 399–404

Little CJL, McNeil PE and Robb J (1991) Hepatopathy and dermatitis in a dog associated with the ingestion of mycotoxins. *Journal of Small Animal Practice* **32**, 23–26

Patel A, Whitbread TJ and McNeil PE (1996) A case of metabolic epidermal necrosis in a cat. *Veterinary Dermatology* **7**, 221–226

Scott DW, Miller WH and Griffin CE (2001) Nutritional skin diseases. In: *Muller and Kirk's Small Animal Dermatology, 6th edn*, pp. 1119–1122. WB Saunders, Philadelphia

White SD, Bourdeau P, Rosychuk RAW *et al.* (2001) Zinc-responsive dermatosis in dogs: 41 cases and literature review. *Veterinary Dermatology* **12**, 101–109

29

Actinic (solar) dermatoses

Mandy Burrows

Solar-induced dermatitis and neoplasia occur in dogs and cats as a consequence of chronic exposure to sunlight and ultraviolet (UV) radiation on white, lightly pigmented or damaged (depigmented or scarred) skin that is unprotected by hair.

The deleterious effects of UV radiation on skin depend upon:

- The duration and frequency of exposure
- The intensity of solar radiation, based on the geographical latitude
- The reactivity of the skin, based on genetically determined skin colour, haircoat density and genetic susceptibility.

Solar-induced skin lesions in dogs and cats are primarily located on unpigmented, or lightly pigmented, sparsely haired regions of skin that are frequently exposed to sun. Lesions are more common in dogs and cats that sunbathe or are housed where there is reflective ground cover (including snow) and little sun protection. This is especially problematical in hot sunny climates such as in Australia, California, Florida, Hawaii and South Africa. The most commonly affected dog breeds are white English Bull Terriers, Dalmatians, Beagles, Fox Terriers, Whippets, white Boxers,

American Staffordshire Bull Terriers and American Bulldogs. White or coloured cats that have white-haired areas on the face and ears with unpigmented skin are also prone. Blue-eyed white cats are most susceptible.

Actinic (solar) dermatitis

Dogs

Clinical features

The earliest clinical signs are patchy to confluent erythema and scaling (Figure 29.1a). With chronic solar exposure, there is marked thickening of erythematous skin, and confluent, erythematous, indurated, linear plaques develop in unpigmented skin that is often found abruptly adjacent to normal, pigmented areas (Figure 29.1b,c). Severely affected dogs also characteristically develop erythematous papules, crusting, comedones and nodules. Actinic comedones are usually multiple grouped dilated hair follicles that are filled with darkly coloured keratinous material (Figure 29.1d). Rupture of comedones releases follicular keratin and hair into the dermis, eliciting a foreign body response that then results in deep furunculosis (Figure 29.1e). Intact haemorrhagic bullae are a distinctive feature secondary to actinic comedonal rupture (Figure 29.1f).

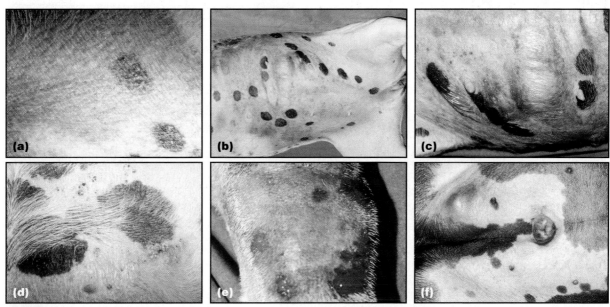

29.1 Canine actinic dermatitis. (a) Erythema and scaling. (Courtesy of G Burton.) (b, c) Erythema, indurated plaques and papules. (d) Erythematous plaque and comedones. (e) Furunculosis. (f) Haemorrhagic bullae.

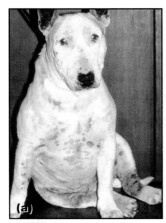 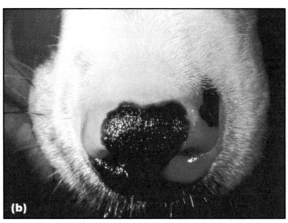 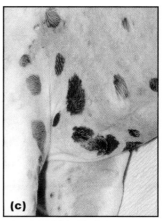

29.2 Canine actinic dermatitis. (a) English Bull Terrier with lesions affecting the face, ventrum and hindlimbs. (b) Lesions on the nasal planum of a dog. (Courtesy of R Muse.) (c) Lesions on the ventral abdomen and hindlimb of a dog.

In dogs that sunbathe in lateral recumbency, lesions are commonly observed on the ventrolateral abdomen and flank, adjacent to normal pigmented skin, although the hock and distal hind limb, bridge of the nose, pinnae, muzzle and tail tip may also be affected (Figure 29.2). Some dogs will lie on one side more frequently and cause more severe lesions on the side with greatest sun exposure. The ventral region, scrotum and perineal skin are often affected in dogs that sunbathe on their backs or are housed on reflective surfaces.

Differential diagnoses

For the early stage of solar dermatitis, differential diagnoses include hypersensitivity dermatitis (atopic, dietary, contact irritant, insect), *Malassezia* dermatitis and primary keratinization disorders. The more chronic lesions need to be differentiated from bacterial folliculitis and furunculosis (including pustular demodicosis) and other nodular tumours (e.g. cutaneous lymphoma, mast cell tumour and metastatic neoplasia).

Cats

Clinical features

The early clinical signs appear on the margin of the sparsely haired pinnae and are characterized by mild erythema and fine scaling (Figure 29.3). Advanced lesions consist of severe erythema, alopecia and thickening of the pinnae with peeling, crusting and erosion that are associated with pain, scratching and twitching of the pinnae. With further progression there is severe crusting, ulceration and haemorrhage, and pinnal margins may curl (Figure 29.4). The margins of the lower eyelids, lips, dorsal aspect of the planum nasale and preauricular region of the face may be similarly affected.

Differential diagnoses

These include immune-mediated diseases that can affect the pinnae and face, including pemphigus foliaceus and erythematosus, systemic and discoid lupus erythematosus, vasculitis and drug reactions. Other diseases that should be ruled out in a pruritic cat

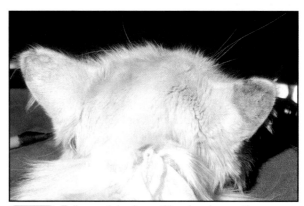

29.3 Feline actinic dermatitis, showing erythema and scaling on the pinnae of a cat. (Courtesy of WT Clark.)

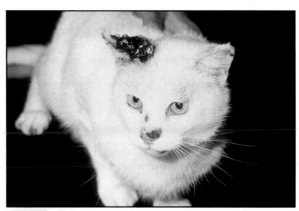

29.4 Feline actinic dermatitis with progression to squamous cell carcinoma. There is crusting, erosion and haemorrhage on the pinna and face.

include dermatophytosis, notoedric and otodectic mange, adverse reaction to food, and feline atopy. In cold climates, cold-agglutinin disease and frostbite also need to be considered.

Diagnosis

The diagnosis of actinic dermatitis in the dog and cat is initially based on the evidence of acute or chronic sun exposure. The presence of erythematous lesions in unpigmented sparsely haired regions and a history of sun exposure are highly suggestive of solar dermatitis. It is useful to compare the adjacent pigmented skin with the lesional unpigmented areas. The pigmented regions are supple on palpation and the skin is a normal thickness, whereas lesional areas are non-pliable and thickened. A history of regression of erythema and other lesions following sun avoidance or topical sunscreen application is also supportive. Some dogs and cats with actinic dermatitis show seasonal variation in clinical signs, with lesions being more severe in the summer.

Definitive diagnosis of actinic dermatitis requires histological evaluation of skin biopsy material. In the early stages of disease there is a mild superficial perivascular dermatitis (hyperplastic and spongiotic). Vacuolated keratinocytes with pyknotic nuclei and eosinophilic cytoplasm or 'sunburn cells' are also scattered throughout the epidermis.

Epidermal hyperplasia, follicular keratosis and mild superficial dermal fibrosis are features of more chronic solar dermatitis. A narrow subepidermal band of homogenous pale-staining condensed collagen is the most frequent dermal histopathological change in dogs with solar dermatitis. It may also be an indicator of early solar damage in clinically normal dogs (Frank et al., 1996; Figure 29.5). Actinic comedones are often multiple, with concentric accumulations of pale-staining collagen surrounding dilated, keratin-filled follicles (Gross et al., 1992). Pyogranulomatous folliculitis and furunculosis are common sequelae to comedonal rupture.

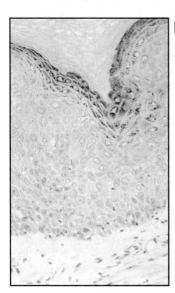

29.5 Histological characteristics of actinic dermatitis. There is epidermal hyperplasia, keratinocyte dysplasia and a subepidermal band of pale-staining collagen. (H&E; X40 original magnification.)

Solar elastosis is well recognized in humans with chronic solar exposure but is rarely identified in dogs or cats with solar dermatitis. In tissue sections stained with haematoxylin and eosin (H&E), elastosis appears as a linear band of indistinct pale-staining fibrils in the superficial dermis and as black tangled thick elastotic material with Verhoeff's–van Giessen elastin stain (Frank et al., 1996). Solar elastosis is not considered a reliable indicator of actinic dermatitis in the dog and cat.

Clinical management

Optimal early therapy includes: limitation of sun exposure; use of sunscreens and protective bodysuits; and the administration of antimicrobial agents to treat any secondary bacterial pyoderma. If this is ineffective, a short course of topical and systemic glucocorticoids may be evaluated. In cases that are refractory, surgery or treatment with a specialized drug or procedure should be considered.

Environmental control

Avoidance of direct or reflected sunlight is of paramount importance. Affected dogs and cats should be kept inside from 9 am to 3 pm and should not be permitted to sunbathe near open doors and windows. Normal window glass does not block UV radiation. Total sun avoidance is recommended but unfortunately is not often achievable. For animals that cannot be kept inside, providing generous shade is highly recommended. White concrete floors should be avoided, due to their ability to reflect sunlight.

A waterproof sunscreen product with an optimal sun protection factor (SPF) of 30 is also recommended. For maximal efficacy, the product should be gently rubbed into the area at least 30 minutes prior to sun exposure. If the solar exposure is unpredictable, the sunscreen should be applied twice daily.

Black ink can be applied to the nasal planum of dogs and cats with nasal solar lesions, using felt-tipped markers or cotton-tipped applicators and permanent laundry or stamp pad ink. The markers are easier to use but the solvents can occasionally irritate the skin. 'Inking' does not negate the requirement for other prophylactic measures, as black skin can still absorb some sunlight. Tattooing is a more permanent technique, but rare adverse reactions to the tattoo ink have made this option unpopular.

Sun-protective clothing, such as a T-shirt or body suit made from cotton and synthetic fabric with a high SPF, can be very useful (Figure 29.6). In our experience, most dogs tolerate the flexible and comfortable protection suits and these have been very successful adjuncts to management in dogs that cannot be confined inside.

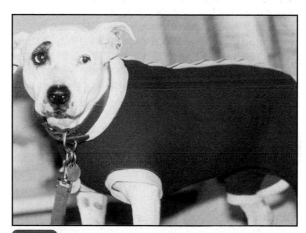

29.6 A sun protection suit.

Drugs

Corticosteroids: Acute solar dermatitis responds well in the dog and cat to the application of topical corticosteroids, using 1–2.5% hydrocortisone ointment or cream every 12 to 24 hours for 7–10 days. If systemic therapy is required to reduce erythema, a short course of oral prednisolone (1 mg/kg every 24 hours for 7–10 days) is usually sufficient.

Beta-carotene: Beta-carotene (30 mg orally every 12 hours for 30 days and then every 24 hours) in combination with prednisolone (0.5–1 mg/kg orally every 24 hours) has also been advocated as a management option. However, oral beta-carotene does not effectively block UVB. The overall therapeutic benefits of carotenes are highly controversial and their use is not currently recommended.

Synthetic retinoids: Isotretinoin and etretinate have been used in canine solar dermatititis with variable results. Isotretinoin at 1–2 mg/kg orally every 12 hours, was ineffective in treating dogs (Rosenkrantz, 1993), whereas etretinate at a dosage of 1 mg/kg orally every 24 hours was effective for actinic keratosis but was of no benefit for solar dermatitis (Power and Ihrke, 1995).

Actinic keratoses

Actinic keratoses are premalignant epithelial lesions that occur in the sparsely haired regions of unpigmented skin in middle-aged to older dogs and cats that are frequently exposed to sunlight. Actinic keratoses are capable of transforming to invasive squamous cell carcinoma (SCC).

Clinical features

Dogs
Lesions are either single or multiple and are classically asymptomatic, erythematous, scaly red to reddish-brown ill-defined macules that progress to indurated crusted plaques, varying in size from 0.5 to 5 cm in diameter, and are rough on palpation. Actinic comedones may be present. Palpation of visibly normal skin may detect irregular firmness and thickening. The glabrous skin of the ventral and lateral abdomen and inner thigh is most frequently affected. Induration, erosion, ulceration or increasing diameter of the keratotic lesion should raise the suspicion of evolution into SCC.

Cats
Lesions consist of erythematous plaques with crusting, erosion and superficial ulceration. They affect the margins of the pinnae, nasal planum, pre-auricular region of the face and dorsal muzzle. The lesions may appear symmetrical.

Diagnosis
It is impossible to differentiate premalignant actinic keratosis from solar-induced malignancy without histological evaluation of an incisional or excisional biopsy. The principal histological diagnostic feature of an actinic keratosis is an irregular epidermal hyperplasia and diffuse dysplasia with marked hyperkeratosis or parakeratosis. Dysplasia is characterized by a loss of normal stratification of the epidermis, nuclear atypia, increased mitotic activity and individual keratinocyte dyskeratosis. In dogs, a dense lymphoplasmacytic dermal infiltrate obscuring the dermal–epidermal interface is common, with superficial to deep laminar dermal fibrosis. In the cat, the dermal infiltrate is usually mild and perivascular. Solar elastosis may be seen in dogs and rarely in cats. Actinic keratosis is differentiated from SCC by absence of dermal invasion.

Clinical management
The principal therapeutic options for actinic keratosis in dogs and cats are excisional surgery, cryosurgery and carbon dioxide laser ablation of the affected epidermis. For optimal success rates with cryosurgery, temperature probes should be used to determine adequate freezing time.

Topical chemotherapy with 0.1–5% 5-fluorouracil cream is widely accepted as a treatment modality for human actinic keratoses but is not often used in dogs and is toxic to cats (Schwartz and Stoll, 1999).

Oral retinoids, however, may have value in the treatment of actinic keratosis in humans, dogs and cats. In one study, some dogs with actinic keratoses exhibited partial to complete resolution of lesions when given etretinate (1 mg/kg orally every 12 hours for 90 days) but lesions in other dogs remained static or progressed to SCC (Marks *et al.*, 1992). Isotretinoin (3 mg/kg orally) was ineffective in feline actinic keratoses (Evans *et al.*, 1985), but more recent studies with etretinate (10 mg orally every 24 hours) have shown more encouraging results (Power and Ihrke, 1995). Etretinate is no longer available in the UK, USA or Australia, but acitretin could be used at a dosage of 5–10 mg per cat every 24 hours.

The combination of a low dose of a systemic retinoid and topical tretinoin has been reported to be beneficial for both treatment and prophylaxis of actinic keratoses and SCC in human renal transplant recipients but has not been evaluated in dogs (Rook *et al.*, 1995). Topical tretinoin is considered to be less effective in the treatment of multiple actinic keratoses in humans but has been used successfully by the author to treat actinic keratoses in dogs.

Laser ablation with a carbon dioxide laser is an effective treatment modality in human actinic keratosis (Spicer and Goldberg, 1996) and is used by some veterinary dermatologists. Cutaneous dermabrasion and chemical peeling with 35% trichloroacetic acid, alpha-hydroxy acid and liquid nitrogen spray are also valuable treatment options in diffuse actinic keratoses in humans (Schwartz, 1996) and have been advocated in dogs (M. Shipstone, personal communication).

Solar protection, including reducing exposure to sunlight and regular use of sunscreen, may prevent the development of new actinic keratoses.

Squamous cell carcinoma

Cutaneous SCC is a malignant proliferation of the keratinocyte of the epidermis and the most frequently reported malignant epithelial neoplasm of the dog and cat. It is associated primarily with exposure to the UV irradiation of sunlight and is usually preceded by actinic (solar) keratoses. Cutaneous SCC is most commonly located in the unpigmented or depigmented skin in the sparsely haired regions of white dogs and cats in geographical regions characterized by long periods of intense sun exposure. Papillomavirus structural antigens have been demonstrated in up to 50% of canine SCC, suggesting a viral aetiological role and abnormalities in tumour suppressor gene p53 expression have been described in dogs and cats with cutaneous SCC (Teifke and Lohr, 1996).

Clinical features

Dogs

Canine SCC occurs at an average age of 9 years, with no sex predilection. Short-coated breeds with white or piebald hair and skin colour, such as the English Bull Terrier, Dalmatian and Beagle, have the highest incidence of solar-induced SCC. Lesions occur most commonly on the trunk, scrotum and hindlimbs and less frequently on the lips, nose and anus. Lesions may be single or multiple. SCC occur as shallow, crusted ulcers that become deep and crateriform or as papillary to nodular masses that vary from several millimetres to several centimetres in diameter (Figure 29.7). Erythema, erosion, ulceration, crusting and haemorrhage are often present.

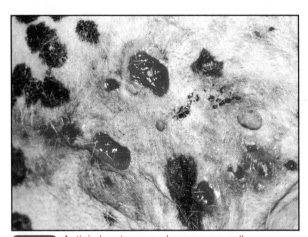

29.7 Actinic keratoses and squamous cell carcinoma. There are multiple ulcerated nodules on the ventrum of this dog.

Cats

Feline SCC occurs at an average age of 11 years, with no breed or sex predilection, and is more frequent in white-haired cats. The most common sites are the pinnae, external nares, preauricular region, eyelids and lips. Feline SCC can be proliferative, but is more commonly an erosive, crusted and indurated lesion that bleeds easily when traumatized. Lesions are multiple in about 45% of affected cats (Figure 29.8).

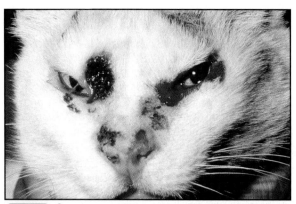

29.8 Squamous cell carcinoma. There is crusting, erosion and haemorrhage on the eyelids, preauricular region and nasal planum of this cat.

Diagnosis

The diagnosis of SCC requires histological examination of skin biopsy material. Histologically, SCC consists of irregular masses or cords of keratinocytes that proliferate downwards and invade the dermis. Frequent findings include keratin formation, atypia, mitotic figures, intercellular bridges and horn pearls. Solar elastosis may occasionally be seen.

Well differentiated and mildly invasive feline SCC exhibit a significantly greater number of CD3[+] T lymphocytes, B lymphocytes and IgG-bearing plasma cells. They also express Class II major histocompatibility complex (MHC) antigens in a higher proportion than in moderately differentiated and invasive tumours, suggesting that a cellular and humoral response may play a role in the down-regulation of tumour growth but does not induce tumour regression (Perez et al., 1999).

Clinical management

SCC is considered a locally invasive, malignant tumour with a low rate of metastasis. However, metastasis to regional lymph nodes and lung is seen with poorly differentiated neoplasms. In cats, the prognosis correlates with the degree of histological differentiation and a correlation between the histological grade and local invasiveness of the tumour has been reported (Perez et al., 1999).

Clinical management of SCC may include: surgical excision; cryosurgery; electrosurgery; hyperthermia; radiotherapy; chemotherapy; photodynamic, and laser therapy.

Surgery or cryosurgery

Surgery and cryosurgery are the most common therapeutic modalities used (Clarke, 1991; Lana et al., 1997) and are the most practical for the general practitioner, although there are numerous reports detailing the use of hyperthermia (Lana et al., 1997), radiotherapy (Theon et al., 1995) and photodynamic therapy (Peaston et al., 1993). In general, the outcome for small, superficial, non-invasive lesions that are treated early is favourable. A combination of surgery with radiation therapy or adjuvant chemotherapy may be the best approach for advanced, infiltrative lesions.

Chemotherapy

In general, systemic chemotherapy with various agents has shown little consistent efficacy for the management of canine and feline SCC. However, the use of intralesional sustained-release cisplatin or 5-fluorouracil has been investigated, with over 50% of dogs and cats with actinic-related SCC achieving a complete response (Kitchell *et al.*, 1992, 1995). In cats, intratumoural administration of carboplatin in sesame oil produced complete remission in 67% of cases of SCC of the nasal planum, with no systemic toxicity reported (Theon *et al.*, 1996).

Environmental control

In all cases avoidance of sunlight is important, as successful management of SCC does not preclude the development of new lesions in other unpigmented sites.

Cutaneous haemangioma and haemangiosarcoma

Cutaneous haemangioma is a benign neoplasm arising from vascular endothelial cells and is common in dogs and rare in cats. Cutaneous haemangiosarcoma is a malignant neoplasm of the same cells and is uncommon in both species. Chronic solar irradiation has been implicated as the cause of haemangioma and haemangiosarcoma in the ventral glabrous skin of lightly pigmented, sparsely haired dogs (Hargis *et al.*, 1992) and as the cause of haemangiosarcoma on the pinnae of white-eared cats (Miller *et al.*, 1992).

Clinical features

Dogs

Cutaneous solar-induced haemangioma and haemangiosarcomas occur in dogs at an average age of 10 years and there is a female sex predilection. Whippets, Dalmatians, Beagles, Bassett Hounds, Salukis, English Pointers, American Staffordshire Bull Terriers and other short-haired and light-skinned breeds are at increased risk. Lesions are usually located on the ventral abdomen and thorax. Solar-induced haemangiomas are usually well circumscribed round blue to red–black lesions 0.5–4 cm in diameter and are dermal to subcutaneous in location (Figure 29.9). Conversely, solar-induced

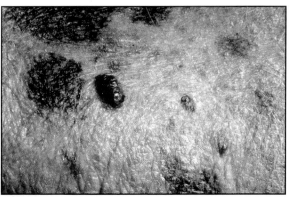

29.9 Solar-induced haemangioma on the ventrum of a dog.

haemangiosarcomas are often multiple, poorly circumscribed, red to blue plaques or nodules, usually less than 2 cm in diameter, and are dermal in location. They are also often associated with haemorrhage and ulceration.

Cats

Feline solar-induced haemangiosarcomas usually occur in male cats older than 10 years, with no breed predilection. White cats are predisposed. Lesions are usually solitary, rapidly growing and occur most commonly on the head and pinnae. Dermal haemangiosarcomas are poorly circumscribed, red to dark blue plaques or nodules that are usually less than 2 cm in diameter.

Diagnosis

Histologically haemangiomas are characterized by a proliferation of blood-filled vascular spaces lined by single layers of well differentiated endothelial cells. Haemangiosarcomas are characterized, however, by an invasive proliferation of atypical endothelial cells with areas of vascular space formation. Solar dermatosis and elastosis may be present.

Clinical management

Clinical management of haemangiomas includes surgical excision, cryosurgery, electrosurgery, and observation without treatment. The therapy of choice for haemangiosarcomas is radical surgical excision. However, the prognosis for both dogs and cats is poor, with local recurrence and metastasis being common.

References and further reading

Clarke RE (1991) Cryosurgical treatment of cutaneous squamous cell carcinoma. *Australian Veterinary Practitioner* **21**, 148–153

Evans AG, Madewell BR and Stannard AA (1985) A trial of 13-cis-retinoic acid for treatment of squamous cell carcinoma and preneoplastic lesions of the head in cats. *American Journal of Veterinary Research* **46**, 2553–2557

Frank LA and Calderwood Mays MB (1994) Solar dermatitis in dogs. *Compendium on Continuing Education for the Practicing Veterinarian* **16**, 465–472

Frank LA, Calderwood Mays MB and Kunkle GA (1996) Distribution and appearance of elastic fibres in the dermis of clinically normal dogs and dogs with solar dermatitis and other dermatoses. *American Journal of Veterinary Research* **57**, 178–181

Gross TL, Ihrke PJ and Walder EJ (1992) *Veterinary Dermatopathology: A Macroscopic and Microscopic Evaluation of Canine and Feline Skin Disease*, pp. 270–271. Mosby–Year Book, St Louis

Hargis AM, Ihrke PJ, Spangler WL *et al.* (1992) A retrospective clinicopathologic study of 212 dogs with cutaneous haemangiomas and haemangiosarcomas. *Veterinary Pathology* **29**, 316–328

Irving RA, Day RS and Eales L (1982) Porphyrin values and treatment of feline solar dermatitis. *American Journal of Veterinary Research* **43**, 2067–2069

Kitchell BE, McCabe M, Luck EE *et al.* (1992) Intralesional sustained-release chemotherapy with cisplatin and 5-fluorouracil therapeutic implants for treatment of feline squamous cell carcinoma (abstract). *Proceedings of the 12th Annual Meeting of the Veterinary Cancer Society*, p. 55

Kitchell BE, Orenberg EK, Brown DM *et al.* (1995) Intralesional sustained-release chemotherapy with therapeutic implants for treatment of canine sun induced squamous cell carcinoma. *European Journal of Cancer* **31**, 2093–2098

Lana SE, Ogilvie GK, Withrow SJ, Straw RC and Rogers KS (1997) Feline cutaneous squamous cell carcinoma of the nasal planum and pinnae: 61 cases. *Journal of the American Animal Hospital Association* **33**, 329–332

Marks SL, Song MD, Stannard AA and Power HT (1992) Clinical evaluation of etretinate for the treatment of canine solar-induced squamous cell carcinoma and preneoplastic lesions. *Journal of the American Academy of Dermatology* **27**, 11–16

Mason KV (1987) The pathogenesis of solar induced skin lesions in Bull Terriers. *Proceedings of the American Academy of Veterinary Dermatology and American College of Veterinary Dermatology* **4,** 12

Miller MA, Ramos JA and Kreeger JM (1992) Cutaneous vascular neoplasia in 15 cats: clinical, morphologic and immunohistochemical studies. *Veterinary Pathology* **29,** 329–336

Peaston AE, Leach MW and Higgins RJ (1993) Photodynamic therapy for nasal and aural squamous cell carcinoma in cats. *Journal of the American Veterinary Medical Association* **202,** 1261–1265

Perez J, Day MJ, Martin MP *et al.* (1999) Immunohistochemical study of the inflammatory infiltrate associated with feline squamous cell carcinoma and precancerous lesions (actinic keratosis). *Veterinary Immunology and Immunopathology* **69,** 33–45

Power HT and Ihrke PI (1995) The use of synthetic retinoids in veterinary medicine. In: *Kirk's Current Veterinary Therapy XII,* ed. JD Bonagura, pp.585–590. WB Saunders, Philadelphia

Rook AH, Jaworsky C, Nguyen T *et al.* (1995) Beneficial effect of low-dose systemic retinoid in combination with topical tretinoin for the treatment and prophylaxis of premalignant and malignant skin lesions in renal transplant recipients. *Transplantation* **59,** 714–719

Rosenkrantz WS (1993) Solar dermatitis. In: *Current Veterinary Dermatology,* ed. CE Griffin *et al.,* pp. 309–315. Mosby, St Louis

Ruslander D, KaserHotz B and Sardinas JC (1997) Cutaneous squamous cell carcinoma in cats. *Compendium on Continuing Education for the Practicing Veterinarian* **19,** 1119–1129

Schwartz RA (1996) Therapeutic perspectives in actinic and other keratoses. *International Journal of Dermatology* **35,** 533–545

Schwartz RA and Stoll HL (1999) Epithelial Precancerous Lesions In: *Fitzpatrick's Dermatology in General Medicine, 5th edn,* ed. IM Freedburg *et al.,* pp.823–840. McGraw-Hill, New York

Scott DW, Miller WH and Griffin CE (2001) *Muller and Kirk's Small Animal Dermatology, 6th edn.* pp. 1073–1081. WB Saunders, Philadelphia

Spicer MS and Goldberg DJ (1996) Lasers in dermatology. *Journal of the American Academy of Dermatology* **34,** 1–17

Teifke JP and Lohr CV (1996) Immunohistochemical detection of p53 overexpression in paraffin wax-embedded squamous cell carcinomas of cattle, horses, cats and dogs. *Journal of Comparative Pathology* **114,** 205–210

Theon AP, Madewell BR, Shearn VI *et al.* (1995) Prognostic factors associated with radiotherapy of squamous cell carcinoma of the nasal plane in cats. *Journal of the American Veterinary Medical Association* **206,** 991–996

Theon AP, VanVechten MK, Madewell BR (1996) Intratumoural adminstration of carboplatin for the treatment of squamous cell carcinoma of the nasal plane in cats. *Journal of the American Veterinary Medical Association* **57,** 205–210

30

Mast cell tumours

David Vail

Mast cell tumours (also known as histiocytic masto-cytoma or mast cell sarcoma) are defined as neoplastic proliferations of mast cells. They are the most commonly encountered skin tumours of dogs (16–21%) and the second most common cutaneous tumours of cats (8–20%) (Hottendorf and Neilson, 1967; Bostock, 1986; Rothwell *et al.*, 1987; Miller *et al.*, 1991; Thamm and Vail, 2001). Cutaneous mast cell tumours are thought to arise from tissue mast cells in the dermis. These tumours can be confined to the skin or can be part of a systemic process referred to as mastocytosis. In both dogs and cats there is a wide spectrum of biological aggressiveness in cutaneous mast cell tumours. Several prognostic factors, in particular histological appearance, will help the clinician determine if a particular case is likely to be biologically more benign or malignant.

Mast cell tumours (MCTs) are primarily seen in older dogs, with a mean age of around 9 years, but have been reported in dogs from 3 weeks to 19 years of age (Patnaik *et al.*, 1984; Bostock, 1986; Thamm and Vail, 2001). Most occur in mixed breeds; however, Boxers, Boston Terriers, Labrador Retrievers, Beagles and Schnauzers have all been reported to be at higher risk. Boxers are at increased risk for MCT development, accounting for nearly half the dogs in one large series. Commonly, they develop the histologically well differentiated form of the disease which usually has a favourable prognosis (Bostock, 1986).

Two distinct forms of cutaneous MCT have been reported in cats:

* Mastocytic MCT – more typical, histologically similar to MCT in dogs
* Histiocytic MCT – less common, with morphological features characteristic of histiocytic mast cells (Wilcock *et al.*, 1986; Chastain *et al.*, 1988).

An overall mean age of 8–9 years is reported for cats with MCT, though the mastocytic and histiocytic forms occur at mean ages of 10 and 2.4 years, respectively (Miller *et al.*, 1991; Thamm and Vail, 2001). Siamese cats appear to be predisposed to development of MCT of both histological types (Wilcock *et al.*, 1986; Chastain *et al.*, 1988). No sex predilection exists in either species.

Aetiology

The aetiology of MCTs in the dog and cat is largely unknown. On rare occasions MCTs have been associated with chronic inflammation or the application of skin irritants. Recently, mutations of the tumour suppressor gene p53 and the proto-oncogene *c-kit* have been found in approximately 50% of canine MCTs and the mutation frequency appears to correlate with histological grade (London *et al.*, 1996; Jaffe *et al.*, 2000). No association with feline leukaemia virus (FeLV), feline immunodeficiency virus (FIV) or feline infectious peritonitis (FIP) has been reported. A genetic predisposition has been proposed due to the high incidence of MCT in the Siamese breed (Wilcock *et al.*, 1986; Chastain *et al.*, 1988).

Histology and staging

Well differentiated mast cells contain cytoplasmic granules (Figure 30.1) that contain a number of bioactive constituents, including histamine and heparin. These granules stain metachromatically with toluidine blue. Complications and associated clinical signs associated with degranulation of MCTs causing release of several vasoactive amines can occur in both species and will be discussed. Highly anaplastic, agranular MCTs may be difficult to diagnose by routine light microscopy, and immunohistochemical techniques may need to be applied to differentiate these from other anaplastic round cell tumours.

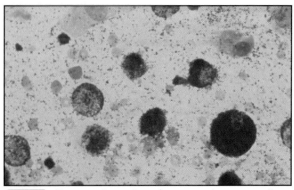

30.1 Fine needle aspirate from a canine mast cell tumour. There are individual round cells with round-to-oval nuclei that are obscured by an abundance of fine basophilic cytoplasmic granules. Numerous mast cell granules are present in the background. (Wright's stain; X1000 original magnification.)

Several histological grading systems have been applied to canine MCTs based on degree of differentiation and have been shown to predict biological aggressiveness (Bostock, 1973; Patnaik *et al.*, 1984). The number grades used in these studies are at odds. For the sake of clarity, the three differentiation groups should be simply referred to as:

- Undifferentiated (high) grade: approximately 20% of cutaneous MCTs
- Intermediate grade: approximately 40%
- Well differentiated (low) grade: approximately 40%.

A similar histological grading system does not exist for the cat, and the system described for canine MCTs provides no prognostic information for feline tumours (Molander-McCrary *et al.*, 1998). Feline cutaneous MCTs occur in two histologically distinct forms (Wilcock *et al.*, 1986; Chastain *et al.*, 1988; Miller *et al.*, 1991):

- Mastocytic
- Histiocytic.

The mastocytic form can be further subdivided on histological appearance into two categories: compact and diffuse. The compact form, comprising 80–90% of cases, is associated with more benign behaviour. The diffuse form is histologically more anaplastic and behaviourally more malignant. Two studies showed that most of the cases that recurred or metastasized were of the diffuse histotype (Holzinger, 1973). The majority of feline cutaneous MCTs are behaviourally benign.

History and clinical signs

Tumour appearance
Cutaneous MCTs have an extremely varied range of clinical appearance and biological behaviour. The majority of tumours are solitary, but 11–14% of dogs and up to 20% of cats present with multiple lesions.

Dogs
In dogs, tumour appearance has been correlated with the degree of histological differentiation (Bostock, 1973). Well differentiated MCTs tend to be solitary, 1–4 cm in diameter, slow growing, rubbery tumours often present for at least 6 months. Typically, they are not ulcerated but overlying hair may be lost (Figure 30.2). Undifferentiated MCTs tend to be rapidly growing, ulcerated lesions that cause considerable irritation and attain a large size (Figure 30.3). Surrounding tissues may become inflamed and oedematous. Tumours of intermediate differentiation fall between these two extremes. In dogs, a subcutaneous form of MCT that is soft and fleshy on palpation is often misdiagnosed clinically as a lipoma (Figure 30.4).

Cats
The typical feline cutaneous MCT is a solitary raised firm well circumscribed hairless dermal nodule 0.5–3 cm in diameter (Figure 30.5) (Wilcock *et al.*, 1986; Miller *et al.*, 1991). The tumours are often non-pigmented, although

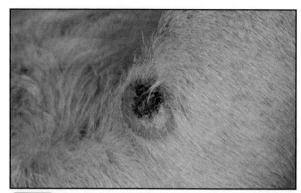

30.2 A solitary, well differentiated mast cell tumour on a 7-year-old mixed breed dog. The overlying hair has been lost and some small degree of excoriation is present.

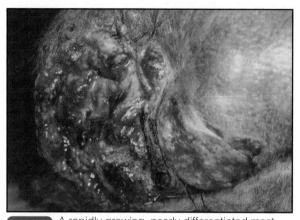

30.3 A rapidly growing, poorly differentiated mast cell tumour on the hip of a 9-year-old black Labrador. The tumour has ruptured, presumably because the rapid growth outstripped the available blood supply and caused necrosis.

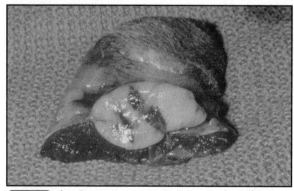

30.4 A subcutaneous mast cell tumour from the shoulder of a 7-year-old Golden Retriever. The tumour extends through the fascia and muscle, and wide surgical excision including the deep muscle layer was necessary to achieve complete 'clean' surgical margins. Based on palpation alone, the mass had originally been misdiagnosed as a lipoma. (Reprinted from Thamm and Vail (1999) with permission.)

a pink erythematous form is occasionally encountered. Superficial ulceration is present in approximately a quarter of cases. Two other clinical forms have been described: one is a flat pruritic plaque-like lesion similar to an eosinophilic plaque, and the other presents as subcutaneous nodules.

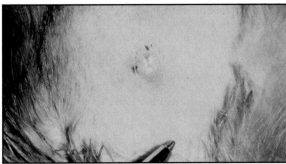

30.5 A typical solitary, raised, well circumscribed hairless dermal cutaneous mast cell tumour on a 10-year-old Domestic Shorthair. Surgical excision was curative in this case. (Reprinted from Thamm and Vail (1999) with permission.)

Degranulation

The history and clinical signs of MCTs in dogs and cats are complicated by signs attributable to release of histamine, heparin and other vasoactive amines from the MCT granules. These include:

- Coagulation disorders
- Gastrointestinal ulceration (with related signs of vomiting (possibly with blood), anorexia, melaena and abdominal pain
- Altered smooth muscle tone
- Hypotensive shock
- Anaphylactoid reactions
- Occasionally, mechanical manipulation during examination of the tumour results in degranulation and subsequent erythema and wheal formation in surrounding tissues ('Darier's sign') (Figure 30.6).

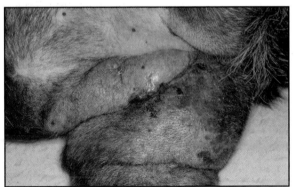

30.6 An inguinal poorly differentiated mast cell tumour on a 8-year-old Golden Retriever. This location is usually associated with a more aggressive biology. There is erythema and oedema (Darier's sign), resulting from degranulation and release of vasoactive amines.

Distribution of lesions

In dogs, MCTs are most commonly found on the trunk; tumours on the limbs account for only one quarter of all sites, and lesions are least common on the head and neck. In contrast, the head and neck are the most common sites for MCT in cats, followed by the trunk, limbs and miscellaneous sites (Miller *et al.*, 1991). Those on the head often involve the pinnae near the base of the ear.

Mast cell tumours have been reported to occur infrequently in other sites in both species, including the conjunctiva, salivary gland, nasopharynx, larynx and oral cavity.

Visceral MCT

A visceral form of MCT, often referred to as disseminated mastocytosis, can also occur. In the dog, an undifferentiated primary cutaneous lesion usually precedes visceral MCT. Consistent physical examination findings include lymphadenopathy, splenomegaly, and/or hepatomegaly as a result of disseminated MCT. Bone marrow and peripheral blood involvement with neoplastic mast cells are common. Pleural and peritoneal effusions containing abundant neoplastic mast cells have been observed in dogs with visceral MCT.

In cats, visceral MCTs often do not represent extension of a primary cutaneous lesion, and purely visceral forms of MCT (e.g. liver, spleen, intestinal tract) can also occur in the dog. These are beyond the scope of this chapter and the reader is referred to reviews on the subject (O'Keefe *et al.*, 1987; Thamm and Vail, 2001).

Diagnosis

Cytology

Mast cell tumours are initially diagnosed on the basis of fine-needle aspiration (FNA) cytology. Romanovsky or rapid haematological type stains used in most practices will suffice. Mast cells appear as small to medium-sized round cells with abundant small uniform cytoplasmic granules that stain purplish red (metachromatic) (see Figure 30.1). A small percentage of MCTs have granules that do not stain readily, giving them an epithelial, 'fried egg', or macrophage-like appearance. In these cases, histological assessment is necessary for diagnosis.

The granules present in feline MCTs stain blue with Giemsa and purple with toluidine blue. They tend to appear more eosinophilic than their canine counterparts with hematoxylin and eosin stains. The uncommon histiocytic form of feline MCT is more challenging to diagnose cytologically as mast cells may comprise only 20% of the cells present; the majority of cells are sheets of histiocytes that lack distinct cytoplasmic granules and are accompanied by randomly scattered lymphoid aggregates and eosinophils. In those cases, histological assessment may be more appropriate.

Histology

If the MCT is in a location amenable to wide surgical excision and none of the negative prognostic indicators (see Figure 30.8) is present, wide surgical excision is performed. Wide surgical excision is not as critical in cats with MCT, as most are biologically benign. The excised tissue is submitted *in toto* for assessment of histological differentiation and completeness of surgical removal (margins). FNA cytology is not sufficient to grade MCT; therefore histological assessment is strongly recommended.

Ancillary diagnosis

In the dog, if the tumour presents at a site that is *not* amenable to wide surgical excision (e.g. distal extremity), or if negative prognostic factors exist in the history or physical examination, ancillary diagnostics to grade the disease are undertaken prior to definitive therapy (Figure 30.7). These include:

- Cytological assessment of regional lymph nodes
- CBC and buffy coat smear to document peripheral mastocytosis
- Abdominal ultrasonography (with cytological assessment of spleen or liver if abnormalities are observed)
- Thoracic radiography (usually negative)
- Bone marrow aspiration
- Incisional biopsy, for determination of histological grade.

It is important to realize that mast cells are also found in normal tissues, including lymph nodes. Peripheral mastocytaemia (1–90 mast cells/μl) is reported in dogs with acute inflammatory disease (in particular parvoviral infections), regenerative anaemia, neoplasia other than MCT, and trauma (Bookbinder *et al.*, 1992; McManus, 1999). One study revealed that peripheral mastocytosis is actually more likely to occur, and may be more dramatic, in dogs with diseases other than MCT. Therefore, the dogma that buffy coat smears are an important diagnostic assessment of MCT patients should be tempered and may be of more benefit if used to assess changes over time in dogs with MCT already confirmed histologically.

Knowledge of the extent of MCT margins prior to surgery can be enhanced with the use of diagnostic ultrasonography or computed tomography (CT). Such information allows more appropriate planning of definitive surgery or radiotherapy. The cost effectiveness of such a study depends on the location of the tumour and whether wide excision is technically simple or difficult.

Visceral MCT

If visceral dissemination is suspected, careful examination of peripheral blood and bone marrow cytology is recommended; bone marrow cytology appears to be superior to both peripheral blood and buffy coat smears in determining systemic involvement.

Prognosis

Figure 30.8 lists the prognostic factors associated with MCT in dogs.

Histological grade

Histological grade is the most consistent prognostic factor available for dogs with MCT. The vast majority of dogs with well differentiated tumours, and approximately 75–85% of dogs with moderately differentiated tumours, experience long-term survival following complete surgical excision. Dogs with undifferentiated tumours treated surgically typically die of the disease within 6 months due to local recurrence or metastasis. Metastatic rates for undifferentiated tumours range from 55 to 96%. The majority disseminate first to local lymph nodes, then to spleen and liver. Other visceral organs may be involved but lung involvement is infrequent. Neoplastic mast cells may be observed in the bone marrow and peripheral blood in cases of widespread systemic dissemination. Recently, silver colloid staining of paraffin-imbedded sections to determine the relative presence of agyrophilic nucleolar organizer regions (AgNORs) has been correlated with histological grade and post-surgical outcome (Kravis *et al.*, 1996).

Location of lesion

Tumours in the preputial/inguinal area (see Figure 30.6), subungual (nail bed) region (Figure 30.9), and other mucocutaneous sites including the oral cavity and perineum are often undifferentiated tumours that metastasize early.

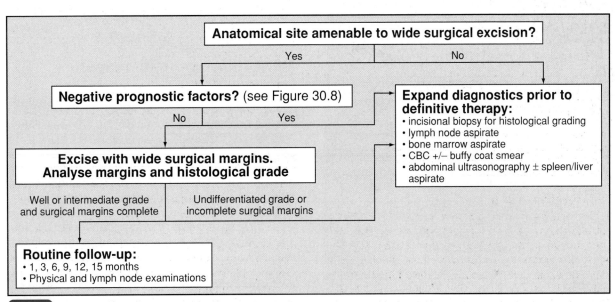

30.7 Suggested approach to diagnosis of canine cutaneous mast cell tumours.

Factor	Comment
Histological grade*	Strongly predictive of outcome. Dogs with undifferentiated tumours typically die of their disease following local therapy. Dogs with well or moderately differentiated tumours are usually cured by appropriate local therapy
Clinical stage*	Stage 0 and I, confined to the skin without local lymph node or distant metastasis, have a better prognosis than higher stage disease
Recurrence*	Recurrent tumours are usually more aggressive biologically
Location*	Peripreputial, subungual, perianal, oral and other mucocutaneous sites are associated with more undifferentiated tumours and poorer prognosis. Visceral or bone marrow disease carries a grave prognosis
Growth rate*	MCTs that remain localized and are present for prolonged periods of time (months or years) are usually benign. Tumours with recent rapid growth are more likely to be undifferentiated
AgNOR count*	Relative frequency of AgNORs (agrophillic nuclear organizer regions) is predictive of post-surgical outcome. The higher the AgNOR count, the poorer the prognosis
DNA ploidy	Trend towards shorter survival and higher stage disease in dogs with aneuploid tumours
PCNA assessment	A higher percentage of positive PNCA immunopositivity is associated with a more guarded prognosis
Systemic signs	The presence of systemic illness (i.e. anorexia, vomiting, GI ulceration, melaena) associated with more aggressive forms
Age	Older dogs may have a shorter median disease-free interval when treated with radiotherapy
Breed	MCTs in boxers tend to be more differentiated and carry a better prognosis
Sex	Male dogs had a shorter survival time than bitches when treated with chemotherapy

30.8 Prognostic factors for canine mast cell tumours. (Modified from Thamm and Vail (2001) with permission.) * = Most strongly predictive.

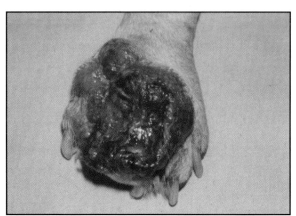

30.9 A subungual mast cell tumour on a 6-year-old English Bulldog. This location is often associated with aggressive undifferentiated tumours.

Clinical appearance

Clinical appearance is also prognostic in dogs; however, at least one study has suggested that there is no difference in outcome between patients with a single MCT and those with multiple cutaneous MCTs (Thamm *et al.*, 1999). Thus, this part of the staging scheme may not accurately correlate with outcome.

Visceral MCT

Systemic signs of anorexia, vomiting, melaena, widespread erythema, and oedema associated with vasoactive substances from mast cell degranulation are more commonly associated with visceral forms of MCT, and carry a more guarded prognosis (O'Keefe *et al.*, 1987; Thamm and Vail, 2001). Median survivals of 60–90 days are reported in dogs with visceral MCT (O'Keefe *et al.*, 1987).

Recurrence

Recurrence of MCT following surgical excision is associated with a guarded prognosis (Figure 30.10). Appropriately aggressive therapy at the time of *first* presentation, rather than at the time of recurrence, may improve the long-term prognosis in patients with MCT.

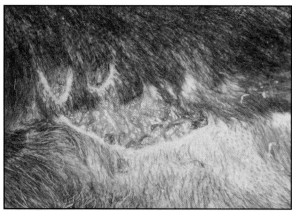

30.10 Recurrence of a mast cell tumour at the site of a previous excisional surgery. Recurrence is usually associated with aggressive biology.

Management and therapeutics

Dogs

Treatment decisions are based on the presence or absence of negative prognostic factors (see Figure 30.8) and on the clinical stage of disease. Figure 30.11 summarizes the treatment recommendations for clinical stage 0 and I, histologically low- or inter-mediate-grade MCT. Surgical excision and radiation therapy are the most successful treatment options described to date.

Following definitive therapy, dogs with low and intermediate grade tumours should be re-evaluated regularly for local recurrence and possible systemic spread. In the author's practice, patients are re-evaluated 1 month after definitive therapy, then every 3 months for 1½ years, then every 6 months thereafter. Local site and regional lymph node evaluation and a

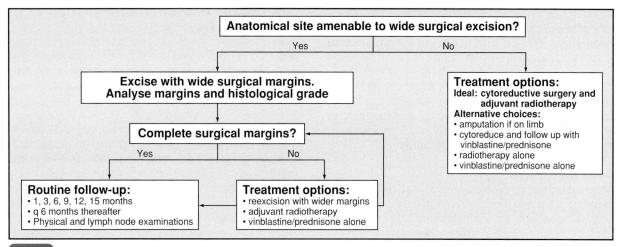

Anatomical site amenable to wide surgical excision?

Yes → Excise with wide surgical margins. Analyse margins and histological grade

No → **Treatment options:**
Ideal: cytoreductive surgery and adjuvant radiotherapy
Alternative choices:
• amputation if on limb
• cytoreduce and follow up with vinblastine/prednisone
• radiotherapy alone
• vinblastine/prednisone alone

Complete surgical margins?

Yes → **Routine follow-up:**
• 1, 3, 6, 9, 12, 15 months
• q 6 months thereafter
• Physical and lymph node examinations

No → **Treatment options:**
• reexcision with wider margins
• adjuvant radiotherapy
• vinblastine/prednisone alone

30.11 Suggested approach to treatment of canine cutaneous mast cell tumours of low or intermediate grade.

complete physical examination are performed at these intervals. More complete staging including abdominal ultrasonography, buffy coat smears and bone marrow aspiration are pursued if warranted.

Tumours amenable to wide excision

Surgery is the treatment of choice for tumours present in areas amenable to wide excision. Surgical excision should be planned to include a 3 cm margin of surrounding normal tissue in dogs (Figure 30.12). Extensive deep margins are as important as lateral margins in this species, and if necessary fascial and muscle layers are removed in continuity with the tumour (see Figure 30.4). Surgical margins should be evaluated histologically for completeness of excision.

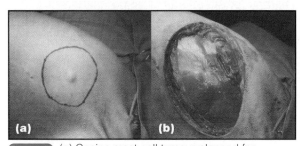

30.12 (a) Canine mast cell tumour planned for surgical excision. (b) Completed excision; note the recommended wide (3 cm) surgical margins. (Courtesy of J. McAnulty.)

A source of controversy is what should be done in a case of MCT of intermediate grade following complete (i.e. clean) surgical excision. Some recommend adjuvant therapy with long-term corticosteroids, others a number of cycles of vinca alkaloids, and still others radiotherapy in the face of complete surgical margins. There is no clinical evidence that any of these strategies is of benefit. In a recent study, the vast majority of intermediate grade MCTs having surgery effecting complete surgical margins had very low rates of recurrence (5%) and distant metastasis (5%) (Seguin et al., 2001). Based on these data and this author's personal experience, no further adjuvant therapy is recommended in this scenario and these animals are placed on the previously mentioned re-evaluation schedule.

Excised tumours with incomplete histological margins

For cases where planned curative excisional surgery is unsuccessful and histological margins are reported as incomplete, further local therapy is warranted. A second excision, with additional wide margins of the surgical scar, or adjuvant radiotherapy is recommended. Not all MCTs with surgically incomplete margins will recur: in one report only 30% of MCTs with histologically confirmed incomplete margins did so (Misdorf, 1987). This figure seems extremely low based on the personal experience of the author, and may reflect confusion with normal cutaneous mast cells at the surgical margin.

Tumours not amenable to wide excision: low or intermediate grade MCT

Tumours in areas not amenable to wide surgical margins, such as distal extremities, should be evaluated by incisional biopsy for histological differentiation prior to definitive therapy. If a distal extremity MCT is of low or intermediate grade differentiation, three primary therapy options exist.

Amputation: The most aggressive option is amputation. This generally guarantees wide margins, but results in the least functional outcome.

Radiotherapy: In the gross disease setting this results in 1-year control rates of only 50% (Allan and Gilette, 1979). Recently, course fraction radiation protocols (3 or 4 weekly 8 Gy fractions) have, anecdotally, resulted in local responses lasting months to even a year or longer.

Surgery and radiotherapy combination: The third and, in this author's opinion the ideal, option for low- or intermediate-grade MCT in areas where wide surgical excision is not possible is a combination of surgery and radiotherapy. The complementary use of surgery to achieve clinical stage 0 disease (i.e. microscopically incomplete margins) and external beam radiotherapy is associated with long-term control

(2-year control rates of 85–95%) of low or intermediate grade differentiation (Al-Sarraf *et al.*, 1996; Frimberger *et al.*, 1997; LaDue *et al.*, 1998). Some authors advocate prophylactic irradiation of cytologically negative regional lymph nodes (LaDue *et al.*, 1998); however, definitive evidence of a survival advantage associated with this practice is lacking. Unfortunately, dogs with undifferentiated tumours do not fare as well, with the majority developing distant metastasis within 4–6 months of therapy.

Other local therapies

Alternative local therapies for confined MCTs have been reported and include hyperthermia in combination with radiotherapy, intralesional brachytherapy, photodynamic therapy, intralesional corticosteroids, cryotherapy, and intralesional deionized water. None of these is as thoroughly investigated, as clinically effective or as practical as surgery, radiation therapy or combinations of the two. Despite its widespread use, there is no clinical evidence that additional adjuvant corticosteroid therapy is of any benefit in cases of intermediate-grade MCTs that have been either excised completely or have been treated with adjuvant local radiotherapy.

High-grade MCT

The management of biologically high-grade MCT remains frustrating for both the client and the practising clinician. This designation includes dogs with undifferentiated tumours as well as those with intermediate-grade tumours that have established regional or distant spread. Client education with respect to prognosis is essential in the decision-making process. Undifferentiated tumours should be treated with aggressive local surgery or radiotherapy *only* if thorough staging fails to reveal dissemination and if the clients are fully informed as to the likelihood of future dissemination. The long-term prognosis for such dogs is not favourable, as regional and distant metastasis are likely, especially in high-risk locations such as preputial and perianal areas.

Poorly differentiated and metastatic MCT will almost invariably kill the host in the absence of effective post-surgical intervention. Systemic adjuvant therapy should be offered in such cases in an attempt to decrease the likelihood of systemic involvement or, at least, potentially improve disease-free intervals. Corticosteroids such as prednisolone have been reported to be of some benefit in primarily preclinical or anecdotal settings. Glucocorticoids may also contribute to apparent antitumour response by decreasing peritumoural oedema and inflammation. The Veterinary Cooperative Oncology Group (VCOG) studied the efficacy of single-agent systemic prednisolone therapy for intermediate- and high-grade canine MCT. Response rates were less than 25% and improvements were short-lived, lasting only a few weeks in the majority of cases (McCaw *et al.*, 1994).

Chemotherapy

Recently, a number of studies have evaluated the response rate of canine MCT to various systemic chemotherapy drugs and protocols (Fig 30.13). Response rates as high as 78% have been reported, and preliminary evidence suggests that multiagent protocols may confer a higher response rate than single-agent therapy. In the author's practice, patients with poorly differentiated MCT receive prednisolone and vinblastine. In this protocol, vinblastine (2 mg/m^2, i.v.) is given weekly for 4 consecutive weeks and then every other week for four additional treatments (a total of eight treatments). Prednisolone is given at 1 mg/kg orally, once daily for 2 weeks, then decreased to 0.5 mg/kg daily for 10 additional weeks before being tapered off. This results in a median survival time of 331 days, with 45% of evaluable patients alive at 1 and 2 years (Thamm *et al.*, 1999). This is an apparent improvement over historical cases employing surgery alone.

Therapy for the effects of degranulation

Ancillary therapy for the systemic effects of MCT related to degranulation is sometimes recommended.

Histamine blockers: Blocking all or some of the effects of histamine release can be accomplished by administering the H$_1$ blocker diphenhydramine (2–4 mg/kg orally bid) and the H$_2$ blockers cimetidine (4 mg/kg orally tid) or ranitidine (2 mg/kg bid). Omeprazole (0.5–1 mg/kg sid), a newer proton pump inhibitor, has yet to be evaluated in dogs with MCT but theoretically should be effective.

Drug(s)	Number treated	CR	PR	ORR	Median response duration	Reference
Prednisone	25	4%	16%	20%	NR	(McCaw *et al.*, 1994)
Vincristine	27	0%	7%	7%	NR	(McCaw *et al.*, 1997)
Lomustine (CCNU)	21	6%	38%	44%	79 days*	(Rassnick *et al.*, 1999)
Prednisone/Vinblastine	41	33%	13%	47%	154 days	(Thamm *et al.*, 1999)
P/C/V	21	0%	78%	78%	NR	(Elmslie, 1997)
COP–HU	17	23%	35%	59%	53 days	(Gerritsen *et al.*, 1998)

CR: Complete response. PR: Partial response. ORR: Overall response rate. P/C/V: Prednisone/Vinblastine/Cyclophosphamide. COP–HU: Cyclophosphamide/Vincristine/Prednisone/Hydroxyurea. NR: Not reported. * Excludes patient that experienced a CR; euthanized without evidence of disease after 440 days.

30.13 Published chemotherapy protocols for canine mast cell tumours. (Modified from Thamm and Vail (2001) with permission.)

It is recommended that the use of these agents is reserved for those cases where:

- Systemic signs are present
- The tumour is likely to be entered or manipulated at surgery (i.e. cytoreductive surgery)
- Treatment is undertaken where gross disease will remain and degranulation is likely to occur *in situ* (e.g. radiotherapy, corticosteroid or chemotherapy for tumours that are not surgically cytoreduced to a microscopic setting).

These agents are not routinely used for cases where wide surgical excision is to occur without excessive manipulation of the tumour itself.

Gastric protectants: For cases with active evidence of gastric or duodenal ulceration, sucralfate (0.5–1.0 g orally tid) and occasionally misoprostol (3 µg/kg orally tid) may be given in addition to histamine blockers.

Heparin antagonist: The use of protamine sulphate, a heparin antagonist, has been recommended by some for use in cases of intraoperative haemorrhage.

Cats

Mastocytic MCT

Surgery is the treatment of choice for the mastocytic form of cutaneous MCT. As previously discussed, most are behaviourally benign and wide surgical margins may not be as critical as in the dog. This is fortunate, as most occur on the head where such margins would be difficult to achieve.

Local recurrence and systemic spread have been reported to occur in 0–24% of cases following surgical excision (Wilcock *et al.*, 1986; Molander-McCrary *et al.*, 1998). More recent studies and the author's experience suggest the number is closer to 5–10% of cases. Recurrence, should it occur, is usually noted within 6 months.

For histologically anaplastic (i.e. diffuse) mastocytic tumours, a more aggressive approach similar to that used for canine MCT may be prudent, as higher rates of recurrence and metastasis are associated with this type.

Histiocytic MCT

Following biopsy confirmation, conservative resection or a 'wait and see' approach may be taken with the histiocytic form in young cats with multiple masses (Figure 30.14), as the majority are reported to regress spontaneously within 1 year (Chastain *et al.*, 1988; Miller *et al.*, 1991).

Adjuvant therapy

Little is known about the effectiveness of adjunctive therapy for cutaneous MCT in the cat. Efficacy trials for corticosteroids, chemotherapeutics or radiotherapy do not exist in the veterinary literature. In the author's practice, prednisolone/vinblastine combinations or lomustine (CCNU) are presently being evaluated for cases with systemic dissemination. Response to steroids in cats with the histiocytic form is equivocal (Chastain *et al.*, 1988).

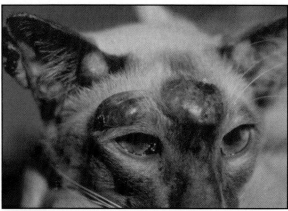

30.14 Histiocytic mast cell tumours on the head of a young Siamese cat. These tumours regressed spontaneously, as is often the case. (Courtesy of K Moriello. Reprinted from Thamm and Vail (2001) with permission.)

References and further reading

Allan GS and Gilette EL (1979) Response of canine mast cell tumors to radiation. *Journal of the National Cancer Institute* **63**, 691–694

Al-Sarraf R, Mauldin GN, Patnaik AK *et al.* (1996) A prospective study of radiation therapy for the treatment of grade 2 mast cell tumors in 32 dogs. *Journal of Veterinary Internal Medicine* **10**, 376–378

Bookbinder PF, Butt MT and Harvey HJ (1992) Determination of the number of mast cells in lymph node, bone marrow, and buffy coat cytologic specimens from dogs. *Journal of the American Veterinary Medical Association* **200**, 1648–1650

Bostock DE (1973) The prognosis following surgical removal of mastocytomas in dogs. *Journal of Small Animal Practice* **14**, 27–40

Bostock DE (1986) Neoplasms of the skin and subcutaneous tissues in dogs and cats. *British Veterinary Journal* **142**, 1–19

Chastain CB, Turk MAM and O'Brien D (1988) Benign cutaneous mastocytomas in two litters of Siamese kittens. *Journal of the American Veterinary Medical Association* **193**, 959–960

Elmslie R (1997) Combination chemotherapy with and without surgery for dogs with high grade mast cell tumors with regional lymph node metastases. *Veterinary Cancer Society Newsletter* **20**, 6–7

Frimberger AE, Moore AS, LaRue SM *et al.* (1997) Radiotherapy of incompletely resected, moderately differentiated mast cell tumors in the dog: 37 cases (1989–1993). *Journal of the American Animal Hospital Association* **33**, 324

Gerritsen RJ, Teske E, Kraus JS *et al.* (1998) Multi-agent chemotherapy for mast cell tumours in the dog. *Veterinary Quarterly* **20**, 28–31

Holzinger EA (1973) Feline cutaneous mastocytomas. *Cornell Veterinarian* **63**, 87–93

Hottendorf GH and Neilson SW (1967) Survey of 300 extirpated canine mastocytomas. *Zentralblatt für Veterinärmedizin* [A] **14**, 272–281

Jaffe MH, Hosgood G, Taylor HW *et al.* (2000) Immunohistochemical and clinical evaluation of p53 in canine cutaneous mast cell tumors. *Veterinary Pathology* **37**, 40–46

Kravis LG, Vail DM, Kisseberth WC *et al.* (1996) Frequency of argyrophilic nucleolar organizer regions in fine-needle aspirates and biopsy specimens from mast cell tumors in dogs. *Journal of the American Veterinary Medical Association* **209**, 1418–1420

LaDue T, Price GS, Dodge R *et al.* (1998) Radiation therapy for incompletely resected canine mast cell tumors. *Veterinary Radiology and Ultrasound* **39**, 57–62

London CA, Kisseberth WC and Galli SJ (1996) Expression of stem cell factor receptor (c-kit) by the malignant mast cells from spontaneous canine mast cell tumors. *Journal of Comparative Pathology* **115**, 399–414

McCaw DL, Miller MA, Ogilvie GK *et al.* (1994) Response of canine mast cell tumors to treatment with oral prednisone. *Journal of Veterinary Internal Medicine* **8**, 406–408

McCaw DL, Miller MA, Bergman PJ *et al.* (1997) Vincristine therapy for mast cell tumors in dogs. *Journal of Veterinary Internal Medicine* **11**, 375–378

McManus PM (1999) Frequency and severity of mastocytemia in dogs with and without mast cell tumors: 120 cases (1995–1997). *Journal of the American Veterinary Medical Association* **215**, 355–357

Miller MA, Nelson SL, Turk JR (1991) Cutaneous neoplasia in 340 cats. *Veterinary Pathology* **28**, 389–395

Misdorf W (1987) Incomplete surgery, local immunostimulation, and recurrence of some tumour types in dogs and cats. *Veterinary Quarterly* **9,** 279–286

Molander-McCrary H, Henry CJ, Potter K *et al.* (1998) Cutaneous mast cell tumors in cats: 32 cases (1991–1994). *Journal of the American Animal Hospital Association* **34,** 281–284

O'Keefe DA, Couto CG, Burke-Schwartz C *et al.* (1987) Systemic mastocytosis in 16 dogs. *Journal of Veterinary Internal Medicine* **1,** 75–80

Patnaik AK, Ehler WJ and MacEwen EG (1984) Canine cutaneous mast cell tumor: morphologic grading and survival time in 83 dogs. *Veterinary Pathology* **21,** 469–474

Rassnick KM, Moore AS. Williams LE *et al.* (1999) Treatment of canine mast cell tumors with CCNU (lomustine) *Journal of Veterinary Internal Medicine* **13,** 601–605

Rothwell TLW, Howlett CR and Middleton DJ (1987) Skin neoplasms of dogs in Sydney. *Australian Veterinary Journal* **64,** 161–164

Seguin B, Leibman NF, Bregazzi VS *et al.* (2001) Clinical outcome of dogs with grade-II mast cell tumors treated with surgery alone: 55 cases (1996–1999). *Journal of the American Veterinary Medical Association* **218,** 1120–1123

Thamm DH, Mauldin EA and Vail DM (1999) Prednisone and vinblastine chemotherapy for canine mast cell tumor: 41 cases (1992–1998). *Journal of Veterinary Internal Medicine* **13,** 491–497

Thamm D and Vail DM (2001) Mast cell tumors. In: *Small Animal Clinical Oncology, 3rd edn,* ed. SJ Withrow and EG MacEwen, pp.261–282 WB Saunders, Philadelphia

Wilcock BP, Yager JA and Zink MC (1986) The morphology and behavior of feline cutaneous mastocytomas. *Veterinary Pathology* **23,** 320–324

31

Acral lick and other compulsive disorders

Soraya Juarbe-Diaz and Linda Frank

A compulsive disorder can be defined as the expression of repetitive ritualized behaviours that are exaggerated in intensity, frequency and duration. They are expressed out of context and to the exclusion of normal maintenance and social behaviours. Many compulsive disorders are an exaggeration of normal locomotive, grooming, oral (foraging) behaviours or they may be sensory in nature. Compulsive grooming behaviours may present with cutaneous manifestations.

Depending upon the severity and progression of the disease prior to presentation, the lesions will vary from partial alopecia with barbering of the hair to full thickness excoriation, inflammation and reactive granuloma formation. Secondary bacterial infections are common, and it sometimes becomes difficult to determine the extent to which behavioural and secondary dermatological components contribute to the skin lesion when the pet is examined. Discoloration of white or light coloured hair due to the effect of salivary amylase may also be noted in compulsive licking behaviours.

The precise pathophysiology of compulsive disorders is not known. Abnormal metabolism of serotonin (5-HT) in the basal ganglia and caudate nucleus of the limbic system, excess dopaminergic function (also in the basal ganglia) and abnormal endorphin levels have all been described in studies of obsessive–compulsive patients. Few studies have been conducted in animals, but at least one has identified abnormal endogenous opiate levels in horses with compulsive disorders, some of which responded to opiate antagonists. In cases of self-mutilation, a sensory neuropathy could also be at work with a possible abnormality of substance-P metabolism.

Common compulsive disorders that can result in dermatological lesions are listed in Figure 31.1.

Syndrome	Status as compulsive disease	Breed/Species
Acral lick dermatitis	Contributing or causative	Large breed dogs
Psychogenic alopecia	Contributing or causative	Any feline breed
Flank sucking	Suspected	Doberman Pinscher
Nail biting	Suspected	Any feline breed
Hyperaesthesia syndrome	Doubtful	Any feline breed

31.1 Dermatological compulsive disorders

Clinical approach

Acral lick lesions often have an inciting cause. Identifying the initiating factor is the first step towards treating the dermatitis. Inciting causes may include:

- Allergies
- Previous trauma
- Prior surgery
- Foreign body
- Infection (pyoderma, dermatophytosis, demodicosis)
- Arthritis
- Neoplasia
- Behavioural abnormalities.

In addition, licking repetitively at a site results in follicular rupture and furunculosis. Secondary infection further perpetuates the desire to lick. For the most successful management of an acral lick lesion, treatment must be directed at eliminating the infection and identifying the underlying cause, together with behavioural modification to break the compulsive itch–lick cycle.

History

The first step when evaluating a dog with an acral lick lesion or a cat with psychogenic alopecia is determining whether or not they are truly pruritic (see Chapters 5 and 10). Allergies are very common causes of focused pruritus as seen with acral lick dermatitis. Usually dogs will have other evidence of an allergy (see Chapter 18). However, some dogs with a single acral lick lesion and no other evidence of pruritus have been diagnosed with a food hypersensitivity/intolerance (Paterson, 1998).

In addition, whenever a psychotropic component needs to be ruled out, information about the pet's behaviour must be collected. Because most behavioural data are 'soft' (consisting of owner-provided descriptions of the behaviours), the manner in which the behaviour history is taken must be such that the owner is not led to give the answer he or she thinks the examiner wants to hear. As an example, the question, 'What percentage of the time when you can see or hear your dog does it spend licking?' as opposed to 'Does your dog lick a lot?' will yield more useful and precise information. The latter question depends upon the owner's concept of 'a lot' while the former asks the owner to think about the actual time engaged in the behaviour.

Examples of behavioural histories can be found in a number of texts (Landsberg *et al.*, 1997; Overall, 1997), and the reader is referred to these for a more thorough coverage of behaviour history taking. It is not unusual to uncover evidence of anxious behaviour in response to what seem to be non-threatening stimuli or situations. The pet may be described as easily frightened, jittery, afraid of people or places, or easily startled. Physiological signs of sympathetic stimulation, such as hypervigilance, pupillary dilation, panting/tachypnoea, tachycardia, vomiting, increased urgency to void or loose stools, are sometimes observed by the owner in response to seemingly benign circumstances. In other cases the compulsive grooming is the only evidence of an anxiety disorder, or it is the first manifestation of other existing problems (e.g. separation anxiety or thunderstorm phobia).

Clinical syndromes

Acral lick dermatitis of behavioural origin

Large breed dogs are affected most commonly and Dobermanns, Rottweilers, Labrador Retrievers and Golden Retrievers are over-represented in some behaviour referral practice caseloads. This list is not exclusive, and mixed breed dogs may also be seen.

Age of onset is variable but most commonly the problem begins during the juvenile period or young adulthood. Similarly, the dorsal aspect of the carpus is a common focus for the licking behaviour, although the dorsal aspects of the fore- and hindlimbs, the lateral aspect of the elbow and tarsometatarsal joints, and the skin over the sacrum and ileum can be targeted. Licking has a *constant and invariant* quality about it not seen in an animal grooming normally (such as pauses and breaks in the licking, changes in posture and the area groomed) or in cases of irritation or pain where chewing also is involved. In the beginning, it may be possible for owners to interrupt the behaviour but typically the behaviour worsens, either because of natural progression of the disorder or because the anxiety created when the behaviour is prevented (particularly if the dog is punished to make it stop) exacerbates the condition.

Flank sucking

Seen almost exclusively in the Dobermann, this may be a similar but attenuated version of acral lick granuloma, or it may be a separate entity. Affected dogs grab a fold of skin in their flank area and perform sucking motions. Typically, owners report that the flank area is frequently moist with saliva. In a few cases, these dogs create dermatological lesions secondary to this behaviour. It is not known what percentage of Dobermanns that suckle on fabric go on to develop flank sucking, but it is not rare for flank suckers to have suckled on fabric prior to sucking on their flanks.

Feline psychogenic alopecia

There does not seem to be a breed predilection for psychogenic alopecia. Excessive grooming may be secondary to social friction in a multi-cat household, secondary to a separate medical condition or due to endogenous anxiety. The latter is sometimes hard to qualify. In some cases the anxiety is triggered by easily identifiable events such as a change in the owner's schedule, an addition to the household, or a move to a new home. In others, the excessive grooming behaviour seems to start spontaneously. The abdominal area, particularly the ventral aspect just cranial to the pubis, is the common target, but severe cases may present with complete body alopecia except for the head and neck where the cat cannot reach to groom itself. The lesions start with barbering of hair and alopecia and can progress through erythema and excoriation.

Feline hyperaesthesia syndrome

Unlike the disorders discussed above, feline hyperaesthesia has not been placed under the compulsive category. The pathophysiology has not been discerned, but is thought to involve neuropathic pain. Also known as 'twitchy cat disease' and 'rolling skin syndrome', cats suffering from this problem do not show methodical grooming, but rather explosive, sometimes violent attacks directed at themselves. Signs can develop suddenly, with the cat acting as if experiencing severe pain or discomfort. The skin over the dorsum may ripple or twitch, and the attack may be directed at this area, or the cat may run as if fleeing an unseen assailant. The cat may vocalize as it runs, try to hide or act aggressively, and may even redirect its aggression. Self-mutilation lesions can be severe and inflicted over a short period of time.

Diagnosis

Examination

Acral lick dermatitis lesions are clinically unique and easily identified on physical examination (Figure 31.2). Lesions are usually single and unilateral over the cranial carpal or metacarpal area or, less commonly, over the tarsal or metatarsal area. They are raised firm alopecic nodules or plaques that have a peripheral rim of hyperpigmentation and an eroded or ulcerated surface.

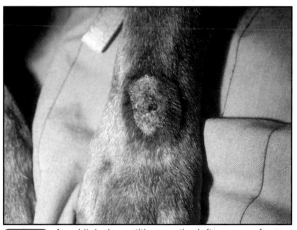

31.2 Acral lick dermatitis over the left carpus of an 8-year-old Dobermann Pinscher.

The clinical presentation of cats with self-induced alopecia is that of alopecia restricted to areas where the cat can groom (Figure 31.3). Because this presentation is similar to that seen with pruritic cats, a systematic approach to the cat with self-induced alopecia is necessary to rule out allergic causes (see Chapter 10).

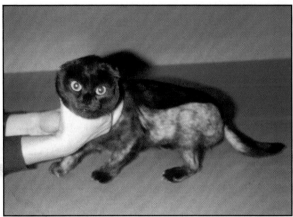

31.3 Psychogenic alopecia in an adult male Scottish Fold cat.

Diagnostic tests

Diagnostic tests are needed to rule out possible inciting and perpetuating factors. The first steps when approaching an acral lick lesion are:

- Multiple deep skin scrapings to rule out demodicosis
- Cytology to identify an infective organism
- 30-day therapeutic antibiotic trial
- Institution of strict flea control.

Biopsy for both histopathology and culture may permit the identification of possible initiating or perpetuating factors. Radiography may reveal an underlying arthritis. Periosteal reaction is commonly seen and thought to be secondary to the inflammatory process (Scott and Walton, 1984). Further allergy work-up should be pursued if the lesion fails to respond to routine therapeutics discussed below or if the lesion responds but recurs.

Management and therapeutics

Initial therapy

The first line of treatment for a dog with acral lick dermatitis is a prolonged course of antibiotics using a broad-spectrum bactericidal antibiotic such as cefalexin. The antibiotic is usually combined with a topical antipruritic/antifibrosing treatment such as fluocinolone in DMSO and a psychotropic drug such as amitriptyline and/or an opioid agonist such as hydrocodone (Scott *et al.*, 2001). In many cases, this approach will resolve the condition. If, however, the inciting cause has not been addressed, the lesion will recur. Also, the more chronic the lesion, the less responsive it is to this basic approach.

Behaviour modification

Psychotropic medication is an important component of treatment but environment and behaviour modification must be part of the plan to maximize response. With the possible exception of feline hyperaesthesia, anxiety plays a major component in the initiation and exacerbation of compulsive disorders, and efforts to minimize stressful elements must be a part of the treatment plan. The scope of this chapter prohibits comprehensive coverage of all the anxiety-based disorders that can confound compulsive disorders and the reader is referred to the suggested reading list for guidance in the management of the behaviour modification aspect of psychogenic disorders.

Pharmacological agents

In human psychiatric medicine, clomipramine (a tricyclic antidepressant, TCA) and fluoxetine (a serotonin specific reuptake inhibitor, SSRI) are the two most successfully used pharmacological agents in the treatment of compulsive disorders and are frequently recommended in dogs and cats for compulsive syndromes. Amitriptyline and doxepin, also TCAs, and other SSRIs such as paroxetine, fluvoxamine or citalopram (Stein *et al.*, 1998) have also been used (Overall, 1997; Luescher, 1998; Shuster and Dodman, 1998) (Figure 31.4).

Given the possible added benefits of tricyclics (antihistaminic and mild analgesic effects via interference with substance-P metabolism), making them the first choice in drug treatment is acceptable. Tricyclics should not be used in patients with a history of glaucoma, seizures, cardiac problems or hepatic disease, and should be used cautiously in patients with thyroid disease.

Figure 31.4 summarizes the properties of these pharmacological agents which can be used as adjunct treatment in the management of the compulsive or anxiety component of dermatological problems. Medication may take 3–4 weeks to show the desired effect, due to adjustment of functional neurotransmitter receptor density which undergoes alternating down- and upregulation until functional homeostasis is achieved. Starting at the low end of the dosing range, the dose may need to be titrated to effect every 2–3 weeks and taken to the maximum dose before the drug is deemed non-efficacious. Slow tapering off over 2–3 weeks can be followed by use of a second or third choice of medication. As most of these drugs are used in extra-label fashion, obtaining a serum chemistry panel, with a thyroid profile, and informed consent in writing, are highly recommended.

At present, there are no established guidelines for the duration of drug treatment. Empirically, a minimum of 4–6 month's duration of resolution of clinical signs should be achieved before an attempt is made to find the lowest effective dose or to wean the patient off the psychotropic agent.

Prognosis

Prognosis is highly variable, from fair to good, contingent upon response to medication and owner compliance with all recommendations.

Drug	Classification	Mode of action	Dog dosage	Cat dosage	Side effects
Amitriptyline	Tricyclic antidepressant	5-HT and NE reuptake inhibitor	1–3 mg/kg orally q8–24h	0.5–1.0 mg/kg orally q12–24h	Hepatic toxicity, sedation, dry mucous membranes, constipation, urinary retention
Clomipramine	Tricyclic antidepressant	5-HT reuptake inhibitor	1–3 mg/kg orally q12h *start at low end*	0.5 mg/kg orally q24h	Hepatic toxicity, sedation
Citalopram	Specific serotonin reuptake inhibitor	5-HT reuptake inhibitor	0.5–1 mg/kg orally q24h	0.25–0.5 mg/kg orally q24h	GI upset, anorexia, sedation
Doxepin	Tricyclic antidepressant	5-HT and NE reuptake inhibitor	3–5 mg/kg orally q8–12h	0.5–1.0 mg/kg orally q12–24h	Hepatic toxicity, sedation Anticholinergic signs
Fluvoxamine	Specific serotonin reuptake inhibitor	5-HT reuptake inhibitor	1 mg/kg orally q24h	0.5–1.0 mg/kg orally q24h	GI upset, anorexia, sedation, paradoxical anxiety
Fluoxetine	Specific serotonin reuptake inhibitor	5-HT reuptake inhibitor	1 mg/kg orally q24h	0.5–1.0 mg/kg orally q24h	GI upset, anorexia, sedation, paradoxical anxiety
Hydrocodone	Narcotic	Opiate agonist	0.25 mg/kg orally q8–12h	0.25–1.0 mg/kg orally q12–24h *start at low end*	Sedation, dry mucous membranes, constipation, GI upset
Paroxetine	Specific serotonin reuptake inhibitor	5-HT reuptake inhibitor	1 mg/kg orally q24h	0.5–1.0 mg/kg orally q24h	GI upset, anorexia, sedation, constipation

31.4 Abridged formulary of drugs useful in the treatment of compulsive or anxiety components of dermatological disease in the dog and cat.

References and further reading

Beaver DV (1999) *Canine Behavior: A Guide for Veterinarians.* WB Saunders, Philadelphia

Beaver DV (1992) *Feline Behavior: A Guide for Veterinarians.* WB Saunders, Philadelphia

Heuson CJ *et al.* (1998) Efficacy of clomipramine in the treatment of canine compulsive disorder. *Journal of the American Veterinary Medical Association* **213,** 1760–1766

Landsberg G, Hunthausen W, and Ackerman L (1997) *Handbook of Behaviour Problems of the Dog and Cat.* Butterworth-Heinemann, Oxford

Luescher UA (1998) Pharmacologic treatment of compulsive disorder. In: *Psychopharmacology of Animal Behavior Disorders,* ed. NH Dodman and L Shuster, pp. 203–221. Blackwell Science, Oxford

Overall KL (1997) *Clinical Behavioral Medicine for Small Animals.* Mosby, St. Louis

Overall KL (1998) Self-injurious behavior and obsessive-compulsive disorder in domestic animals. In: *Psychopharmacology of Animal Behavior Disorders,* ed. NH Dodman and L Shuster, pp. 223–

254. Blackwell Science, Oxford

Paterson S (1998) A placebo-controlled study to investigate clomipramine in the treatment of canine acral lick granuloma. In: *Advances in Veterinary Dermatology, 3,* ed. KW Kwochka *et al.,* pp. 436–437. Butterworth Heinemann, Boston

Scott DW and Walton DK (1984) Clinical evaluation of a topical treatment for canine acral lick dermatitis. *Journal of the American Animal Hospital Association* **20,** 565–570

Scott DW, Miller WH and Griffin CE (2001) Canine psychogenic dermatoses. In: *Muller & Kirk's Small Animal Dermatology, 6th edn,* ed. DW Scott et al., pp. 1058–1064. WB Saunders, Philadelphia

Shuster L and Dodman DH (1998) Basic mechanisms of compulsive and self-injurious behavior. In: *Psychopharmacology of Animal Behavior Disorders,* ed. NH Dodman and L Shuster, pp.185–202. Blackwell Science, Oxford

Stein DJ *et al.* (1998) Use of the selective serotonin reuptake inhibitor citalopram in a possible animal analogue of obsessive–compulsive disorder (OCD). *Depression and Anxiety* **8,** 39–42

Wynchank D and Berk M (1998) Fluoxetine treatment of acral lick dermatitis in dogs: a placebo-controlled randomized double blind trial. *Depression and Anxiety* **8,** 21–23

32

Eosinophilic dermatoses

Karen A. Moriello

'Eosinophilic dermatoses' are a group of skin diseases in which eosinophils are the predominant cell type in skin lesions. These diseases can occur in both cats and dogs but, for reasons that are unclear, are more common in cats. Over the years veterinary dermatologists have come to appreciate the fact that 'eosinophilic dermatitis' is a reaction pattern and not a final diagnosis. The challenge is finding the underlying primary cause.

Eosinophils are granulocytes and have a number of important functions. These cells are best known for their role in hypersensitivity reactions and their participation in the regulation of inflammation and host reactions to extracellular parasites. Eosinophils are phagocytic and will engulf immune complexes, mast cell granules, aggregated immunoglobulins, and certain bacteria and fungi (Scott *et al.*, 2001). They play an important role in the immune system because of their ability to communicate with other cells via surface receptors and the secretion of cytokines. Eosinophil granules secrete preformed mediators and, unlike other inflammatory cells, newly synthesized leucotrienes and a variety of cytokines when activated. Major basic protein, eosinophil cationic protein, eosinophil-derived neurotoxin and eosinophil peroxidase are potent toxic mediators. These substances have been shown to kill parasites. In addition, eosinophil proteases can cause host tissue damage, delay wound healing and degrade types I, II and XVII collagen. In summary, eosinophil degranulation results in the release or formation of toxic granule proteins, cytokines, lipid mediators, enzymes and reactive oxygen intermediates, all of which can cause collateral damage during a host response to an allergic, parasitic or inflammatory reaction.

The exact pathogenesis of eosinophilic skin diseases is unknown. Presumably there is an initial insult (allergic, inflammatory and/or parasitic). Humoral and cellular defence mechanisms are triggered which include granulocytes and mast cells. Mast cells are often seen in association with eosinophils. Mast cells play a key role in the chemotaxis and activation of eosinophils. The joint release of mast cell and eosinophil proteolytic enzymes and pro-inflammatory mediators cause tissue damage and a further influx of inflammatory cells. Collagen granuloma formation is believed to occur as a result of collagen necrosis from mast cell and eosinophil degranulation and a subsequent influx of macrophages. These foci have specific organizational patterns and have been called palisading granulomas. The necrotic collagen acts as a foreign body and may calcify. Secondary infections are common.

The major causes of eosinophilic skin diseases in dogs and cats are allergic and parasitic skin diseases. Eosinophilic dermatoses are less common in dogs and often the underlying trigger is unknown. In cats, the underlying triggers may include irritant reactions, foreign body reactions (e.g. cacti spines, insect parts), genetic predispositions and infections. Recently the author has seen unilateral eosinophilic lip ulcers form at the exact site where there was a small dermatophyte infection.

Clinical approach

As mentioned above, eosinophilic skin disorders are not a diagnosis; rather, they represent a specific reaction pattern to an underlying skin disease. The underlying skin disease may be a chronic skin disease (e.g. atopy) or it may be an acute trigger that is no longer present at the time the pet is examined. The first step in the clinical approach to these disorders is familiarity with the clinical features of some of the commonly recognized syndromes.

Canine eosinophilic dermatoses

Canine nasal folliculitis/furunculosis syndrome
Canine nasal folliculitis syndrome is an acute skin disease that develops on the dorsal nasal skin and muzzle. The aetiology is unknown but bites and stings from wasps, bees, biting flies and spiders are thought to be involved in some cases. Typically, lesions develop acutely and lesion severity peaks in approximately 24 hours. Clinically, dogs present with papules, nodules, plaques and varying amounts of ulceration, exudation, haemorrhage and crusting on the nose. Pruritus is variable. Lesions tend to start on the distal haired region of the nose and spread to the muzzle and periocular region. Some dogs develop similar lesions on the trunk, ventral abdomen and thorax. Most dogs are healthy but a few may be depressed, febrile and anorexic.

Canine eosinophilic granuloma
Canine eosinophilic granulomas occur most commonly in the oral cavity as ulcerative plaques in the oral mucosa (Figure 32.1) or on the soft palate, or as

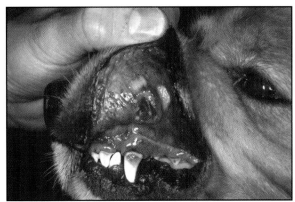

32.1 An ulcerative lesion in the mouth of a 3-year-old Cocker Spaniel cross. The lesions developed over several weeks and the dog was presented for evaluation of mouth odour.

vegetative masses under the tongue. Cavalier King Charles Spaniels have been reported to develop lesions on the soft palate or near the tonsillar crypts (Scott *et al.*, 2001). Although less common, papular to nodular, haired to ulcerative lesions may occur on the ventral abdomen, prepuce and penis, digits, trunk and face. This disorder is rare and any age, sex or breed may be affected. The majority of lesions occur in male dogs under 3 years of age, and there appears to be a breed predilection for the Siberian Husky. The cause is unknown; however, some lesions are seasonal suggesting an allergic aetiology. The breed predilection for Siberian Huskies suggests a genetic predisposition or trigger.

Canine eosinophilic dermatitis and oedema
Canine eosinophilic dermatitis and oedema is a rare disease. Four of the nine reported cases were in Labrador Retrievers (Holm *et al.*, 1999). Clinically the dogs presented with an acute onset of erythematous macules that coalesced into plaques on the ears, abdomen and thorax. Tissue oedema varied in severity from facial oedema to generalized pitting oedema. The cause is unknown but may include allergies, drug reactions, dietary hypersensitivity, arthropods and immune-mediated skin diseases. The author has observed one case of this disease which occurred in a mixed breed dog (Figure 32.2). The only change in the dog's environment was exposure to lawn pesticides approximately 6 hours before lesions developed. This exposure may have been the trigger or simply a coincidence.

Canine eosinophilic proliferative otitis externa
Canine eosinophilic proliferative otitis externa is a rare inflammatory disorder of the ear canal. Affected dogs have a history of unilateral otitis externa. Otoscopic examination reveals solitary or multiple masses on stalks in the ear canal. Histological examination of tissue specimens reveals eosinophilic dermatitis and/or eosinophilic granuloma. Surgical excision may be curative or lesions may recur. The underlying aetiology is unknown; the unilateral nature of the lesions is atypical of allergic diseases. It is possible that these lesions are the result of foreign body reactions to parasitic and/or vegetative material in the ear canal.

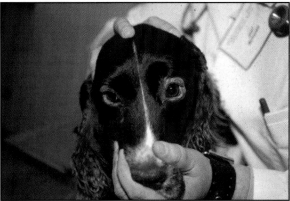

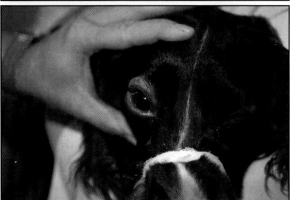

32.2 Eosinophilic cellulitis and oedema around the eyes in a 5-year-old Springer Spaniel. Recent exposure to lawn pesticides may have been a factor but this is not certain.

Canine sterile eosinophilic pinnal folliculitis
Canine sterile eosinophilic pinnal folliculitis is an uncommon bilateral (or unilateral in the author's experience) pinnal skin disease. The cause is unknown and it appears to be non-seasonal, although all of the cases seen by the author have occurred during the warm summer months. Lesions may have a slow or rapid onset of development and pruritus is variable; in the author's experience the pruritus has been severe. Clinically, erythematous papules that crust develop on the inner pinnae. The earflap may become very oedematous and papules may spread to the haired region of the pinnae. Lesions tend to recur.

Canine eosinophilic pustulosis
Canine eosinophilic pustulosis is a rare idiopathic pustular skin disease. There is no age, sex, or breed predisposition. There is a rapid onset of pruritic, follicular to non-follicular papules and pustules on the trunk or generalized over the entire body. The lesions develop into erosive lesions and epidermal collarettes. The lesions may resemble those of a bacterial pyoderma. Dogs may be clinically healthy or they may be febrile, depressed and anorexic and have a peripheral lymphadenopathy.

Feline eosinophilic dermatoses
In this author's opinion, there have been two great stumbling blocks that have slowed the study and advancement of feline dermatology. The first was the discovery that many feline skin diseases are exquisitely

sensitive to glucocorticoids (diseases tend to be investigated only if there is no treatment) and the second was the coining of the term 'eosinophilic granuloma complex'. The latter refers to a triad of clinical signs (indolent ulcers, plaques, granuloma) that could occur individually or in combination on the same patient. The fact that these lesions were glucocorticoid-responsive only further added to what is commonly referred to as the 'eosinophilic confusion complex'.

The following is a brief summary of the clinical reaction patterns in cats associated with a tissue eosinophilia. These reaction patterns vary in clinical appearance but share many of the same underlying aetiologies. Definitive diagnosis of the underlying cause is made by obtaining a good history, and conducting a thorough physical examination and a methodical diagnostic evaluation.

Miliary dermatitis

'Miliary dermatitis' is more accurately described as a papulocrusting dermatitis. It is not a specific disease but rather a reaction pattern. Clinically, lesions are characterized by small erythematous crusting papules (Figure 32.3). Lesions may be generalized or localized. In some cats, these lesions may be secondary foci of bacterial or yeast dermatitis due to an underlying allergy, similar to allergic dogs with secondary bacterial infections. See Chapter 6 for a list of differential diagnoses.

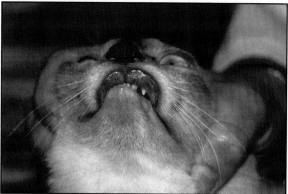
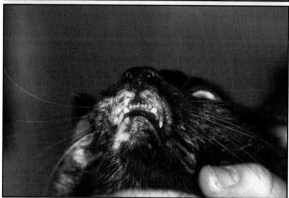

32.4 Bilateral indolent lip ulcers in two cats, caused by allergic skin disease. Despite their severity, the lesions did not appear to affect the cats.

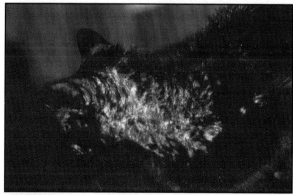

32.3 Miliary dermatitis on the head and neck of an adult Domestic Shorthair.

Indolent ulcer

An indolent ulcer is an ulcerated lesion on the upper lip. It may be unilateral or bilateral, extending from either side of the philtrum (Figure 32.4). Early lesions tend to start as foci of erythema and develop into well circumscribed areas of ulceration and alopecia. The border of the lesion tends to be slightly raised. Lesions appear to be non-painful and non-pruritic. There is no breed predilection but some clinicians have observed that females may be predisposed. There is some evidence that there may be a genetic predisposition for some cats to develop lesions when exposed to appropriate triggers, e.g. fleas. The author has observed unilateral indolent ulcers in cats with dermatophytosis. In those cats, one or two infected hairs were observed at the site prior to the development of the lesion. In some cats, particularly young kittens, lesions may develop and resolve without treatment and not recur.

Eosinophilic plaques

Eosinophilic plaques are intensely pruritic, erosive, exudative, raised lesions varying from small foci to large, well circumscribed plaques resembling skin tumours (Figure 32.5). Lesions are commonly seen in areas of self-trauma: face, abdomen, inguinal region, medial and caudal thigh areas and neck. These lesions are most commonly triggered by an itch–scratch event and recurrent lesions are the hallmark of an underlying allergic disease, but not always. The author has seen eosinophilic plaques develop as a result of a pruritic case of dermatophytosis.

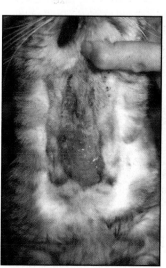

32.5

An eosinophilic plaque on the ventral neck of a 2-year-old Domestic Shorthair. This lesion was triggered by clipping the haircoat for venepuncture and was completely responsive to oral antibiotic treatment. On cytology, neutrophils and cocci outnumbered eosinophils.

Eosinophilic plaques may be the feline equivalent of canine pyotraumatic lesions ('hot spots') and many respond better to aggressive antimicrobial therapy than glucocorticoid therapy, not unlike hot spots in dogs. Cytological examination of the exudate may help determine the most appropriate treatment. Eosinophils are typically found on impression smears. If there is a marked neutrophilic component with or without intra- or extracellular cocci present, a course of antibiotic therapy may be the best treatment approach.

Eosinophilic granuloma
Eosinophilic granulomas are the only 'true granuloma' variant of the archaic 'eosinophilic granuloma complex'. The granulomas are caused by collagen necrosis and have a wide variety of clinical presentations. This author recognizes two major variations in clinical appearance. The first is an ulcerated, proliferative lesion often present in the oral cavity. Depending upon the location of the mass, dysphagia, drooling, abnormal mastication and coughing may be present. The other form is characterized by a hard non-inflammatory swelling. Alopecia is variable and the cat seems unperturbed by the lesion.

Clinical presentations include:

- Linear pencil-thick lesions on the caudal thigh of young cats (Figure 32.6a)
- Linear lesions on limbs
- 'Fat lips'
- Asymptomatic chin swelling (Figure 32.6b)
- Firm 1–5 mm papular lesions on the ears
- Interdigital masses.

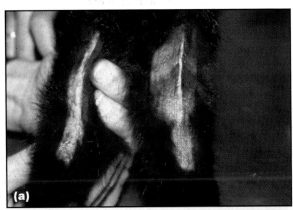

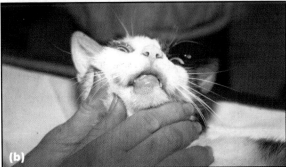

32.6 Eosinophilic granuloma. (a) Linear lesions on the backs of the hind legs of a 6-month-old Domestic Shorthair kitten. (b) Firm chin swelling on a 7-year-old Domestic Shorthair. Both lesions resolved without therapy.

Insect bite hypersensitivity
Hypersensitivity to mosquito bites and other insect bites and stings is characterized by a papular erosive eruption on the face, ear tips, nose (Figure 32.7) and footpads. Lesions tend to start in the thinly haired areas and may be more common in dark-coated cats. The lesions are intensely pruritic, and depigmentation, crusting and exudates may occur. The lesions were first noted in cats exposed to mosquitoes but can result from the bites of other small flying insects such as black flies and *Culicoides*. Typically the cat has access to the outdoors, especially during the early morning or evening hours when the insects are feeding. It is important to remember that many of these biting insects are small enough to get through the holes used to screen outdoor porches and windows.

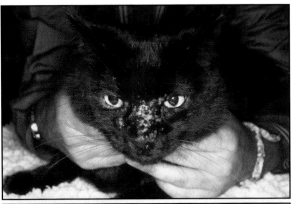

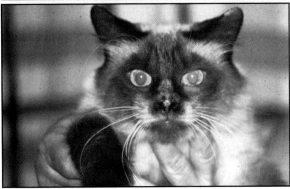

32.7 Mosquito bite hypersensitivity in a Domestic Shorthair and a Siamese cross. Note the distribution of lesions on the face and ear tips in both cats. The lesions also show a predisposition for areas with dark hair.

Familial eosinophilic lesions
Familial eosinophilic lesions have been described in specific pathogen-free laboratory cats by at least two investigators (Power and Ihrke, 1995; Colombini *et al.*, 2001). These cats developed lesions at between 4 and 18 months of age. The lesions tended to recur until the cats were approximately 4 years old and to be most common during the spring and summer, suggesting possible seasonal allergen, insect, hormonal or reproductive triggers. To date, none has been documented. A hereditary predisposition to eosinophilic lesions is not unexpected. The predisposition to develop atopic dermatitis in dogs has long been known to be heritable and feline atopy has recently been described in three littermates (Moriello, 2001).

Hypereosinophilic syndrome

Feline hypereosinophilic syndrome is a rare disease of middle-aged to older cats. These cats may present with a generalized maculopapular eruption, severe pruritus, excoriations, wheals (Figure 32.8) and limb oedema. It is more common for affected cats to present with weight loss, diarrhoea, vomiting, anorexia and often lymphadenopathy. The disease is caused by a massive tissue infiltration of mature eosinophils causing multiple organ failure/dysfunction. The bone marrow, lymph nodes, spleen and gastrointestinal tract are involved. Feline hypereosinophilic syndrome is difficult to treat and the prognosis is poor. The survival time for patients is short and, unfortunately, cats respond poorly to treatment. Cats with cutaneous lesions may have a short but beneficial response to large doses of prednisone or prednisolone (4.4–6.6 mg/kg).

Diagnosis

There are two aspects of diagnosis with respect to eosinophilic skin diseases. The first is the clinical recognition of the syndrome. Key diagnostic findings for canine and feline eosinophilic dermatoses are summarized in Figures 32.9 and 32.10. The second is the identification of the underlying cause. In some cases, the underlying trigger is no longer present, e.g. insect bite hypersensitivity. Figure 32.11 lists the common primary causes of eosinophilic dermatoses in cats.

Core diagnostic tests for the initial identification of an eosinophilic syndrome include:

- Skin scrapings
- Impression smears
- Skin biopsy
- Dermatophyte culture (cats).

Diseases with a clearly pustular nature should have samples cultured, especially if appropriate antibiotic therapy has failed.

Secondary diagnostic tests for identification of the primary cause or trigger are indicated in, but not limited to, cases where:

- An underlying cause is suspected
- Lesions are non-responsive to treatment
- Lesions are clearly recurrent and chronic.

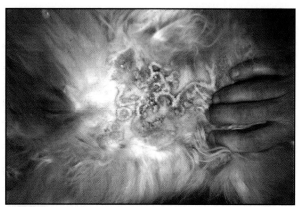

32.8 Hypereosinophilic syndrome in a 5-year-old female Domestic Longhair. The lesions were initially attributed to flea allergy dermatitis. A diagnosis of hypereosinophilic syndrome was made after the lesions did not respond to flea control or therapy with low-dose glucocorticoids.

Skin disease	Dermatological clinical signs	Systemic clinical signs	Major differential diagnoses	Focused diagnostic testing	Key diagnostic findings
Nasal folliculitis/ furunculosis syndrome	Acute development of papules, nodules Exudation on nose Rarely, concurrent lesions on body	Uncommon but some dogs become depressed, febrile and anorexic	Staphylococcal nasal folliculitis/ furunculosis Fungal kerion	Impression smears Complete blood count	Eosinophilic inflammation with occasional degenerate neutrophils and rare intracellular cocci Peripheral eosinophilia is common
Eosinophilic granuloma	Oral nodular to plaque-like lesions Skin nodules possible Most common in Siberian Huskies	Rare	Granulomatous and neoplastic skin diseases	Skin biopsy	Eosinophilic and histiocytic infiltration Granuloma formation
Eosinophilic dermatitis and oedema	Erythematous macules that develop into plaques Variable facial and limb oedema	Rare	Drug eruption Immediate hypersensitivity reaction Any differential for limb oedema	Skin biopsy	Superficial and deep perivascular eosinophilic dermatitis with oedema and vascular dilation
Eosinophilic proliferative otitis externa	Unilateral otitis with solitary or multiple masses in ear	Rare	Foreign body Atypical presentation of pemphigus	Biopsy	Papillomatous, proliferative eosinophilic dermatitis Eosinophilic granuloma Eosinophilic microabscesses

32.9 Key diagnostic findings for canine eosinophilic dermatoses. (continues) ▶

Skin disease	Dermatological clinical signs	Systemic clinical signs	Major differential diagnoses	Focused diagnostic testing	Key diagnostic findings
Sterile eosinophilic pinnal folliculitis	Typically bilateral, erythematous papular eruption on inner pinnae, with variable pruritus	Rare	Bacterial pyoderma Drug reaction Allergic reaction	Impression smear Biopsy Bacterial culture	Sterile eosinophilic inflammatory infiltrate Eosinophilic folliculitis and/or furunculosis Sterile bacterial cultures
Eosinophilic pustulosis	Acute local to generalized eruption of pustules, target lesions and epidermal collarettes	Uncommon but some dogs are febrile, anorexic, depressed and may have lymphadenopathy	Staphylococcal pyoderma Pemphigus foliaceus Drug eruption Subcorneal pustulosis	Impression smear of pustule Complete blood count Bacterial culture of pustule Skin biopsy	Peripheral eosinophilia Eosinophilic exudates with rare acantholytic cells Sterile bacterial culture Intraepidermal eosinophilic pustulosis

32.9 (continued) Key diagnostic findings for canine eosinophilic dermatoses.

Skin disease	Dermatological clinical signs	Systemic clinical signs	Major differential diagnoses	Focused diagnostic testing	Key diagnostic findings
Miliary dermatitis	Erythematous papular to crusted lesions	Rare	Infectious agents that can cause folliculitis Mast cell tumours	Usually a clinical diagnosis. The syndrome is a clinical sign of an underlying skin disease. Skin biopsy may be warranted early in some cases to rule out mast cell tumour	
Indolent ulcer	Unilateral or bilateral, well circumscribed mucocutaneous erosions on the lip	Rare	Trauma Infectious ulcers Neoplasia	Usually a clinical diagnosis. Refractory cases warrant biopsy; care must be taken when obtaining tissue to maintain a cosmetic appearance. Definitive diagnosis is often made via response to therapy	
Eosinophilic plaque	Well circumscribed, raised, round to oval, pruritic exudative lesions Older lesions may show matting of the haircoat	Rare Lesions may occur on the conjunctiva and cornea	Infections that can cause non-healing wounds Mast cell tumours Lymphoma	Impression smears Complete blood count Skin biopsy	Peripheral eosinophilia Superficial to deep perivascular eosinophilic dermatitis Spongiosis Impression smears may reveal primary eosinophilic inflammation or a mixed infiltrate of eosinophils and neutrophils
Eosinophilic granuloma	Two major variants: (a) oral proliferative lesion (b) hard firm painless lesion that may be papular, nodular or linear	Rare	Bacterial or fungal granuloma Insect bite reaction Injection site reaction Neoplasia	Skin biopsy Complete blood count	Nodular to diffuse granulomatous dermatitis with collagen degeneration Peripheral eosinophilia is variable
Insect hypersensitivity	Papular to erosive lesions on the face, ear tips, nose and footpads	Rare Footpad lesions may cause lameness	Pemphigus complex Dermatophytosis Drug eruption	Skin biopsy	Biopsy similar to eosinophilic plaque or granuloma Regression of lesions during cold weather or indoor housing
Familial eosinophilic lesions	Eosinophilic skin lesions in related cats	Rare	Infections or parasites triggering lesions	Rule out contagious diseases Confirm eosinophilic reaction pattern via skin biopsy	Strong history of familial lesions, difficult to confirm in cats as this history is often lacking

32.10 Key diagnostic findings for feline eosinophilic dermatoses. (continues) ▶

Skin disease	Dermatological clinical signs	Systemic clinical signs	Major differential diagnoses	Focused diagnostic testing	Key diagnostic findings
Hypereosinophilic syndrome	Generalized macular–papular crusting, erythema, severe pruritus, excoriations	Weight loss Diarrhea Vomiting Anorexia	Flea allergy dermatitis Allergic dermatitis Food allergy/ eosinophilic gastroenteritis Mast cell tumours Eosinophilic leukaemia	Rule out other skin diseases Direct smear of skin Bone marrow biopsy Complete blood count Skin biopsy Ultrasound-guided biopsy	Marked to moderate peripheral eosinophilia Eosinophilic inflammation on impression smears Superficial to deep perivascular to diffuse eosinophilic dermatitis Organ eosinophilia

32.10 (continued) Key diagnostic findings for feline eosinophilic dermatoses.

Allergic and other immunological causes

Feline atopy/Aeroallergens
Flea bite hypersensitivity
Insect bite hypersensitivity
Adverse food reaction
Intestinal parasites
Drug reactions

Foreign body reactions

Mite or insect particles
Plant material (e.g. cactus spine)

Infections

Dermatophytosis
Bacterial infections (primary or secondary to allergies)

Parasites

Cheyletiella
Fleas
Otodectes cynotis
Notoedres cati
Demodex
Lice

Miscellaneous

Hereditary predisposition
Contact allergy or contact irritant reaction
Neoplasia
Idiopathic

32.11 Common primary causes of eosinophilic dermatoses in cats.

Management and therapeutics

There are two approaches to the treatment of eosinophilic dermatoses: symptomatic relief; and treating the underlying aetiology.

Canine eosinophilic dermatoses

The underlying aetiology of these diseases is unknown. With the exception of eosinophilic pustulosis, it is possible that these diseases represent unusual manifestations of hypersensitivity disorders. If the lesions are recurrent or become refractory to symptomatic treatment, a more aggressive approach involving flea control, food elimination diets and allergy testing is indicated. If impression smears of the lesions reveal an overwhelming bacterial infection, treatment with oral antibiotics for 14–21 days may be warranted prior to the use of glucocorticoids. In general however, this in not needed.

Oral glucocorticoid therapy is preferred over the use or injectable or repositol glucocorticoids. Oral prednisone or prednisolone 0.5–2.2 mg/kg once daily for 10–20 days is generally recommended until the lesions resolve. Alternate-day therapy is then used for an additional 10–20 days before gradually tapering the dose.

Canine eosinophilic proliferative otitis externa: This condition usually requires surgical removal of the lesions. Concurrent use of glucocorticoids may be helpful in reducing the size of the lesions preoperatively and/or preventing them from recurring.

Sterile eosinophilic pinnal folliculitis: Some dogs with this condition have responded to topical glucocorticoids. The severity and extent of the lesions and other patient factors will help determine if this is the best treatment option.

Canine eosinophilic pustulosis: This requires lifelong glucocorticoid therapy. The dosage required to induce remission of clinical signs is much higher than that used in other eosinophilic dermatoses, 2.2–4.4 mg/kg orally once daily. The patient should receive a high dose of glucocorticoids until lesions are in remission. This can take anywhere from 5 to 20 days. If the drug dose is stopped or tapered too quickly, the patient can relapse. Long-term alternate-day therapy is required to maintain a good quality of life for the patient, and intermittent relapses are to be expected.

Feline eosinophilic dermatoses

Miliary dermatitis, indolent ulcers, eosinophilic plaques, eosinophilic granulomas and insect bite hypersensitivity have similar treatment approaches. It is important to remember that there is always some underlying trigger causing these lesions. The major question at the time of examination is whether or not the trigger is still present, and if so, does it require aetiology-based treatment. It cannot be stressed enough that core diagnostic tests (skin scrapings, flea combings, dermatophyte cultures, impression smears) should be done to rule out parasitic and infectious aetiologies before pursuing expensive and time-consuming aetiology-based treatments/diagnostics.

Aetiology-based treatment

Aetiology-based treatment requires the identification of the underlying trigger or primary cause of the eosinophilic dermatosis in question. In some cats, the eosinophilic skin disease may be a one-time occurrence or it may occur infrequently. In those situations, it is appropriate to rely upon symptomatic therapy to resolve the relapse. In other situations, the owner may be unwilling or unable to pursue the necessary diagnostics needed to identify the primary cause. In these situations, the clinician must find the optimal symptomatic therapy for the patient. The most common underlying triggers for the above diseases include fleas and flea allergy dermatitis, food allergies/dietary intolerances and feline atopic dermatitis. Diagnostic and therapeutic approaches for these disorders are discussed in detail in other chapters.

Symptomatic therapy

Symptomatic therapy is always indicated, even during the pursuit of an underlying cause. Care must be taken to avoid drugs that may be contraindicated for certain diagnostic testing. Drug treatments are addressed here in the order in which the author uses them to manage symptoms.

Antimicrobial therapy: The author has found antibiotic therapy to be useful in two situations:

- Indolent ulcers where glucocorticoids cannot be used or have not been beneficial
- Eosinophilic plaques.

The author has found and treated many cats with lesions colonized by bacteria and *Malassezia* organisms which respond to combination antimicrobial therapy. Many of these cats do not require follow-up glucocorticoid therapy. In the case of cats with eosinophilic plaques that are non-responsive to glucocorticoids, the author always treats them with concurrent systemic antibiotics and itraconazole before using alternative drugs.

Recommended therapies include itraconazole (5–10 mg/kg for 15–30 days) for the treatment of yeast infections and trimethoprim/sulphonamide (30 mg/kg orally bid), cefalexin (20 mg/kg orally tid or 30 mg/kg orally bid) or doxycycline (10 mg/kg orally sid) for 30 days. Response to antibiotic therapy may indicate that the lesion was perpetuated by a secondary bacterial infection or it may be due to the anti-inflammatory properties of the drug.

Glucocorticoid therapy: Without a doubt, glucocorticoid therapy is the most common symptomatic therapy used for these patients. Methylprednisolone acetate 4 mg/kg i.m. every 2–3 weeks until the lesion resolves is the author's first choice therapy for indolent ulcers and cats with insect bite hypersensitivity. It is also the author's first choice for eosinophilic granulomas. It is not always necessary to treat these granulomas, however. In some cases the lesion is more worrisome and annoying to the owner than to the cat. In general, cats tend to respond to injectable glucocorticoids more favourably than to oral forms. This may be artefactual since the problem may not be with the formulation but rather with difficulties in medicating the patient. Oral prednisone or prednisolone can be used at a dose of 1–3 mg/kg orally once daily for 3–4 weeks and then on an alternate-day basis. Since cats are nocturnal predators, it may be appropriate to medicate them in the evening to match their diurnal rhythm. Oral glucocorticoid should be administered with food since the drug is very irritating to the gastric mucosa.

Antihistamines: Cetirizine is an antihistamine that has been shown to have significant effects on eosinophil migration in humans. It is used in human cases of insect bite hypersensitivity and has been shown in a double-blind study to decrease wheal formation and pruritus (Townley, 1991). This drug may be beneficial in the long-term management of cats with eosinophilic skin disorders, either alone or in combination with glucocorticoids. The oral dose is 5 mg per cat once or twice daily. The author uses fexofenadine 2 mg/kg orally once or twice daily in cats with pruritus and has found this to be useful adjuvant therapy for cats with recurrent eosinophilic plaques or miliary dermatitis.

Ciclosporin: Ciclosporin is an oral immunosuppressive drug used to prevent organ transplantation rejection. Recently it has been found to be helpful in the treatment and management of non-responsive feline indolent ulcers, eosinophilic plaques and oral eosinophilic granulomas. The dose is 5–8 mg/kg divided and given twice daily until lesion remission (14–21 days) and then it is used on an alternate-day treatment plan. Vomiting is the only adverse effect noted by the author. This drug should not be given to patients that are receiving ketoconazole, itraconazole, fluconazole erythromycin or methlyprednisolone because these drugs may potentiate toxicity.

Chlorambucil: Chlorambucil is an orally administered alkylating immunosuppressive drug that is more commonly used to treat autoimmune skin diseases. It has been used alone or in combination with glucocorticoids to treat refractory eosinophilic lesions. The oral dose is 0.1–0.2 mg/kg once daily or every other day. The adverse effects include anorexia, vomiting and diarrhoea. Serum chemistries and complete blood counts should be monitored every 2 weeks for the first several months of therapy and monthly thereafter.

Miscellaneous: Other treatments for refractory indolent ulcers include:

- Aurothioglucose: 1 mg/kg i.m. once weekly until remission and then every 2–4 weeks
- Megestrol acetate: has potent anti-inflammatory effects and can be a useful therapy for intractable indolent ulcers. The dose is 2.5–5.0 mg per cat orally every 48 hours until the lesion resolves and then weekly or biweekly to maintain remission. This drug has serious adverse effects, including diabetes mellitus, polyphagia, mammary hyperplasia, pyometria, behavioural changes and suppression

of adrenal function. This drug should be considered a drug of last resort where euthanasia is being considered. Many clients are often willing to treat cherished pets when other therapies for disfiguring indolent ulcers have failed.

References and further reading

Colombini S, Hodgin EC, Foil CS *et al.* (2001) Induction of feline flea allergy dermatitis and the incidence and histopathological characteristics of concurrent indolent lip ulcers. *Veterinary Dermatology* **12,** 155–161

Holm KS, Morris DO and Gomez SM (1999) Eosinophilic dermatitis with edema in nine dogs compared with eosinophilic cellulitis in humans. *Journal of the American Veterinary Medical Association* **215,** 649–651

Mason I (1993) Pustules and crusting papules. In: *Manual of Small Animal Dermatology*, ed. PH Locke *et al.*, pp. 60–64. BSAVA Publications, Cheltenham

Mason K and Burton G (2000) Eosinophilic granuloma complex. In: *A Practical Guide to Feline Dermatology*, ed. E Guaguère and P Prélaud, pp. 12.1–12.9. Mérial, Lyon, France

Moriello K (2001) Feline atopy in three littermates. *Veterinary Dermatology* **12,** 177–181

Patterson S (2000) *Skin Diseases of the Cat*. Blackwell Science, Oxford

Patterson S (2000) *Skin Diseases of the Dog*. Blackwell Science, Oxford

Power HT and Ihrke PJ (1995) Selected feline eosinophilic skin diseases. *Veterinary Clinics of North America: Small Animal Practice* **25,** 833–850

Scott DW, Miller WH and Griffin CE (2001) *Muller and Kirk's Small Animal Dermatology, 6th edn.* WB Saunders, Philadelphia

Townley RG (1991) Cetirizine: a new H₁ antagonist with antieosinophilic activity in chronic urticaria. *Journal of the American Academy of Dermatology* **25,** 668–674

33

Rabbits and rodents

David H. Scarff

Diseases of the skin and its appendages are common reasons for presentation of small mammals to a veterinary surgeon. For accurate diagnosis and treatment, a similar approach is necessary to the one taken every day for canine and feline dermatoses: a diagnostic approach followed by specific therapy. However, as in much of small mammal medicine, the limitations imposed by financial considerations are of importance. This increases the need for accurate diagnosis from the outset.

General approach

It is important for the veterinarian to have some knowledge of the correct husbandry of the species presented, or to be equipped with an adequate source of information. Many owners are quite ignorant of the dietary and management needs of small mammals. The assessment of husbandry is important in the diagnosis and therefore successful treatment of small mammal dermatoses.

History
Careful history-taking is essential for assessment of any disease situation. This can be made more difficult when an adult rarely looks at the animal in question. Many small mammal consultations start with the history 'We found it like this'. If the owner is a child, involve the child in answering questions, as they may be more knowledgeable than their parents.

Initial questions should request information on basic husbandry of the animal:

- Breed, age and sex of the patient?
- Length of time owned and source – petshop, private breeder?
- Size of group; sex of other animals in group?
- Other species in direct contact or sharing environment?
- Type of housing (cage, hutch, indoors or out, outbuilding, house rabbit, hamster in complicated maze of tunnels)?
- Type of flooring – wire or wooden?
- What bedding is used; does the animal eat the bedding?
- How is the hutch or cage cleaned and with what? How frequently is this done?
- What foodstuffs are given, including supplements?
- What sort of water bowl or bottle is used?

- Is the environment protected against insect vectors of disease, such as mosquitoes? Do wild rabbits enter the garden at all? If so, do they look healthy?
- How is the general health of the animal? Owners are reluctant to dwell on this, as they are keen to discuss the problem as they see it.

At this stage it is appropriate to consider the presenting problem:

- What is the problem that the owners are worried about?
- How long has it been noticed?
- Are any other animals affected? Are they in contact or housed close by?
- Are any other species affected? Include careful questions about the people who handle the pet. If possible do not induce alarm about zoonotic disease at this stage
- What treatments (including proprietary medications) have been used, and with what success?
- Is the condition pruritic?
- Have any parasites been seen?
- If this is a house rabbit, are there cats or dogs in the same environment, and what flea control is practised?

General clinical examination
Many small mammals will be presented in a cardboard box stuffed with hay or shavings, or other containers, and are often in a stressed state. This is not ideal, as observation of the animal at rest can give a useful idea of general health. In particular, signs of respiratory disease should be noted.

A full examination of the animal is necessary, even if the problem appears to be obvious. For example, *Trixacarus* infestation in the guinea pig can be the consequence of underlying disease such as respiratory infection. Underlying disease will interfere with the ability to provide a successful outcome, and stressful treatments such as dipping can be risky in a debilitated patient.

Examination of the oral cavity and dental arcade is of specific importance to some skin disorders, such as moist dermatitis and subcutaneous abscesses, and should be undertaken carefully, especially in the rabbit. Likewise, careful examination of the respiratory system, including the nares and conjunctivae for signs of discharge, is important.

Test	Notes on technique	Indications
Acetate strip samples	Clip affected area carefully. Apply strip several times. Use fresh tape – more adhesive	Ectoparasites; dermatophytes; assessment of self-trauma
Skin scraping	Clip affected area carefully. Moisten skin with liquid paraffin. Scrape gently – avoid excessive trauma	Ectoparasites; dermatophytes
Fine-needle aspirate	Clip and clean lesion. Use 21G needle as exudate may be thick	Subcutaneous abscesses; possible neoplasia
Bacterial culture	Standard aerobic culture	Possible *Pseudomonas* or *Staphylococcus* infection
Wood's lamp examination	Allow lamp to warm up. Perform test in dark room. Allow enough time to examine carefully	*Microsporum canis* only – less common in small mammals than *Trichophyton mentagrophytes*
Fungal culture	Take plenty of hairs or use Mackenzie brush technique	Dermatophytes including *Trichophyton mentagrophytes* and *Microsporum canis*
Skin biopsy	Sedation or general anaesthesia usually required. 4—6 mm punch often used	Possible neoplasia

33.1 Diagnostic tests.

Examination of the skin

Complete examination of the skin should be undertaken, even if the dermatosis appears to be localized.

Diagnostic tests

The diagnostic tests for various indications are considered in Figure 33.1.

Dermatoses

Congenital/hereditary

Due to the relative in-breeding of many small mammals and their short reproductive cycles, congenital defects are not uncommon.

Congenital dermatoses including hereditary alopecia and cutaneous asthenia (Harvey *et al.*, 1990) have been reported in the rabbit (Figure 33.2).

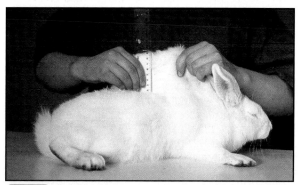

33.2 Rabbit with cutaneous asthenia. The skin had increased extensibility and was easily torn. Electron microscopy revealed disorganization and variability in size of collagen bundles. (Courtesy of R. Harvey)

Viral diseases

Myxomatosis

The most important viral dermatosis of the rabbit is myxomatosis. A poxvirus, this disease is endemic in rabbit populations in South America. It was introduced into Australia in the 1950s to help control the rabbit population. Myxomatosis virus was then accidentally introduced into Europe, where it nearly eradicated the wild rabbit population. The disease is still endemic in wild populations of rabbits in Europe, although there is some variation in virulence.

Insect vectors, including mosquitoes and the rabbit flea, spread the myxomatosis virus. Several clinical syndromes occur depending upon the virulence of the virus, including a fatal peracute infection, widespread skin tumour production and a temporary papillomatous condition in partially immune rabbits (Figure 33.3).

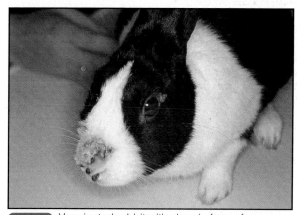

33.3 Vaccinated rabbit with chronic form of myxomatosis.

In France a respiratory form of the disease occurs that is spread by direct contact. An unusual variant of this disease occurred in recently depilated Angora rabbits, where multiple cutaneous papules and plaques appeared in the area which had been depilated. These lesions progressed to become necrotic and haemorrhagic. The disease was not usually fatal, and most rabbits recovered spontaneously (Ganière *et al.*,1991).

Various vaccines are available around the world. In the UK the only vaccine available is a heterologous vaccine derived from Shope fibroma virus. This is variably successful, the efficacy being increased if the vaccine is partially injected intradermally.

In acute cases rabbits are lethargic, febrile and depressed. Oedema of the ears, lips, eyes, genitalia and anus is present, and the disease rapidly progresses to death. In less virulent strains, skin tumours are produced in large numbers. These sometimes regress spontaneously, although affected rabbits are predisposed to respiratory infection.

In the acute form of the disease, the clinical signs are diagnostic. In the early stages the disease resembles venereal spirochaetosis, but the true diagnosis is soon apparent. In subacute forms, biopsy is diagnostic in samples with intact epidermis.

There is no treatment for this disease. Rabbits with subacute disease can recover but this requires intensive nursing and maintenance of a high environmental temperature. Antibacterial treatment to prevent secondary respiratory infection is wise. Vaccination and screening from insect vectors are helpful in reducing the incidence of the disease.

Bacterial dermatoses

Rabbits

Bacterial dermatoses present variously in the rabbit, with the most common presentation being subcutaneous abscess. Abscesses are often associated with underlying disease, particularly that affecting the dental arcade (Figure 33.4).

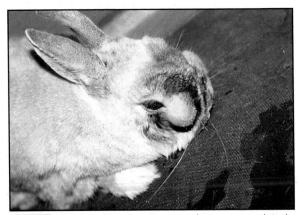

33.4 Rabbit with subcutaneous abscess associated with dental disease.

Rodents

Bacterial skin diseases are common in rodents. Cutaneous abscesses are most frequent. These often involve oral flora and are commonly caused by fights.

Chinchillas kept in humid environments are prone to bacterial skin infections.

Bacterial dermatoses will be discussed here by causative organism, but it must be remembered that mixed infections often occur. Antibiotics suitable for use in rabbits and rodents are listed in Figure 33.5. Some antibiotics can cause a fatal enterotoxaemia in hamsters and other small rodents.

Pasteurella multocida

Rabbits: Most rabbits carry *Pasteurella multocida* asymptomatically in the nasal cavity. When stressed, clinical disease can occur. Subcutaneous abscesses are caused as an extension of a penetrating wound (including bite wounds), septicaemia or dental disease. Extension of disease to underlying bone may occur. Subcutaneous abscesses present as firm to fluctuant subcutaneous swellings. Commonly found around the head and lower jaw, abscesses can occur in any site and may appear to be fixed to underlying structures. Careful examination sometimes reveals a penetrating wound. Other clinical presentations include mastitis in lactating does and skin disease at the medial canthus of the eye associated with chronic conjunctivitis and epiphora.

Diagnosis is achieved by examination of fine needle aspirates. Aspiration is difficult unless a 21G needle is used, as the exudate is very thick. Examination following staining with a rapid Romanowsky or Gram stain reveals the causative organisms.

Examination for underlying disease is important, especially examination of the dental arcade. Unless an underlying disease is identified and resolved, the abscess is likely to recur, whatever treatment is used. If a mixed infection is present, bacterial culture is wise, including examination for anaerobic bacteria. If underlying bone is thought to be involved, radiographic examination is indicated to determine the extent of disease.

The treatment of choice is the complete surgical excision of the abscess in its surrounding capsule but this is often extremely difficult and can be impossible if there is underlying dental disease. If excision is not possible, then surgical opening of the abscess

Drug	Route	Dose rate	Indication
Enrofloxacin (licensed for use in the rabbit)	s.c.	5 mg/kg bid—sid	Pasteurellosis; spirochaetosis; staphylococcal disease
	drinking water	50—100 mg/l	
Trimethoprim–sulphonamide	s.c.	30 mg/kg sid	Moist dermatitis; pasteurellosis
Tetracycline HCl	s.c., orally	20 mg/kg bid	Pasteurellosis; spirochaetosis
Chloramphenicol	orally	50 mg/kg bid	Pasteurellosis; spirochaetosis
Penicillin (procaine or benzathine) **RABBIT ONLY**	i.m.	42,000 IU/kg weekly for 3 weeks	Venereal spirochaetosis

33.5 Common antibacterials used in rabbits and rodents.

together with flushing and the use of topical or systemic antibiotic preparations will help. However, such cases are likely to recur, as are those with underlying bone or dental disease.

Staphylococcus aureus

Rabbits: Diseases caused by staphylococcal bacteria present with a number of different clinical syndromes, from a highly fatal disease of neonatal rabbits to subcutaneous abscesses and an exudative dermatitis resembling impetigo. Mastitis and pododermatitis are also associated with this organism. Underlying factors include the age when affected, concurrent disease or stress, and the virulence of the strain of *S. aureus* seen. It would appear that phage group II strains are the most virulent, and contain genes for the production of epidermolytic toxins (Noble, 1989). A virulent rabbit biotype of *S. aureus* has been reported in Belgian rabbitries (Okerman *et al.*, 1984).

Neonates suffer from two specific patterns of staphylococcal disease: septicaemia and sudden death, or exudative dermatitis. Both can be associated with poor husbandry and are most often reported from commercial rabbit rearing units. Examination of swabs taken from rabbits with exudative dermatitis reveals the causative organism. Culture samples are necessary in septicaemic animals and allow the typing of the staphylococcal strains involved.

Systemic antibiotics are needed to control and prevent this condition. This may not be an economic option in commercial units, where the culling of affected rabbits followed by disinfection of the premises and re-stocking may be necessary. If this is not done, the problem is likely to recur, as the causative organism is endemic in affected groups.

Rodents: Staphylococcal skin diseases often occur in rodents, especially young animals, either as septicaemia or in more chronic forms including generalized pyoderma. Poor nutrition and housing contribute to this. The treatment of such diseases must address deficiencies in husbandry, as well as controlling the bacterial infection.

Pseudomonas aeruginosa

Rabbits: *P. aeruginosa* is responsible for a moist dermatitis. The condition is predisposed by constant wetting of the affected skin, either due to dribbling secondary to dental disease (slobbers) or by faulty drinking apparatus. Moist dermatitis occurs on the ventral neck (dewlap) area or flanks. The fur is matted or clumped and often stained blue–green by the production of pyocyanin pigment. The skin in affected areas is almost always wet.

The clinical signs are diagnostic in their own right. Bacterial culture may be helpful due to the multiresistant nature of *Pseudomonas.*

Clipping and cleaning of affected skin is important. Topical or systemic antibiotics may be used, although unless the underlying cause of wetting is not addressed, the condition is likely to recur. The use of drinking bottles rather than open water containers is recommended.

Fusobacterium necrophorum

Rabbits: Clinical signs include inflammation, erosion, ulceration or necrosis of skin, particularly around the head and neck. Subcutaneous abscesses may be seen.

Direct smears reveal the organism, although anaerobic culture is necessary to confirm the cause. Mixed infections can occur, and so aerobic culture should always be undertaken at the same time.

Clipping, cleaning and surgical debridement, together with topical or systemic antibiotics, are needed for successful treatment.

Treponema cuniculi

Rabbits: Venereal spirochaetosis is an uncommon dermatosis of the rabbit. Transmission is by direct contact and, due to the rabbit's grooming practices, auto-transmission to skin other than that of the genitalia is common.

Vesicles, papules, oedema, erosion and crusting may be seen on the genitalia and also on the lips, face, eyelids, ears and paws. Lesions are sometimes mistaken for early signs of myxomatosis or, if limited to scaling on the face, may be confused with dermatophytosis.

Diagnosis may be difficult as the organism is difficult to culture, but examination of biopsy samples stained with silver stains or the demonstration of the organism in dark-ground microscopy examination confirms the diagnosis. In some countries, serological tests are available.

Penicillin injected at weekly intervals for 3 weeks is the treatment of choice. All affected and in-contact animals need to be treated, whereupon the prognosis is good. Tetracycline and chloramphenicol treatments are also effective.

Pododermatitis (sore hocks)

Rabbits and guinea pigs: This condition is one of the most frustrating for the practitioner, and affects rabbits and guinea pigs (Figure 33.6). Whilst bacteria are involved in this condition, other factors are needed to initiate disease. Predisposing factors include heavy body size, thin metatarsal pad fur, damp or soiled bedding and housing on wire.

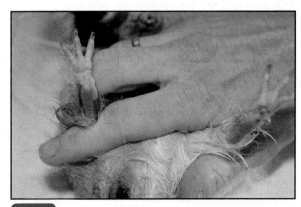

33.6 Sore hocks on a guinea pig.

Swelling of the metatarsal or metacarpal area follows scaling and erosion of the volar surfaces. The swellings may be very large with necrotic centres. The clinical signs are highly suggestive of the diagnosis. *S. aureus* is isolated in most cases.

Treatment will not be successful if the underlying factors are not identified and improved. Heavy rabbits (> 5 kg) should not be housed on wire, and bedding should be changed regularly. Management of the lesions involves the application of topical antibacterial ointments such as mupirocin 2% ointment. This product is not licensed for use in these species. Severe lesions should be cleaned, debrided and, if possible, bandaged. Recurrence is common and the prognosis in severe cases is guarded.

Fungal disease

Rabbits and rodents

There are two dermatophytes of significance in small mammals, of which *Trichophyton mentagrophytes* is carried asymptomatically in the coat of many. Rabbits in contact with cats and dogs are rarely infected with *Microsporum canis*. Whilst the latter is usually considered to be of more zoonotic significance, its pathogenicity in the fur of a paratenic host is unknown. *T. mentagrophytes* is more likely to cause zoonotic disease when carried by a small mammal than when it is infecting a dog or cat.

Owners are often worried about the zoonotic significance of dermatophytosis in small mammals. Most people who become infected are predisposed in some way (atopic or immunosuppressed). In most cases the risk appears to be very slight, although it is wise to limit the owner's contact with known infected animals, especially if the owner is a child.

Clinical signs: T. mentagrophytes may be carried asymptomatically. Clinical disease for both dermatophytes is essentially similar. Scaling, crusting and alopecia with some pruritus are found. Usually the bridge of the nose is affected, together with the eyelids, ears and paws. Occasionally widespread disease is found (Figure 33.7). Broken hairs may be found on close examination and these should be collected for fungal culture.

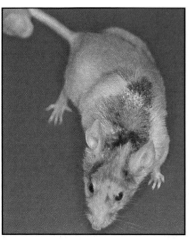

33.7 Crusting lesions on a mouse due to *Trichophyton mentagrophytes*.

Diagnosis: Fungal culture is the test of choice for diagnosis. Wood's lamp examination is useful in *Microsporum canis* infections, although not all strains will fluoresce. *Trichophyton* spp. do not fluoresce.

Treatment: Griseofulvin treatment at 25–50 mg/kg sid is the treatment of choice. However, it must be remembered that this drug is unlicensed for small mammals. It is highly teratogenic and so must not be used in breeding animals. Owners must take care in handling griseofulvin. Treatment should be continued until the clinical signs have resolved. In a group, all in-contact animals should be treated. Topical enilconazole (0.2% w/v solution) has also been used with success.

Clipping of the haircoat can be useful in longhaired breeds; clipped hair should be disposed of by burning. However, from experience in the cat, close clipping may increase the severity of clinical disease.

Parasitic diseases

Parasites affecting rabbits and rodents are listed in Figure 33.8.

Parasite groups	Examples	Hosts
Flies	Blowfly larvae	Rabbit, guinea pig
Fleas	*Ctenocephalides felis*	Rabbit, rat
	Spilopsyllus cuniculi	Rabbit
Lice	*Haemodipsus ventricosus*	Rabbit
	Gliricola porcelli	Guinea pig
Fur mites	*Leporacarus gibbus; Cheyletiella parasitovorax*	Rabbit
	Chirodiscoides caviae	Guinea pig
	Mycoptes musculinus	Mouse
Sarcoptic mites	*Sarcoptes scabiei*	Rabbit, rat, mouse
	Notoedres muris	Rat, mouse
Demodectic mites	*Demodex cuniculi*	Rabbit
	Demodex merioni	Gerbil
	Demodex criceti; Demodex aurati	Hamster
Ear mites	*Psoroptes cuniculi*	Rabbit

33.8 Parasite groups found on rabbits and rodents.

Myiasis

Rabbits: Unfortunately the presentation of a flyblown rabbit is a common occurrence in most veterinary practices in the summer months. This is a distressing condition for patient, owner and clinician alike. Whilst there is always some degree of lack of care involved, this condition can develop rapidly.

Affected animals are usually somewhat depressed, with skin disease initially focused on the perineum and tail fold. Alopecia is often present, and the skin may be eroded or even necrotic. Careful examination and exploration (for which anaesthesia may be required) will often reveal blowfly larvae (Figure 33.9). It is important to examine for entry into body cavities: this worsens the prognosis.

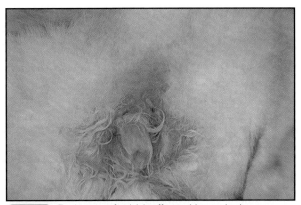

33.9 Perineum of rabbit affected by myiasis. (Reproduced from the *BSAVA Manual of Rabbit Medicine and Surgery*.)

Careful examination will usually reveal evidence of underlying disease, including dental disease, precluding adequate grooming; locomotor disease, including hindlimb paresis and diseases of the digestive system resulting in diarrhoea or lack of coprophagia and subsequent soiling of the perineum.

Clinical signs and demonstration of fly larvae are adequate for diagnosis. Treatment requires careful clipping and cleaning of affected areas. The removal of *all* fly larvae is necessary. Systemic antibiotics are sometimes necessary in severely affected animals. Following initial treatment, the use of insecticidal powders and sprays have been suggested; however, these should not be necessary if the underlying disease and husbandry problems are sorted out. A preventive treatment containing cyromazine (Rearguard) has recently been licensed for the rabbit in the UK.

In the USA the larvae of *Cuterebra* flies affect rabbits housed outdoors. The larvae develop subcutaneously and are treated by surgical removal.

Rodents: Guinea pigs may also be affected by myiasis.

Fleas

Rabbits: Two types of flea affect rabbits: the commonest is *Ctenocephalides felis*, the cat flea. *Spilopsyllus cuniculi*, the rabbit stick-tight flea is sometimes found, especially where wild rabbits enter the garden. The latter is of particular significance as a possible vector of myxomatosis virus. In the USA, rabbits can be infested with *Cediopsylla simples* (common eastern rabbit flea) and *Odontopsyllus multispinosus* (the giant eastern rabbit flea).

Fleas are rarely found in other species of small mammal living outside, but *C. felis* is occasionally found in coat brushings from domestic rats and chinchillas.

House rabbits sharing an environment with cats or dogs may pick up newly emerged adult *C. felis*. These sometimes cause pruritus. *S. cuniculi* is usually found attached to pinnal margins, although the fleas can attach and feed on any part of the rabbit's skin. *Spilopsyllus* may cause pruritus and tightly adherent crusts at the site of attachment.

With *C. felis* often the only clinical sign is the finding of flea faeces in the coat of a normal or pruritic rabbit or rodent; faeces are not found with rabbit fleas. Demonstration of adult fleas is diagnostic for *S. cuniculi* infestation.

The eradication of *C. felis* requires attention to the environmental stages, as well as to the adult fleas. If the house does not contain cats or dogs, then topical environmental control alone is often enough. If the household does contain cats or dogs with access to outdoors, then the use of an adulticide together with environmental control may be necessary. Pyrethrum-containing flea powders suitable for puppy or kitten use have been recommended, although their efficacy without environmental control is limited. A recent study demonstrated that imidacloprid was both effective and safe for the treatment of cat flea infestation in the rabbit (Hutchinson *et al.*, 2001). A good residual action was seen for 1 week, with some action persisting for 30 days.

The control of *S. cuniculi* relies upon two measures: the control of attached adult fleas and the prevention of future infestation. This is achieved either with pyrethrum-containing flea powders or by manual removal. Prevention is best achieved by either screening of the rabbit hutch or by limiting access to the garden by wild rabbits.

Lice

Rabbits: Lice are uncommon causes of skin disease in the rabbit. Rabbit lice (*Haemodipsus ventricosus*) are of the sucking type; heavy infestations result in anaemia. Affected rabbits may be severely pruritic, although this is uncommon. Anaemic animals can be depressed and lethargic, and scaling and crusting on the dorsal trunk may be seen. Lice or their eggs are usually easily demonstrated. The eggs are larger than those of *Cheyletiella* or *Leporacarus* and are attached along most of the length of the egg. The administration of pyrethrum-containing insecticidal powders is usually effective. Ivermectin injected at 200–400 µg/kg s.c. on three occasions at intervals of 2 weeks is effective for sucking lice.

Rodents: Lice are also found on mice, rats and guinea pigs. Whilst most species found are biting lice, skin irritation may occur. In the guinea pig, the resemblance of the lice to human head lice can give rise to concern (Figure 33.10). Reassurance may be given, as these parasites are all highly species-specific. Ivermectin and selenium sulphide washes are effective in reducing lice numbers.

Fur mites

Rabbits: Two types of fur mite are found inhabiting the pelage of the domestic rabbit. These are the true fur mites, *Leporacarus (Listrophorus) gibbus* (Figure 33.11), and the more surface living *Cheyletiella*

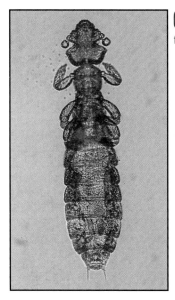

33.10 *Gliricola porcelli* louse from a guinea pig.

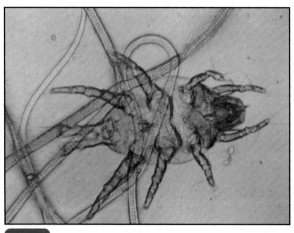

33.11 Male *Leporacarus gibbus* mite from a rabbit.

parasitovorax. The former is often spotted incidentally, and can be carried with no clinical disease, sometimes in large numbers, though severe pruritus has been reported (Patel and Robinson, 1993). *Cheyletiella* is more frequently associated with disease and has zoonotic significance. Lesions in owners consist of pruritic erythematous papules on contact sites such as arms and the trunk. The parasites do not persist on humans once the affected rabbits are treated.

Rabbits affected with either species of fur mite may present with no skin disease at all. Conversely, significant pruritus can be associated with small numbers of mites. Cheyletiellosis is often associated with severe scaling, especially on the dorsum. When pruritic disease is caused by *L. gibbus*, the most important signs are self-trauma and associated hair loss. Clinical cheyletiellosis is more likely in rabbits suffering from concurrent illness.

Demonstration of these mites, which sometimes both occur in the same rabbit, is best achieved with the examination of acetate strip samples. In some cases superficial skin scrapings are required to demonstrate *Cheyletiella*.

Both of these parasites respond to ivermectin injections at the same dose rate suggested for lice infestation. Concurrent washing with 2% selenium sulphide may help. Neither of these preparations is licensed for use in the rabbit. If treatment does not solve the problem, asymptomatic carriers (including dogs or cats) or survival of parasites off the host must be suspected.

Rodents: Pelage mites are also found frequently in rodents. Mites in the same group as *Lepoacarus* are adapted to a life in the pelage, with a pair of limbs adapted to facilitate moving from hair to hair. Whilst rarely the cause of clinical disease, alopecia and pruritus have been reported in the guinea pig, mouse and rat. Members of the group include *Chirodiscoides caviae* (guinea pig) (Figure 33.12), *Mycoptes musculinus* and *Psoregates simplex* (mouse) and *Ornithonyssus bacoti* (rat). Treatment with ivermectin is not always successful, as the mites live in the pelage. Topical washes with selenium sulphide are often effective.

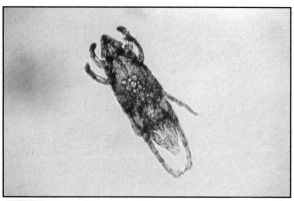

33.12 Male *Chirodiscoides caviae* mite from a guinea pig.

Cheyletiellid parasites in rodents include *Myobia musculi* and *Radfordia affinis*. Clinical signs in these animals (Figure 33.13) are mainly limited to pruritus. Mites may be small in number and sometimes only their eggs can be demonstrated (Figure 33.14). Treatment of these mites is suggested using ivermectin systemically and selenium sulphide washes.

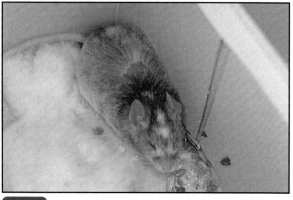

33.13 A pruritic mouse affected by pelage mites.

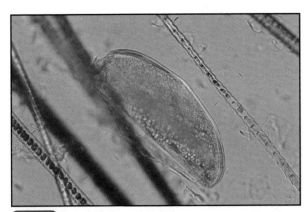

33.14 Egg from pelage mites in a mouse.

Sarcoptic mites

Rodents: Sarcoptic mites are frequently the cause of pruritic skin disease in small mammals. Varieties of *Sarcoptes scabiei* affect rats, although the species-specific *Notoedres muris* in the rat and mouse, and *Trixacarus (caviacoptes) caviae* in the guinea pig (Figure 33.15) are of greater clinical significance. Indeed guinea pigs affected with *T. caviae* probably represent 50% of all rodent dermatology presentations. Clinical signs include alopecia, crusting and extreme pruritus. Some guinea pigs show neurological signs including seizure. Skin scrapings make the diagnosis, although mites are scarce in some guinea pigs. Treatment in all species is by ivermectin (200–400 μg/kg). Three administrations at an interval of 2 weeks are usually effective. Whilst reportedly zoonotic, human lesions caused by *Trixacarus caviae* are surprisingly rare.

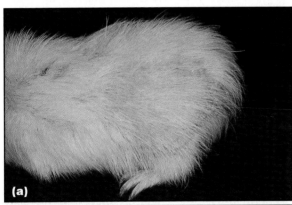

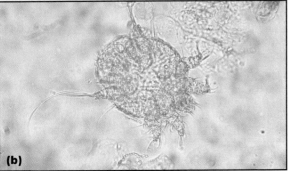

33.15 *Trixacarus caviae.* (a) A guinea pig infested by *Trixacarus caviae* mites. (b) Adult male *Trixacarus caviae* mite.

Demodectic mites

Rabbits: Demodectic mites have been reported rarely in the rabbit (Harvey, 1990).

Affected rabbits exhibited variable pruritus, although the pathological significance of the demodectic mites is unknown (Figure 33.16).

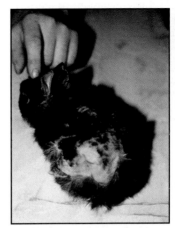

33.16 A rabbit affected by *Demodex cuniculi* mites. (Reproduced from Harvey (1990) with the permission of the *Journal of Small Animal Practice.*)

Rodents: Demodicosis affects gerbils, hamsters and guinea pigs (*Demodex merioni, D. criceti* and *aurati,* and *D. caviae* respectively). Clinical demodicosis is usually an indicator of concurrent illness or old age. The diagnosis is made on careful skin scrapings; these mites are all smaller than *Demodex canis.* Treatment is difficult and often not appropriate.

Ear mites

Rabbits: *Psoroptes cuniculi,* the rabbit ear mite, is a common ectoparasite of the rabbit. Infestations can occur some time after the last contact with another rabbit and clinical disease is sometimes initiated by concurrent stress. Mites survive for up to 3 weeks off the host, with shed scale carrying large numbers of mites.

Clinical signs: Clinical signs include severe crusting and pain of the external ear canal and medial surface of the pinna (Figure 33.17). Tightly adherent crusts are present in most cases and leave bleeding erosions when removed. Curiously, only one pinna may be

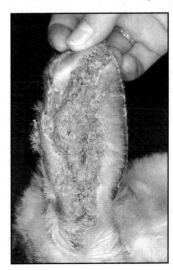

33.17 Crusts on the medial aspect of the pinna of a rabbit infested with *Psoroptes cuniculi* mites. (Reproduced from the *BSAVA Manual of Rabbit Medicine and Surgery.*)

affected. Affected rabbits are often pruritic and will rub at their ears. Secondary bacterial infection of crusted surfaces is common and may lead to otitis media.

Diagnosis: Demonstration of mites on examination of crusts taken from the pinna is usually straightforward as large numbers of mites are often present. Removal of crusts is painful, and so the minimum amount of material necessary should be taken.

Treatment: Ivermectin at 200–400 µg/kg injected on three occasions at intervals of 2 weeks is usually curative. Removal of crusts should not be attempted. One study demonstrated that the use of a phyto-aromatic gel was highly efficacious in the treatment of rabbit otoacariasis (Mignon and Losson, 1996). The gel was applied for two periods of 5 consecutive days, 6 days apart.

Behavioural dermatoses

Behavioural diseases in small mammals may present in the form of over-grooming. These behaviours are often the result of stresses, often due to overcrowding or from territorial disputes. Solitary animals sometimes over-groom, although this is less common than one individual having hair removed by other members of the group (barbering). Barbering of hair by dominant rabbits occurs when rabbits are housed in groups. Separation of the rabbits is the only successful management.

The only treatments for these behaviours are either to provide some form of environmental enrichment, or to remove one or more of the affected group.

Does in the breeding season pluck hair from the dewlap area to line their nests; this may occur in non-pregnant does. If excessive amounts of hair are removed and swallowed, hairballs occur.

Nutritional dermatoses

Poor understanding of the specific nutritional requirements of small mammals can lead to hypovitaminosis and general malnutrition. This can lead to specific skin signs, such as alopecia or scaling, or may be important in the pathogenesis of diseases caused by infectious organisms such as *Trixacarus caviae* infestation in the guinea pig. Guinea pigs also have a specific need for vitamin C, deficiency of which may result in predisposition to infections, together with keratinization defects.

Contaminated foodstuffs are also a potential hazard. Ergotism can cause sloughing of the distal extremities, including digits, pinnae and the tail.

Neoplastic disease

Rabbits

Spontaneous cutaneous neoplasms are rare in the domestic rabbit. Those most frequently found are the lipoma and papilloma. In the USA the oncogenic viruses Shope papilloma virus and Shope fibroma virus are found uncommonly in domestic rabbits, but are endemic in wild rabbit populations. Other neoplasms seen in the rabbit include squamous cell carcinoma, trichoepithelioma and basal cell tumour.

Subcutaneous lymphoma has also been reported, and may be diagnosed by the examination of fine needle aspirates. Recently epitheliotropic lymphoma has been reported in the rabbit (White *et al.*, 2000a). Clinical signs included erythroderma and alopecia. Diagnosis was confirmed on fine needle aspirates and skin biopsies. Lymphoma infiltrates were found in other organs, and the infiltrate was demonstrated to be of T cell origin. No effective treatment was demonstrated.

Rodents

Neoplastic skin diseases appear commonly in rodents. Due to the lack of specific diagnoses in many cases, the true incidence is unknown in pet species.

A full examination for signs of metastasis is important in animals with skin masses, although financial constraints limit the opportunities for histopathology.

Common skin masses include fibromas and adnexal tumours, but many other types are encountered. Sebaceous gland tumours are often found on the 'scent gland' areas of small mammals, especially in the gerbil. It is important to differentiate this from simple hyperplasia. Surgical resection is the most effective treatment.

Miscellaneous dermatoses

Rabbits

Seborrhoea: Seborrhoea of the skin surrounding the scent glands lateral to the anogenital line is occasionally a problem. The use of mild antiseborrhoeic shampoos is usually helpful. Recently sebaceous adenitis was reported in four rabbits (White *et al.*, 2000b). Affected rabbits showed extensive alopecia and crusting. Diagnosis was made by skin biopsy, which demonstrated signs similar to those found in the dog; however, addition pathology included mural and interface folliculitis. There was no effective treatment.

Moulting problems: Rabbits are occasionally presented with disorders of seasonal moulting. Such rabbits may have patches of retained telogen coat and patches of fur at different lengths. This occurs more frequently in older rabbits. Careful grooming and attention to husbandry help.

Dewlap overgrowth: Excessive size of the dewlap can make the rabbit prone to infection in the area, and may also prevent coprophagy. This can lead to faecal soiling and myiasis. Dewlap reduction is achieved by removing an elliptical area of skin and underlying adipose tissue under anaesthesia.

Urine scalding: Urine scalding of the perineal region may occur in rabbits housed in unsanitary conditions. Affected skin is moist and excoriated. This problem is exacerbated if rabbits are obese or have locomotor disease.

Frostbite: Rabbits suddenly exposed to very cold weather may suffer from frostbite, presenting as necrosis of the pinnal margins and tip.

Rodents

Fur slip in chinchillas: The chinchilla has the ability to lose focal areas of fur when handled roughly. This affects areas of fur 2–5 cm in diameter, which will regrow slowly over several months.

Seborrhoea: Rats are frequently presented for this problem. Males are affected more frequently than females, and castration and/or regular bathing helps. Localized seborrhoeic accumulations occur in the tail fold of guinea pigs, especially males.

Bald or sore nose in the gerbil: This condition, whilst occasionally representing mechanical trauma, is usually due to excessive secretion of the Harderian glands. The accumulated porphyrin-rich secretion on the nasal skin causes a contact irritant problem (Figure 33.18). Secondary staphylococcal infection is common. Recommended treatments include control of the secondary infection and surgical removal of Harderian glands.

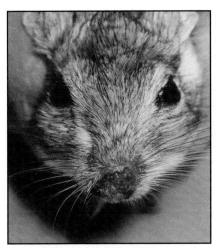

33.18
Sore nose in a gerbil. (Reproduced from the *BSAVA Manual of Exotic Pets, 4th edition.*)

Endocrine diseases: The true incidence of endocrine disease in rodents is largely unknown, due to the lack of simple, affordable diagnostic tests. Cystic ovaries are commonly encountered in the guinea pig, often associated with symmetrical alopecia. The ovaries in affected animals can often be palpated through the flanks. Endometrial hyperplasia or uterine neoplasia may accompany cystic ovaries. Ovariohysterectomy is the treatment of choice, although 'scientific neglect' is the best option in elderly animals.

References and further reading

Baker AS (1999) *Mites and Ticks of Domestic Animals: An Identification Guide and Information Source.* The Stationery Office, London

Brown SA and Rosenthal KL (1997) *Self-assessment Colour Review of Small Mammals.* Manson, London

Collins BR (1987) Dermatologic disorders of common small nondomestic animals. In: *Dermatology,* ed. GH Nesbitt, pp. 235–295. Churchill Livingstone, New York

Ganière JP *et al.* (1991) Myxomatosis of the depilated Angora rabbit. A preliminary study. *Veterinary Dermatology* **2,** 11–16

Harvey RG (1990) *Demodex cuniculi* in dwarf rabbits (*Orcytologus cuniculus*). *Journal of Small Animal Practice* **31,** 204–207

Harvey RG, Brown PF, Young RD *et al.* (1990) A connective tissue defect in two rabbits similar to the Ehlers–Danlos syndrome. *Veterinary Record* **126,** 130–132

Hillyer EV (1997) Dermatologic diseases. In: *Ferrets, Rabbits and Rodents: Clinical Medicine and Surgery,* ed. EV Hillyer and KE Queensbury, pp. 212–219. WB Saunders, Philadelphia

Hutchinson MJ, Jacobs DE, Bell GD *et al.* (2001) Evaluation of imidacloprid for the treatment and prevention of cat flea (*Ctenocephalides felis felis*) infestations on rabbits. *Veterinary Record* **148,** 695–696

Meredith A and Redrobe S (2002) *BSAVA Manual of Exotic Pets, 4th edn.* BSAVA Publications, Gloucester

Mignon BR and Losson BJ (1996) Efficacy of a phyto-aromatic gel against auricular mange in rabbits and carnivores. *Veterinary Record* **138,** 329–332

Noble WC (1989) Bacterial skin infections in domestic animals and man. In: *Advances in Veterinary Dermatology, 1,* ed. C von Tscharner and REW Halliwell, pp. 311–326. Baillière Tindall, London

Okerman L (1988) *Diseases of Domestic Rabbits.* Blackwell, Oxford

Okerman L, Devriese LA, Maertens L *et al.* (1984) Cutaneous staphylococcosis in rabbits. *Veterinary Record* **114,** 313–315

Patel A and Robinson KJE (1993) Dermatosis associated with *Listrophorus gibbus* in the rabbit. *Journal of Small Animal Practice* **34,** 409

Paul-Murphy J and Moriello K (1995) Skin diseases of small mammals. In: *Handbook of Small Animal Dermatology,* ed. K Moriello and I Mason, pp. 245–253. Pergamon Press, Oxford

Scarff DH (2000) Dermatoses. In: *BSAVA Manual of Rabbit Medicine and Surgery,* ed. P Flecknell, pp. 69–80. BSAVA Publications, Gloucester

Scott DW, Miller WH and Griffin CE (2001) Dermatoses of pet rodents, rabbits and ferrets. In: *Muller and Kirk's Small Animal Dermatology, 6th edn,* ed. D W Scott *et al.,* pp. 1415–1458. WB Saunders, Philadelphia

White SD, Campbell T, Logan A *et al.* (2000a) Lymphoma with cutaneous involvement in three domestic rabbits (*Oryctolagus cuniculus*). *Veterinary Dermatology* **11,** 61–67

White SD, Linder KE, Schultheiss P *et al.* (2000b) Sebaceous adenitis in four domestic rabbits (*Oryctolagus cuniculus*). *Veterinary Dermatology* **11,** 53–60

34

Ferrets

Karen L. Rosenthal

Only a few diseases cause the great majority of skin problems in ferrets and almost all skin disease in ferrets is secondary to a primary problem. Ferrets almost never have skin lesions such as pustules or papules or keratinization disorders. Although one is always on the lookout for a 'new' ferret skin disease, most dermatological disease in ferrets can be diagnosed by history, signs and a few diagnostic tests. To avoid assuming the cause of ferret dermatological disease, diagnostic testing, including taking biopsies, should always be recommended to clients.

Figure 34.1 lists the most common pet ferret skin disorders along with a simplified list of signs. Figure 34.2 lists skin diseases that are common in dogs and cats but rarely, if ever, seen in ferrets. This list is intended for the veterinary surgeon who does not see ferrets regularly in their practice and is unfamiliar with the diseases that ferrets do NOT get. If one were to use the common dog and cat dermatological disease rule-outs on ferret dermatological disease, many wrong diagnoses would be made. Tumours reported in ferrets are listed in Figure 34.3. The few diseases that are fairly well characterized will be described in this chapter.

Mast cell tumour

Cutaneous mast cell tumours (MCTs) are the most common cause of skin masses in ferrets. This is almost always a benign disease in ferrets as MCTs rarely metastasize. In fact, MCTs usually appear as a singular mass on the skin. The pathogenesis of this disease is not known.

	Rare	Not reported
Demodicosis	✓	
Self-barbering		✓
Hypothyroidism		✓
Allergic skin disease		✓
Nutritional deficiency		✓
Dermatophytosis	✓	

34.2 Uncommon ferret skin disorders.

	Common	Uncommon
Mast cell tumour	✓	
Sebaceous gland tumour		✓
Basal cell tumour		✓
Squamous cell carcinoma		✓
Adenocarcinoma		✓
Adenoma		✓
Myxosarcoma		✓
Fibrosarcoma		✓
Haemangioma		✓
Haemangiosarcoma		✓
Lymphosarcoma		✓

34.3 Reported skin tumours in ferrets.

	Alopecia	Pruritic	Positive skin scrape	Skin changes	Area of the body
Adrenal gland disease	Yes	Yes	No	Yes	Whole body
Canine distemper virus infection	No	No	No	Yes	Feet/face
Fleas	Yes	Yes	No	Yes	Whole body
Mast cell tumours	Yes	Uncommon	No	Yes	Discrete areas
Sarcoptes	No (unless generalized form)	Yes	Yes	Yes	Feet or whole body

34.1 Common ferret skin disorders.

Clinical approach

Ferrets with MCT have an unremarkable history and there is no particular predisposing factor associated with this disease. Owners often do not realize the mass is present and MCT is usually an incidental finding on a yearly physical examination. In ferrets with white fur, the owner may notice a 'reddened' area of the fur from dried blood from the MCT.

Although MCTs usually appear as individual skin masses, a ferret can have one or a few nodules on different skin areas. It is most common to find these masses on the dorsum and trunk. MCTs are usually round and can vary in diameter from a couple of millimetres to up to 3 cm. Typically, the MCT is erythematous, often eroded and may produce scant bleeding. MCTs can either be flat or slightly raised and both types can appear at the same time on the same ferret. They are non-painful, although, occasionally the area around the MCT is pruritic. Infrequently, localized alopecia will accompany the MCT. Ferrets with cutaneous MCT have no other signs of disease as these tumours rarely spread to distant areas, nor do they cause paraneoplastic syndromes.

Diagnosis

The diagnostic test of choice for a ferret MCT is biopsy. The minimum database to collect before taking a biopsy depends on the age and overall health of the ferret. Since the ferret will need to be sedated or anaesthetized for the biopsy, it is always best to recommend a complete blood count and plasma biochemistry profile along with urinalysis, although these tests are not affected by the tumour itself. The biopsy should be excisional with clean margins. On histopathology, cutaneous MCTs have the characteristics of MCTs in other animals. The mast cells are well differentiated, round to oval, and are usually arranged in sheets. Since this is most commonly a benign disease, mitotic figures are rare.

Management and therapeutics

Surgical removal of the cutaneous MCT is the treatment of choice. These tumours do not require chemotherapy, radiation therapy or follow-up surgery. If the entire lesion is removed, it is thought that surgery is curative.

Prognosis

The prognosis for ferrets with cutaneous MCT is excellent. Even without surgery, these cutaneous tumours do not appear to metastasize. Removal is still indicated, however. If the nodules are pruritic, removal will improve the quality of life. Although it has not been shown that metastasis from cutaneous to systemic disease occurs, prevention by removal of the tumours is warranted for precautionary reasons.

Sarcoptic mange

Sarcoptic mange is not commonly seen in pet ferrets and therefore has not been studied extensively. *Sarcoptes scabiei*, which affects dogs and may secondarily infect cats, is the cause of sarcoptic mange in ferrets. Ferrets do not have to be housed with dogs to be infected with this parasite. In the generalized form, this is likely to be a secondary disease process and the existence of a primary disease should be investigated. Little is known about scabies in ferrets, but it is anticipated that it is likely to be self-limiting.

Clinical approach

Sarcoptic mange in ferrets is not a subtle disease. Whether a ferret has the localized or generalized form, they have obvious skin disease. In the localized form, only the feet are affected. The feet are swollen and erythematous, the pads may be cracked and bleeding, and the ferret may exhibit pain while walking. In the generalized form, there are isolated patches of alopecia and the ferret is intensely pruritic. The skin may be erythematous and ulcerated due to the pruritus.

Diagnosis

As with many other ferret diseases, the diagnosis of sarcoptic mange is not difficult as the signs and diagnostics are not equivocal. There are no other diseases that have the same history and clinical signs.

The disease is diagnosed by a skin scrape revealing either the mite or ova, although in chronic cases it may be difficult to demonstrate the mite on skin scrapes. A biopsy of the skin may be a more consistent diagnostic test as it reveals evidence of the mites and/or severe inflammation.

If diagnostic funds are limited, one can use response to treatment as a diagnostic test for sarcoptic mites. The complete blood count may exhibit a relative and absolute eosinophilia. Plasma biochemistry findings are not affected by this disease. If secondary bacterial dermatitis is present due to the intense pruritus, neutrophilia may be present.

Management and therapeutics

Sarcoptic mite infestation is treated with ivermectin at 0.2–0.4 mg/kg s.c. once, repeated after 2 weeks. This, alone, may not cure the ferret. If other animals in the house are carriers of *Sarcoptes*, they may need to be treated too. This includes other ferrets, dogs and cats. Also, the environment the ferret lives in should be cleaned. If the generalized form is present, treatment with ivermectin will not be likely to cure this disease as one needs to search for a primary problem. Although immune suppression has been suggested as a cause for the generalized form, it is very rare to see this disease in ferrets that are on high doses of prednisolone.

Prognosis

The prognosis for a cure is excellent in the localized form. In the generalized form, unless the primary problem is resolved, the prognosis is more guarded.

Canine distemper virus

Canine distemper virus (CDV) infection is fatal in ferrets. One manifestation of this disease is skin and footpad abnormality. In this condition, the dermatological signs are minor but are nonetheless important for diagnostic purposes. The fatal aspects of CDV infection include pathology of the respiratory, gastrointestinal and neurological systems in the ferret. Inclusion bodies can be found in all tissues on post mortem but are most common in the epithelium of the gastrointestinal tract, bladder and skin.

Very rarely, ferrets will develop atypical CDV infection. In these ferrets, which are potential sources of infection to others, the only sign of disease may be the dermatological changes. These may be ferrets that develop the disease from an inappropriate vaccine. In these instances, a detailed history and skin biopsy may allow for the diagnosis of CDV.

Clinical approach

The dermatological clinical signs of CDV are mainly observed on the chin and footpads. The first signs of this disease are a mild upper respiratory infection including ocular and nasal discharges. In some cases, the dermatological changes follow the upper respiratory signs, or the skin changes can appear first. A chin rash characterized by crusts is common. The crusts can be reddish or yellow in colour. The skin in this area can become swollen. No other areas of the body exhibit these signs.

As the disease progresses, hyperkeratosis of the footpads ensues. The footpads become hard, swollen and crusted. In most cases, other clinical signs of disease accompany hyperkeratosis of the footpads including neurological signs and severe lower respiratory disease. It is most likely that ferrets with CDV will exhibit at least one of the skin lesions, either the chin rash or hyperkeratosis of the footpads.

Ferrets with CDV have a history of being exposed to an animal carrying CDV. This includes other ferrets, dogs or raccoons. Ferrets which contract CDV are usually not vaccinated or have been vaccinated improperly.

Diagnosis

The diagnosis of CDV infection is not difficult in most cases. The history is an important element in the diagnostic pathway: Has the ferret been properly vaccinated? Has the ferret been exposed to CDV?

The skin and footpad changes are accompanied by severe whole body disease, which eventually kills the ferret. The complete blood count may be elevated, reflecting the secondary bacterial pneumonia that accompanies canine distemper virus. Depending on the progression of the disease at the time of venipuncture, various biochemical abnormalities can be exhibited that represent organ dysfunction due to CDV infection.

The definitive diagnosis of canine distemper virus is usually made on post-mortem examination. Inclusion bodies are found in epithelial cells on histopathology. Plasma antibody tests and fluorescent antigen tests aid in the diagnosis. Taking a biopsy of the affected areas of the skin is usually not practical, as the skin problems are a minor aspect of this fatal disease.

Management and therapeutics

There is no treatment for CDV. Antibiotics can be used to treat the secondary bacterial infections but the disease is ultimately fatal.

Prognosis

The prognosis for a ferret with CDV infection is extremely grave, as this is a fatal disease. In the rare instance where an atypical infection occurs, a ferret may survive with long-term dermatological disease (i.e. hyperkeratotic footpads).

Prophylaxis

Two vaccines are available in the USA for use in ferrets: Purevax and Fervac-D.

Fleas

In severe household flea infestations, ferrets can be affected by the dog or cat flea. Ferrets are usually only affected when they are in a house that is overrun with fleas or when they are in contact with dogs or cats that have a severe infestation.

Clinical approach

Ferrets infested with fleas appear as dogs and cats do with this problem, although there is no one particular area of the body that is affected. Ferrets may be pruritic with resulting hair loss and erythema of the skin. It is an obvious disease and owners usually report seeing the fleas on the ferret; flea excrement is also apparent. There is no particular predisposing factor associated with this disease. Flea allergy dermatitis is not recognized in ferrets, although in a severe infestation there is always the possibility it could occur.

Diagnosis

The diagnosis of flea infestation is not difficult. Fleas are easily observed on the ferret's skin along with flea excrement. The history of exposure to a cat, dog or house infested with fleas is common. Ferrets are usually kept indoors and the fleas are brought inside by other animals or people. In mild to severe infestations, there may be an eosinophilia evident in the white blood cell count. In severe and chronic infestations, anaemia is a possible complication.

Management and therapeutics

The management of a flea infestation in ferrets is similar to that for dogs and cats (see Chapter 19). Both the pet and its environment need to be treated. It may be easier to treat the ferret than other animals since ferrets are usually kept indoors; once the flea population is reduced, ferrets are no longer affected. The environment should be treated. If chemicals are used, it is recommended that ferrets are removed from the area unless it is known that the chemicals are safe for ferrets. It is more difficult to recommend individual animal treatment. There are no anti-flea products labelled for use in ferrets. Anecdotally, veterinary surgeons have used fractions of cat doses to treat ferrets. This can be risky and is not recommended. Ivermectin (0.2–0.4 mg/kg s.c.) can be given once and repeated once or twice, 2 weeks apart. Ivermectin may help reduce the flea population on the ferret and, if used with proper environmental treatments, may cure the ferret of this problem. Imidacloprid and fipronil may also be used.

There is a report of using diazinon 20% w/v on ferrets, at a dose range of 0.1 ml on the skin for ferrets with a bodyweight between 0.6 kg and 1.5 kg, and 0.15 ml on the skin for ferrets >1.5 kg bodyweight.

Prognosis
If appropriate controls are used and the ferret is treated appropriately, the prognosis for a cure is excellent.

Adrenal gland disease

Adrenal gland disease is a very common disease in pet ferrets over 3 years of age in the United States. One or both adrenal glands can be affected. Alopecia is a common sign (Figure 34.4) and is due to the over-production of adrenal androgens from the diseased adrenal gland(s). One or more of these compounds is known to be elevated in ferrets with adrenal gland disease: oestrogen, androstenedione, 17-OH-pro-gesterone and dehydroepiandrosterone sulphate (DHEAS). Cortisol is usually not elevated in ferrets with adrenal gland disease.

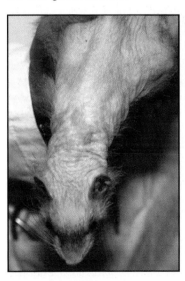

34.4 Generalized alopecia in a 2-year-old female spayed ferret with hyperadrenocorticism. (Courtesy of AP Foster; case material from K Benson)

Clinical approach
The most common sign in ferrets with this disease is alopecia. Hair loss typically starts at the base of the tail or on the tail. Over a period of weeks or months, the alopecia progresses in a symmetrical fashion to include the rump, thigh area, ventrum and, finally, along the dorsum to the shoulder blade area. In extreme cases, only guard hairs are left on the entire body. In females, an enlarged vulva is another common sign. In both males and females, pruritus may be present in approximately 30% of cases. Ferrets do not have to have alopecia to be pruritic in this syndrome.

Diagnosis
The complete blood count and plasma biochemistry findings are usually within the normal range with this disease. Typical tests for adrenal gland disease in dogs such as the ACTH stimulation test, dexamethasone suppression and the urine cortisol:creatinine ratio do not diagnose this disease.

Abdominal ultrasonography can detect an enlarged adrenal gland in some cases. Not all diseased adrenal glands are enlarged, however. Measurement of adrenal androgen concentrations is the most consistent method to diagnose this disease. In ferrets with adrenal gland disease, one or more adrenal androgens will be elevated above the normal range. These compounds include oestrogen, androstenedione, 17-OH-proges-terone and DHEAS. In the UK, some clinical pathology laboratories will measure 17-OH-progesterone in ferret serum samples.

Management and therapeutics
Surgical removal of the diseased adrenal gland is the preferred treatment at present. If both adrenal glands are diseased, the clinician has the option of removing both glands or one whole gland and part of the other. If both glands are entirely removed, then glucocorticoid supplementation is likely to be required. In some ferrets, mineralacorticoid supplementation may also be needed. If one whole gland and part of the other is removed, then supplementation may not be necessary. However, the signs of disease may not entirely dissipate if some diseased gland remains.

Mitotane administration appears to cause signs to regress in some ferrets and appears to work best in younger ferrets with this disease. However, this is not a recommended treatment as it can exacerbate insulinoma hypoglycaemia in ferrets.

Recently, other drugs have been used with some success to treat adrenal gland disease in ferrets. These include leuprolide, anastrozole and flutamide. Leuprolide can be given as a depot injection at 100–150 μg/kg, monthly or every few months. As with anastrozole and flutamide, ferrets may respond to these medications, and signs of adrenal gland disease can dissipate. Most ferrets require lifelong treatment with these medications and, over time, the amount of medication necessarily to depress signs of adrenal gland disease may increase. In some cases, the pruritus from adrenal gland disease may only respond to removal of the diseased adrenal glands.

Prognosis
The prognosis of adrenal gland disease in ferrets is usually excellent if the disease is treated properly. Once the diseased adrenal gland is removed, the clinical signs resolve. If the entire gland cannot be removed, signs may fully or only partially resolve, depending on the amount of diseased gland remaining.

References and further reading

Brown SE and Rosenthal KL (eds) (1997) *Self Assessment Colour Review of Small Mammals.* Manson Publishing, London

Orcutt C (1997) Dermatologic diseases. In: *Ferrets, Rabbits, and Rodents*, ed. EV Hillyer and KE Quesenberry, pp. 115–125. WB Saunders, Philadelphia

Rosenthal K (1997) Endocrine diseases. In: *Ferrets, Rabbits, and Rodents*, ed. EV Hillyer and KE Quesenberry, pp. 91–98. WB Saunders, Philadelphia

35

Birds

Neil A. Forbes

Dermatology in birds is more varied than in any other group of domestic pets because of the great number of species and the variation in size, natural habitat and method of locomotion. A dermatological examination of any bird should include the study of representative feather tracts, skin, beak and cere, ears, legs and claws, preen gland, and cloaca. Thorough history taking, microscopic examination of samples, haematological and biochemical screens serve the avian dermatologist well. One aspect of avian dermatology that is foreign to the small animal clinician is that which relates to aberrant behaviours unique to birds. Avian dermatology cases are typically multifactorial and often reflect underlying or contributory systemic disease. Nutritional deficiencies, poor management, lack of exercise and environmental stimulation are frequent contributory causes.

Anatomy and physiology

The anatomy and physiology of the skin and feathers is well covered in various texts (e.g. Lucas and Stettenheim, 1972; King and McLelland, 1984; McLelland, 1990).

Skin

Avian skin is thinner and more delicate than that of mammals and has skeletal attachments. The epidermis is divided into deep living and superficial dead layers, in total just 10 cells thick. The living layer is divided into the basal layer (adjacent to the dermis), the intermediate layer and the transitional layer (stratum corneum) (mainly keratin and keratin-bound substances).

Avian skin is aglandular except for the uropygial gland and the holocrine glands of the external auditory canal. The bilobed uropygial (preen) gland is located on the dorsal aspect of the insertion point of the central tail flight feathers. There is interspecies variation in gland size, and the gland may be absent (e.g. ratites, many pigeons, Amazon parrots). The gland drains an oily sebaceous secretion in a dorsal direction through two or more ducts. During preening, oil is spread over the plumage, providing additional waterproofing and durability to the feathers. The external ear canal is situated caudolateral to the lateral canthus of the eye and secretes a waxy material comprising predominantly desquamated cells.

Incubation (brood) patches are modified areas of skin that lose their plumage and become oedematous with an increased blood supply; they are used to maintain egg temperature during incubation.

Feathers

Details of individual feather anatomy are shown in Figures 35.1 and 35.2. Feathers are arranged in tracts called pterylae. The featherless areas in between are called apteria and are useful to the clinician, especially in providing access to the jugular vein.

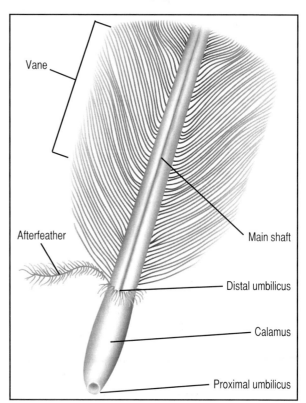

35.1 The parts of a typical feather. (Redrawn after Romagnano and Heard, 2000.)

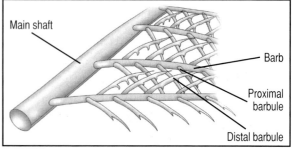

35.2 Interlocking barbules of the barbs of a flight feather. (Redrawn after Romagnano and Heard, 2000.)

Feather types

- Contour feathers: the wing (remiges) and tail (retrices) flight feathers and body feathers. The remiges are divided into primary and secondary (Figure 35.3). *Primary feathers* are attached to the periosteum of the metacarpus laterally on each wing and are responsible for 'forward propulsion' in flight. *Secondary feathers* insert on to the periosteum of the ulna and are responsible for 'lift' in flight. There are typically 12 *retrices* (tail flight feathers), numbered bilaterally from lateral to medial
- Covert feathers: cover the bases of the flight feathers
- Semi-plume feathers: have a long rachis and entirely plumaceous vane; are located along contour feather tracts or in feather tracts of their own; and assist with insulation
- Down feathers: small fluffy plumaceous feathers with a short or absent rachis; provide an undercoat to maintain warmth
- Powder down feathers: specialized down feathers that disintegrate to produce powder spread throughout the plumage as a preening and waterproofing agent. Loss or absence of powder down is an important clinical finding

- Other feathers include hypopenae (after feathers), filoplumes (fine hair-like feathers) and bristles (stiff, usually with no barbs).

Colour
Feather coloration is determined by pigments (melanins, carotenoids and porphyrins) as well as physical structure.

Feather development
As a new feather develops, it originates from the dermal papilla (as a layer of living epidermal cells). As the new calamus and rachis grow, they are filled with a loose reticulum of mesoderm plus an axial artery and vein. At this stage, the feather is described as a 'blood feather'. If this feather should become broken or damaged it will bleed profusely. As the feather matures, the blood vessels degenerate and are resorbed back to the umbilicus; the rachis then takes up a transparent appearance and is termed 'hard penned'. The shape of each feather is established during its development, and does not alter except by wear.

Moulting
All feathers of adult birds are replaced regularly during moulting. Moulting is stimulated by change in day length and typically occurs after breeding. The loss of old feathers is stimulated by passive force applied by

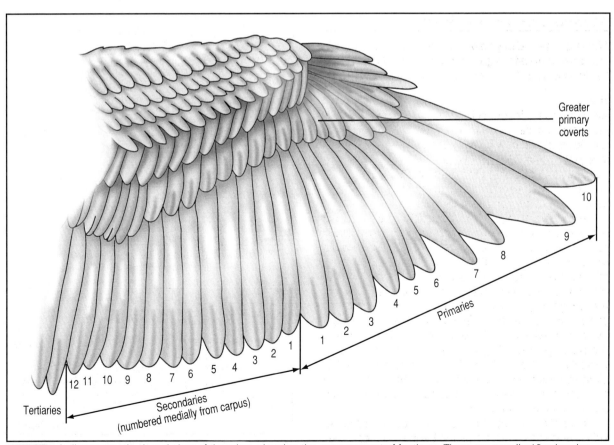

35.3 A diagrammatic dorsal view of the wing, showing the arrangement of feathers. There are usually 10 primaries, though some birds (e.g. canaries) have only 9. There are usually up to 14 secondaries, though some birds have more. (Redrawn after Romagnano and Heard, 2000.)

the new feathers as they grow down. Birds hatch with a 'natal down', which they lose after their first moult. One moult cycle is the period from when a particular feather is moulted to the time when the same feather is moulted again. Many species moult twice a year (having a summer and winter plumage), whilst others (e.g. eagles) take 2–3 years before they complete a single moult cycle.

Approach to the dermatological case

History
The following should be addressed:

- What is the origin of the bird?
- What is the species, sex and age of the bird?
- How long has the owner had the bird?
- Does the owner have other birds? Does the bird live, or has the bird ever lived, with other birds? Does the bird ever go to stay with other birds?
- Husbandry and housing (including other avian and non-avian members of the family): Is the bird's cage adequate in size and position (lighting, seclusion, not in direct sunlight)? Is the bird situated in an active part of the house, e.g. living room? What type of cage does the bird live in?
- How much time does the owner spend with the bird? How long does the bird spend without human contact?
- Is the bird truly imprinted?
- Has the bird's reaction to owner or any other member of the household (including animals) changed recently?
- Is the bird handled; is the bird trained; are the owners dominant to the bird?
- Has previous diagnosis or treatment been administered?
- Has the bird been subjected to any viral or *Chlamydophila* spp. (psittacosis) tests?
- What food is the bird offered? What food does the bird actually eat ? (Any bird on a sunflower- or peanut-based diet will be vitamin A and calcium deficient)
- Has there been any change in food or water consumption?
- What type of toys does the bird have? Are the toys changed? Does the bird entertain itself, e.g. playing with toys?
- For how much of the day is the bird out of the cage?

If the bird is showing evidence of feather picking:

- How long has the bird been plucking? How old was the bird when it started plucking? What month of the year did the plucking start?
- Has the bird picked in the past and started re-picking, is it a seasonal plucker? Is there any seasonal link with moulting or sexual behaviour?

- Does the bird pick when the owner is present, absent or both?
- How does the owner react to the bird if they see it plucking?
- If the bird plucks when the owner is present how does the owner react? Is the bird itchy? Does it scream or vocalize when plucking? Does it interrupt its favourite behaviour to pluck? Is there a certain time of day when it plucks?
- How does the owner describe the bird (one or more of the following): relaxed, anxious, playful, fearful, aggressive, loving, demanding?

Physical examination and collection of diagnostic samples

Examination
A systematic examination of the beak, cere, feet, ears, preen gland, skin and cloaca should be made. In particular, one should assess body condition, colour and nature of plumage, durability of feathers, stage of or interval since last moult (check all feather types).

The feathers should be checked for 'fret' lines or bars which indicate that the bird was stressed by some concurrent disease, nutritional deficiency, trauma, steroid administration or other episode at the time of the previous moult.

Check the skin (face, apteria, inguinal, under wing, legs and feet, cloaca).

Basic tests
Complete blood count, serum chemistries, *Chlamydophila* spp. serology or antigen PCR, faecal microscopy and blood tests for heavy metal (lead and zinc) should be performed on all cases (contact laboratory for sample requirements).

Additional tests
Following examination of the skin and plumage, additional tests may be performed:

- *Feather pulp cytological examination:* A squash preparation is prepared from a fresh feather pulp and stained (e.g. Diff-Quik, Wright's, Giemsa). Slides are examined for inflammatory cells and the presence of pathogens or inclusions. A Gram-stained slide is examined to ascertain type and numbers of bacteria and yeast. If relevant, microbiological culture and sensitivity testing is performed
- *Feather biopsy:* A biopsy may be performed for histological examination
- *Viral tests:* Samples of feather pulp and blood may be collected to test for psittacine beak and feather disease (PBFD) and polyoma virus.

Differential diagnosis
Infectious skin conditions are described in Figure 35.4, and skin conditions related to particular body sites are discussed in Figure 35.5.

Condition	Clinical signs	Differential diagnosis, investigation and treatment
Papillomata	Commonest around palpebrae, commissure of beak or feet (finches) or cloaca or choana of psittacines (especially Amazonia and Macaws) (see Figure 35.6). Hyperkeratosis, hyperplasia with folding of dermis	Considered to be virus-induced and oncogenic, progressing to billary adenocarcinoma. Treatment is by high antigen-loaded autogenous vaccines, laser surgery or cloacal stripping of the lesions. 2% capsicum in the diet may lead to remission
Poxvirus	Different serovars affect different species. Infection transmitted by biting insects. Dry form characterized by dry nodular lesions on non-feathered areas around face, cere and feet. Wet form affects similar areas plus mouth, pharynx and viscera. Lesions self-limiting and normally heal in 6–8 weeks.	Diagnosis by intracytoplasmic 'Bollinger bodies' on histopathology.
	Canary pox is highly infectious, causing 20–100% mortality occurring in autumn and winter. Cutaneous, diphtheritic or septicaemic (including respiratory) forms occur	Vaccination against canary pox is recommended during the summer
Herpesvirus	Dry, white to grey, occasionally crusty, lesions on toes and feet of cockatoos. Herpesvirus may also cause significant liver damage leading to plumage defects	Appear as papillomas but electron microscopy may show inclusions
Localized bacterial papule or granuloma	Frequently around the site of a bite wound, foreign body, trauma or penetration	Typically caused by *Staphylococcus* spp., *Aeromonas* spp. Bacteriology and sensitivity testing should be performed
Mycobacterial granuloma	Caused by *Mycobacterium avium* or *M. tuberculosis*. Commonest in Amazon, Blue and Gold, and Green Wing Macaws (Romagnano and Heard, 2000). Localized lesions, often around the head or face	Skin lesions most likely caused by *M. tuberculosis* (as *M. avium* grows at a higher temperature); may also affect the owner. Long-term (>6 months) therapy required but not generally recommended in view of zoonotic risks
Periarticular infection	*Salmonella* spp. polyarthritis	Localization of septicaemia, common in pigeons. Grave/hopeless prognosis
Fungal	*Candida* spp. or aspergillosis. Localized raised or, more commonly, extensive ulcerative lesions	

35.4 Infectious skin conditions: viral, bacterial and fungal.

Condition	Features	Differential diagnosis, investigation and treatment
Beak		
Trauma	Intraspecies (especially cockatoos) aggression commonly results in acutely painful crush injuries to beaks. If beaks are cut excessively short during trimming such that they bleed, the bird will suffer extreme pain and will require analgesia for several days	
Abnormal growth	Often associated with liver pathology, e.g. hepatic lipidosis. Commonly a sequel to excessive dietary fat content	Scissor beak and brachygnathism (short upper beak) should be treated with physiotherapy when bird still very young. In severe cases dental acrylic ramps (as an extension to the maxilla or to one side of the mandible) may be used to force the beak into the correct position each time it closes
	Fungal (e.g. *Aspergillus, Candida;* Figure 35.7) and viral (PBFD) infections occur	
	Neoplasia (chondroma (Figure 35.8) and chondrosarcoma) cause irregular excessive beak growth	
Crop	Thermal trauma from giving overheated foods to baby parrots gives rise to crop and skin necrosis, with crop leakage to the outside	
Feather cysts	Any species. May present as localized swellings (see Figure 35.14)	Remove cystic follicle and dermal papilla completely
Toe lesions	Pododermatitis is principally a consequence of pressure necrosis, initiated by walking or abnormal weight-bearing on poor surfaces. Initial signs are the loss of normal plantar superficial architecture of the foot, giving rise to pressure necrosis, secondary granuloma or cellulitis	Avoid smooth, hard, and rough perches. Perch surfaces should distribute pressure evenly
	Waterfowl from warmer climates may suffer from the effects of a cold environment during the winter. Cracking of pedal skin and cellulitis may occur. Frost bite or dry necrosis due to aflotoxicosis may give rise to loss of foot web	

35.5 Skin conditions related to particular body sites. (continues) ▶

Condition	Features	Differential diagnosis, investigation and treatment
Toe lesions continued	Constricted toe syndrome is seen predominantly in greys, macaws and eclectus, arising as a consequence of an excessively dry rearing environment. Circumferential fibrous constrictions lead to venous engorgement of distal toes	Treatment of constricted toe syndrome is by surgical cutting of the constricting tissue and environmental changes
Articular gout	Commonest in psittacines (Figure 35.9). Presents as white paste or gritty swellings around the intertarsal or metatarsal joints	Diagnosis is by cytological demonstration of uric acid crystals. Treatment rarely indicated. Allopurinol or uricase may be used to lower blood uric acid levels but lesions will not regress and are typically very painful. Euthanasia is generally indicated on welfare grounds
Keel injuries	Typically in African greys. Most common in feather-clipped birds. Sequel to repeated traumatic crash landings in birds with severe wing clips.	Lesions should be debrided, sutured closed across the carina, and a padded hydrostatic dressing sutured in place over the wound (e.g. Granuflex). Repair or replacement of flight feathers in clipped birds to give a functional wing will prevent recurrence

35.5 (continued) Skin conditions related to particular body sites.

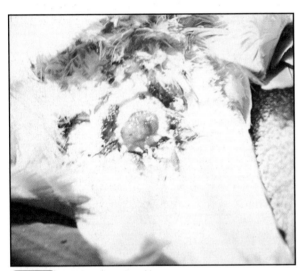

35.6 Cloacal papilloma in an Amazon Parrot.

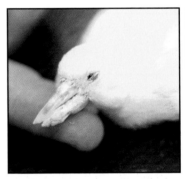

35.8 Canary (*Serinus canaria*) with lower beak affected by a chondroma.

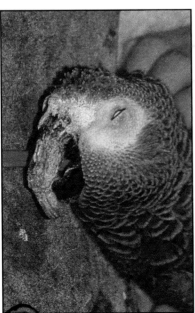

35.7 African grey (*Psittacus erithacus erithacus*) with severe *Candida* spp. infection of the upper beak.

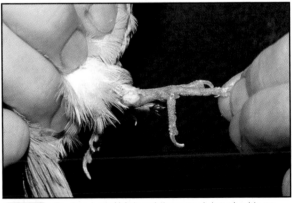

35.9 Budgerigar (*Melopsitticus undulatus*) with an articular gout lesion on the intertarsal joint.

Feather plucking and feather loss

Feather loss is a common problem and is often associated with excessive plucking (Figure 35.10). Plucking can be a major challenge for the veterinary surgeon and the owner because it is a complicated multifactorial problem and may be refractory to therapy. The majority of cases require detailed investigations, which may take some time, and birds may need to be seen several times. Some cases may be best approached by referral to a specialist. The key is to rule out all medical causes prior to accepting that there is a psychological problem.

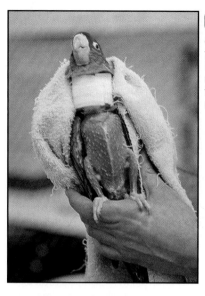

35.10 Typical pattern of feather loss due to picking. The body feathers are missing but head feathers are normal.

The approach to a feather plucking case can be used as a model for the investigation of many skin conditions.

Medical causes

Allergies

There is good evidence for the involvement of allergy in avian dermatology (Macwhirter and Mueller, 1998). However, eosinophils do not play the same role as in mammals (Johnson-Delaney, 1989) and IgG, not IgE, appears to be involved in allergic reactions. Although mast cells and basophils can release histamine, a true mammalian anaphylaxis is not well documented. Insect bite hypersensitivity is documented (Romagnano & Heard, 2000).

Many allergy patients are seasonally itchy, although others (e.g. food allergy) will itch all year round. If allergies are suspected, intradermal skin testing can be performed (Macwhirter and Mueller, 1998; Colombini *et al.*, 2000). The identification of potential avian allergens is in its infancy and, as testing will invoke a response only against the allergens tested for, many other undetected allergens may still be present. Many birds respond to housedust mites, *Aspergillus* spp., sunflower, maize, grain mill dust and various tree, plant or grass pollens. These are all good reasons for eliminating sunflower from the diet and increasing ventilation in the house, plus encouraging daily baths. Test medication using omega fatty oils and antihistamines can be used for a period of 4–8 weeks. A positive response indicates allergy but a negative response does not rule it out.

Ectoparasites

Ectoparasites are often blamed in cases of feather plucking. They are rarely responsible but must be ruled out. A white sheet should be hung around the cage at night; in the morning the inside of the sheet should be studied for mites or lice, often resembling moving grains of sand.

Feather loss in birds with ectoparasite infestation most commonly affects the medial aspects of the thighs, the neck and the covert feathers covering the base of the flight feathers. The following can all play a role: quill mites; *Cnemidocoptes* spp.; *Dermanyssus gallinae*; *Ornithonyssus* spp.; lice (e.g. *Mallophaga* spp.); and ticks (Forbes & Simpson 1993). Infested birds may be treated readily and safely with fipronil. Fipronil can be sprayed on to larger birds; for smaller birds it is measured out and applied directly to the skin; the dose is 3–6 ml/kg. Ectoparasites should be identified, so that the life cycle is known and one can be certain whether the environment as well as the bird requires treatment. If necessary the environment may be treated with permethrin and pyriproxifen.

Scaly face, commonly affecting budgerigars (Figure 35.11), and scaly leg, commonly affecting canaries and backyard poultry, are caused by *Cnemidocoptes* spp. These conditions are characterized by proliferative lesions of the affected area and are confirmed by identification of mites by microscopic examination of tissue in potassium hydroxide. The disease may affect all of a group or only individuals; however, all in-contact birds should be treated with topical ivermectin 200 µg/kg, preferably diluted with propylene glycol at 1:10, once weekly for 3 weeks.

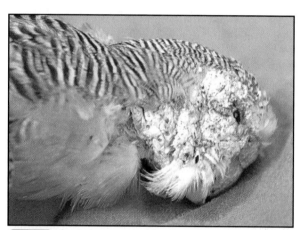

35.11 Scaly face caused by *Cnemidocoptes* spp. on a budgerigar.

Endoparasites

Endoparasites (i.e. enteric worms or protozoa) frequently cause problems, especially in cockatiels, and should be excluded in all species. A microscopic faecal examination (using iodine stains or carbolfuschin) should be performed, as enteric *Giardia* spp. have been recorded to cause a significant incidence of hypersensitivity affecting the wing web of cockatiels and lovebirds, leading to self trauma, typically under the wing (see Superficial Chronic Ulcerative Dermatitis, below).

Environmental problems

Tobacco smoke and too dry an environment (often triggered by central heating being turned on), can lead to itching or poor quality feather growth resulting in brittle feathers, which break as the bird plucks them. Many psittacines are developed for rain forest living and will benefit from a daily water spraying and at least weekly bathing. A continually dry environment may lead to premature wear on the plumage resulting in tatty feathers prior to the subsequent moult.

Poor nutrition during a moult will also result in poor feathers, which wear prematurely. A parrot with poor or damaged feathers may attempt to remove them. Low light intensity, an inability to bathe, or inadequate rest will also cause plucking.

Excessive daylight (>12 hours/day) can lead to a tired irritable bird. It is often best to cover a bird at night and remove the cover in the morning. The bird's cage should not be left in direct sunlight.

Metabolic/systemic disorders

Hypothyroidism: Hypothyroidism has been proven in a very small number of cases (Ogglesbee, 1992; Romagnano and Heard, 2000). Thyroxine is important to initiate a moult. Normal T4 values range from 1.3 to 14.16 nmol/l in Amazons and from 2.57 to 55.3 nmol/l in lovebirds (see also Greenacre *et al.*, 2001). A thyroid stimulation test using TRH is the diagnostic method of choice (Orosz *et al.*, 1997). Such cases will demonstrate a non-pruritic alopecia, thickened skin, cessation of moulting and obesity.

Liver disease: Any form of liver disease may lead to itchy skin and hence plucking. Liver disease may also cause abnormal feather coloration and excessive beak growth. Liver disease in neonates may prevent fledging.

Lead and zinc toxicity

Low level chronic lead or zinc toxicity, acquired from the bird's environment, will cause feather plucking. All birds should have their blood tested for zinc and lead. Zinc toxicity is considered a common cause of feather plucking and the author's own data (unpublished) indicate a 10% incidence of toxicity in caged parrots in the UK. Birds with high levels of zinc in their blood may, on occasions, show abnormal feather coloration.

Infection

Psittacosis: Psittacosis (also known as chlamydophilosis or 'parrot fever') is a common finding in plucking cases and should always be excluded. *Chlamydophila* is the commonest cause of psittacine liver disease, also causing septicaemia and air sacculitis, which may in itself trigger plucking. All affected cases should have a haematological, biochemical and *Chlamydophila* screen. Diagnosis may not be straightforward, and treatment will be prolonged (Tully, 1993). Psittacosis is a common disease in birds and its presence should not be considered the main cause of any skin or feather abnormalities, although it should be tested for and treated if found.

Folliculitis/pulpitis: Clinical signs of folliculitis are typically erythema, swelling, necrosis and exudate formation, although these signs are not universally present. Flight feathers may be 'pinched off' in growth; this may occur due to current trauma, stress, infection or prior damage to the dermal papilla. In relation to folliculitis, cause and effect may be difficult to differentiate. Is the bird picking at its feathers or skin because they are infected, or is the infection present as a consequence of the plucking and physical trauma of plucking?

Folliculitis is an uncommon cause of plucking, but the feather follicles should be examined for any signs of swelling, discharge or exudate.

Causative agents include *Aeromonas* spp., *Pseudomonas* spp., *Staphylococcus* spp., *Streptococcus* sp. and, rarely, *Mycobacterium* spp. Infection may even be present in the absence of swelling, redness or exudate formation. A biopsy to include a follicle is valuable.

Fungal infection: Dermatitis or folliculitis due to fungal infection is rare but clinical signs may not be indicative. *Candida* is commonest in gallinaceous birds in the vent area and in some pet birds around the head. Typically there is follicular involvement with white crusting around the affected follicles. *Aspergillus* is seen as feather or skin lesions and is commonest in pigeons but may well be underdiagnosed. Dermatophytes cause patchy feather loss especially on head, neck and breast.

Polyfolliculitis: In polyfolliculitis, multiple feathers erupt from one follicle. It is a common cause of self-trauma specific to lovebirds (Figure 35.12). Surgical removal of affected follicles is efficacious, although further polyfollicles may form. The condition may be of viral aetiology. A significant proportion of such cases are polyoma seropositive.

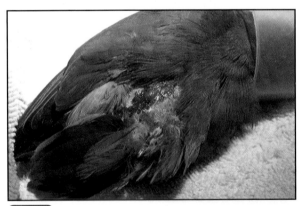

35.12 Polyfolliculitis in a lovebird (*Agopornis*).

Viral infection: Psittacine beak and feather disease (PBFD, caused by a circovirus) and budgerigar fledgling disease (caused by a polyoma virus) both lead to feather dystrophy, poor plumage, feather loss and occasional plucking. The pattern of feather abnormalities is typically different from the standard 'pattern picker' feather plucking case, whose head plumage is normal. These viruses should be excluded where relevant. Bent, weak and distorted short club-like feathers or growing feathers that fail to exsheath are indicative of viral infection. Loss of powder down (so that the beak becomes shiny) (Figure 35.13) is frequently the first sign. Haemorrhage into feathers or under the skin is indicative but not pathognomonic.

The clinical signs of PBFD are dependent on the species and the age at which the viraemia occurred:

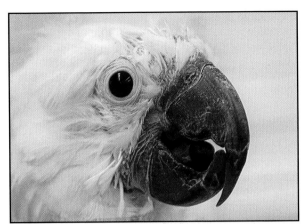

35.13 Psittacine beak and feather disease. Shiny beak (loss of powder down) and dystrophic crest feathers in a cockatoo (*Cacatua alba*).

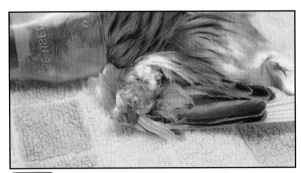

35.14 Canary affected by feather cysts.

- The *chronic form* occurs in mature birds. Feathers erupt from the follicle then quickly stop developing (dystrophic). The numbers of affected feathers increase at successive moults. Powder down feathers are affected first (initially over the hips), as a result the powder is not generated and the beak becomes shiny as opposed to dusty. The disease progresses to affect the contour feathers and finally the flight feathers. In PBFD cases, the head feathers are typically affected, in feather picking cases they are not. Dystrophy is roughly symmetrical and may present as sheath retention, haemorrhage into the pulp cavity and fracture of the proximal rachis. Short deformed clubbed feathers, stress ('fret lines or marks') lines on the vanes or circumferential constrictions around the rachis may be evident

- The *acute form*, referred to as 'French moult', has identical presenting signs to those caused by polyoma virus. The condition is commonest in budgerigars and is typically seen at the first moult when birds change their neonatal down to the first set of feathers. Clinical signs are characterized by sudden changes, including deformed feathers, necrosis, pulp haemorrhage, bending or broken feathers and premature loss of feathers. These signs develop 25–40 days after exposure. Diagnosis is by submission of blood and feather pulp for DNA PCR analysis.

Polyoma virus (Ritchie, 1991) may cause feather abnormalities in large parrots. Presenting signs depend on the age and condition of the bird at the time of infection. Neonates may have reduced down and contour feathers. Juveniles surviving initial infection may have symmetrical feather abnormalities (primary and tail feathers), plus a lack of body down feathers and head and neck filoplumes. Subcutaneous haemorrhage is a common feature. Diagnosis is by submission of blood and feather pulp for DNA PCR analysis.

Genetic causes

'Feather dusters' and 'straw feather' are two genetic abnormalities affecting budgerigars. The names are descriptive of the visual appearance of affected birds.

Feather cysts are common in certain breed lines of canaries (Figure 35.14). A genetic susceptibility is postulated. Many other psittacines suffer feather cysts.

Malnutrition

Malnutrition is the single most significant contributory factor to feather plucking in pet birds. It may be caused by a dietary deficiency, a digestive abnormality, a lack of access to unfiltered natural light, or an allergy to something in the traditional diet.

Nutritional deficiencies are frequently seen in birds fed on sunflower- or peanut-based diets, as hypovitaminosis A is inevitable. Clinically, birds present with dry flaky skin (often most obvious on the feet) and poor wound healing. Choanal atresia is a common finding. Sublingual salivary gland abscessation due to squamous metaplasia may be seen occasionally.

These birds must receive vitamin A supplementation (pure vitamin A should be administered 20,000 IU/kg i.m. once a week for 3 weeks) and be converted on to a better diet (e.g. a quality pelleted diet or a wet/chopped mixed 'sprouted seed/vegetable/rice mix' diet) (Hawley *et al.*, 2000). Vitamin powder applied on top of seed diets is totally ineffective. Sweet corn, apricots and other highly coloured vegetables are excellent sources of vitamin A (Scott, 1996). Vitamins may be given mixed with a soft food, or with some treat e.g. toast and honey, or, less ideally, dissolved in water.

Superficial chronic ulcerative dermatitis

Feather plucking may occur over the site of a skin cancer, or the trauma of repeated plucking may cause such a lesion (most associated with chronic ulcerative dermatitis) (Figure 35.15). Superficial chronic ulcera-

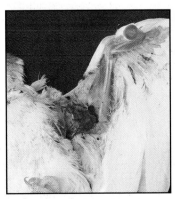

35.15 Superficial chronic ulcerative disease (SCUD) occurring concurrently with a squamous cell carcinoma (SCC) in a cockatiel (*Nymphicus hollandicus*).

tive dermatitis (SCUD) is associated with septicaemia, contact thermal or caustic trauma, occasionally with fungal dermatitis, neoplasia, xanthoma, polyfolliculitis, mycobacteriosis and enteric giardiasis. Lesions are highly pruritic. Surveys of avian neoplasia (Forbes *et al.*, 2000) give valuable data on age, sex, morphology and distribution.

Psychological causes

The typical pet parrot has the mental age of a 4-year-old child but never grows up. Much information can be gained by finding when the bird plucks, who is present or absent at the time, time of day, season of year and how it reacts when it is plucking.

Attention seeking

Feather plucking can be an excellent way of attracting the owner's attention. The owner often gives positive reinforcement for the bad behaviour by 'telling the bird off'. If the bird plucks, the owner should go to the cage, not address the bird, but cover it up, initially for a 3-minute period, increasing to as much as 15 minutes if necessary.

Boredom

Boredom or lack of routine is a very common cause of feather picking. A captive bird does not have to hunt for food, often has no flock mates to play with, and hence will fill more of the day with preening which may then become compulsive. This should be addressed by environmental enrichment. If the bird can be kept occupied and active, these problems are less likely to arise.

Separation anxiety

It is possible that the bird starts to pluck when left alone because it is anxious. Keeping the bird busy will help. Medication can be of value (clomipramine, 0.5–1.0 mg/kg orally bid, fluoxetine, 1–2 mg/kg orally bid or haloperidol, 1–2 mg/kg i.m. every 10 days), but is not a solution unless combined with behavioural modification training. The training should be geared to break down the anxiety triggers and to increase the parrot's confidence so it can cope for short periods alone.

Stressors

Stressors may be many, varied and different from what a human would expect to be stressful. A bird's normal reaction to fear or threat is to flee; if it is unable to escape it may redirect its energy to a 'fear response', which may include plucking or self-mutilation. Causes of stress or fear should be identified and eliminated. Increasing confidence (behavioural modification training) and facilitating controlled flight is beneficial. Haloperidol, 0.02–0.20 mg/kg orally bid or 1–2 mg/kg i.m. every 10 days, clomipramine and fluoxetine can be used in the initial stages of retraining.

Overcrowding

Too many birds together, social stress or too small an environment can lead to plucking.

Environmental change

Birds should be accustomed to a varied life; if variety is normal they will be stimulated and will enjoy it.

Excessive preening

Excessive preening may start as normal preening (in particular at the start of a moult) and then become obsessive, in particular if there is insufficient environmental enrichment or the bird is sexually frustrated and feels a need to build a nest using plucked feathers.

Sexual aggression or frustration

Aggression is commonest in cockatoos and lovebirds. Passerine birds (e.g. finches, lovebirds) are most likely to demonstrate female plucking by the male mate during the breeding season, or plucking of a subordinate male by another male. Feather loss most commonly affects the back, head and occasionally trunk.

In parrots, sexual frustration is, in the author's opinion, responsible for many of the behavioural problems experienced, especially in cockatoos and African greys. Parent-reared birds mature at 5–6 years, but hand-reared birds can become sexually active from the age of 6 months. Some birds will regurgitate to a family member, or present their cloacal region. These birds perceive they are human and on becoming sexually active they request sexual favours from their owners. Signals from the birds are misread and not reciprocated. Such cases require a multifaceted approach.

The birds may be injected intramuscularly every 2 weeks on three occasions with leuprolide acetate (100 µg/kg). This stimulates the pituitary gland, such that the messages from the pituitary instructing the gonads to produce more sex hormones are turned off. At the same time the owner to whom the bird has been making advances must not 'fraternize' with, handle or go near the bird for a period of at least 6 weeks. The daylight is also reduced to 6–8 hours per day so that the bird believes winter is coming and that it would be a bad time to breed anyway. Although these treatments will defuse the situation temporarily, a long-term solution is required.

Behavioural modification training must be used to gain a 'parent–child' or 'leader–follower' relationship, (rather than a 'partner–partner' relationship) between the owner and the bird. This is achieved primarily by gaining a dominant relationship over the bird. This must comprise height advantage at all times, but also the bird must be prepared to obey commands without question. If this is achieved, further sexual problems are unlikely.

Having two birds in separate cages but within each other's view can also lead to sexual frustration and may trigger plucking.

Compulsive behaviour

If a bird suddenly stops in the middle of its favourite activity just to pluck, it is either very itchy or is suffering from obsessive compulsive disorder. Such behaviour is akin to stereotypic behaviour, which is seen in certain badly housed zoo exhibits. Medical therapy is often required to break the disorder (clomipramine, fluoxetine or haloperidol), whilst serious environmental enrichment is implemented. A major change in lifestyle is required. Other causes of severe itch should be eliminated before assuming this diagnosis.

Feather clipping

A poorly or unevenly clipped wing can stimulate a bird to start plucking. The cut-off ends of the primaries or secondaries may be sharp and may irritate the abdominal wall, when the wing is closed against the body. Clipping may be justified only where a bird's dominance needs reducing and training alone has already failed.

The author's opinion is that feathers should never be clipped until after the bird has already learned to fly. In particular, if young grey parrots have their wings clipped they will commonly crash land, causing significant costal pain and ulceration over the carina. Wing clipping should not be used to prevent escape. If a clinician clips a wing, they must stress it is no guarantee that the bird cannot fly (on a windy day, or once any feathers have been replaced at the moult). Replacement of the short, sharp or tatty feather ends by 'imping' may be palliative. Imping involves gluing a suitably trimmed replacement feather on to a peg fixed within the shaft of the remnant of the damaged feather. Imping back a complete set of feathers is better.

Clipping should always be bilateral. Depending on the species, if clipping is essential, either the tip of each wing may be clipped, taking a diagonal line from the tip of the fourth primary to a point one-third from the tip of the first primary, or the outer three or four primaries are left and the next four or five primaries are removed at the level of the covert feathers (Figure 35.16).

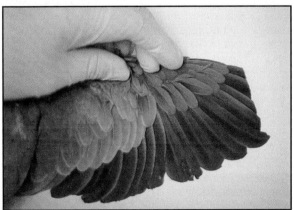
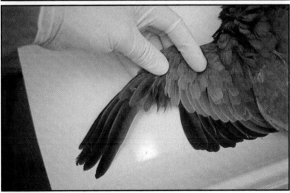

35.16 Acceptable forms of wing clipping. Clipping should be carried out bilaterally, after the bird has learned to fly, in order to restrict but not prevent safe flight.

Trauma

Any bird that has had a traumatic injury (recent or historic) or internal pain may pluck over the focus of pain. Traumatic injuries of the extremities may lead to the development of xanthomas, non-neoplastic nodules which are typically yellow waxy and highly vascular. Surgical removal is possible on occasions but one should be aware of the likelihood of significant intraoperative haemorrhage.

Management of feather loss or plucking

Actions to be taken by the owner

- If the parrot is alone by itself all day whilst everyone is out at work, consider re-homing the bird
- Improve the diet
- If possible, put the bird outside in a flight enclosure
- Improve the bird's environment: no smoking, not too dry, no direct sunshine, no excessive daylight
- Spray the bird lightly each day with warm water, preferably allow access to a bath, most parrots appreciate this
- Take the bird out of the cage as much as possible
- Environmental enrichment. Remind the client that the average parrot has a mental age of a 4-year-old child; you would no more shut a 4-year-old child into a small cage and ignore it all day than you should a parrot. Stimulate the bird mentally. For example, use 12 toys, but only 4 at time, changing them every 3 days. Toys may be divided into climbing, chewing, foot and puzzle toys
- Consider behavioural modification training.

Therapeutic options

Apart from the behavioural, husbandry and nutritional changes recommended above, medication is also required on occasions:

- If a specific pathogen is indicated, relevant systemic antibiotics or antifungals should be administered
- If ectoparasites are incriminated, fipronil may be applied and the environment cleaned and treated with permethrin and pyriproxiphen
- If mites are present, systemic avermectins should be administered
- Metronidazole for giardiasis.

Psychotropic drugs may also be administered (see Compulsive behaviour). These are not a solution but will give an opportunity for training or other techniques to be used to overcome behavioural problems.

Therapeutics

Therapy should be dictated by the aetiology or, if unknown, by the symptoms:

- Trauma: Treat as for any open wound and prevent further trauma (application of a neck brace if necessary)

- Viral infection: Supportive care is needed. Herpesvirus infections may be treated with topical and systemic aciclovir
- Bacterial infection: Perform culture and sensitivity testing. Administer parenteral therapy. Topical washing is often highly effective
- Fungal infection: Long-term systemic and topical antifungal therapy (itraconazole, diflucan, enilconazole, amphotericin) are required.
- Parasitic infestation: Topical treatment with fipronil or avermectins may be given. Treat the environment as necessary.

Drugs

Doseages

A number of avian formularies have been published (e.g. Carpenter *et al.*, 2001; Ritchie and Harrison, 1997; Moore and Rice, 1998). Figure 35.17 summarizes doseages that have been recommended for a range of therapeutic agents.

Safety and contraindications

Safety of a preparation in one species does not imply safety in all avian species. **In particular all birds are very sensitive to the toxic effects of local anaesthetic compounds.** This is of relevance when such compounds are included as minority constituents in other products. For example: Borgal 5% (trimethoprim–sulfadoxine, licensed for dogs and cats) contains 1 mg/ml of lidocaine; Aureomycin Topical Powder contains 1% benzocaine. Either compound might be used without further thought in avian skin cases with potentially fatal consequences. All local anaesthetic-based topical preparations are contraindicated in birds.

All oil-based topical preparations are contraindicated in birds as they destroy the functional integrity of the feathers.

Steroids are generally contraindicated in birds as they are more sensitive to side-effects (e.g. immunosuppression) than are mammals and may then be susceptible to infections such as aspergillosis (Carpenter *et al.*, 2001).

Drug	Dose rate and comments	References
Antiviral agents		
Aciclovir	80 mg/kg orally tid for 7 days	Norton *et al.* (1991)
Antibacterial agents		
Amoxicillin	100 mg/kg tid	Bauck and Hoefer (1993)
Amoxicillin/clavulanate	125 mg/kg orally bid	Moore and Rice (1998)
Cefadroxil/cefalexin	100 mg/kg orally bid for 14–21 days for deep pyoderma	Harlin (1994)
Ceftazidime	75–100 mg/kg i.m., i.v. qid	Rupley (1998)
Clindamycin	25 mg/kg orally tid	Flammer (1998)
Doxycycline	25–50 mg/kg sid may cause vomiting	Flammer (1998)
Enrofloxacin	10–20 mg/kg orally sid, 15–25 mg/kg i.m., s.c. bid	Dorrestein (1993)
Trimethoprim	100 mg/kg orally bid, 75 mg/kg i.m. bid	Bauck and Hoefer (1993)
Antifungal agents		
Fluconazole	20 mg/kg orally q48h for 14–60 days	Flammer (1996)
Itraconazole	10 mg/kg orally bid **Do not use in African grey parrots**	Orosz and Frazier (1995)
Terbinafine	10 mg/kg orally bid	Dahlhausen *et al.* (2000)
Antiparasitic agents		
Carnidazole	30–50 mg/kg orally once; repeat after 14 days For trichomoniasis, giardiasis	Johnson-Delaney and Harrison (1996)
Fenbendazole	20–50 mg/kg orally once **Do not use during moulting**	Marshall (1993)
Fipronil	7.5–15 mg/kg (3–6 ml/kg) once only	
Ivermectin: as anthelmintic	0.2 mg/kg s.c., orally, i.m. once only As an anthelmintic	Stadler and Carpenter (1996)
Ivermectin: as ectoparasiticide	Dilute 1:11 with water for immediate use 0.2 ml/kg orally, s.c., topical on skin, weekly for 3 weeks Preferable to dilute with propylene glycol to give a stable solution	Stadler and Carpenter (1996)
Metronidazole	30 mg/kg orally bid for 10 days For giardiasis	Murphy (1992)
Permethrin + pyriproxifen or cyromazine	For safe environmental control of ectoparasites	

35.17 An avian formulary derived from numerous sources. (continues) ▶

Drug	Dose rate and comments	References
Sedatives and anaesthetic agents		
Butorphanol	1–2 mg/kg i.m.	Clyde and Paul-Murphy (1999)
Diazepam	2.5–4 mg/kg orally, 0.6 mg/kg i.m.	Ritchie and Harrison (1997)
Isoflurane	4–5% induction, 2.0–2.5% maintenance	
Medetomidine	150–300 mg/kg i.m., i.v. Combine with 3–5 mg/kg ketamine for 30 minutes of general anaesthesia; reverse with atipamezole	Forbes (1999)
Midazolam	2–3 mg/kg i.m.	Johnson-Delaney and Harrison (1996)
Hormones		
Chorionic gonadotropin	500 IU/kg i.m. on days 1, 3, 7, 14, 21 For hypersexuality	Carpenter (2001)
Leuprolide acetate	100 µg/kg i.m. 3 times at 2-wk intervals	Millam (1993)
Levothyroxine	0.02 mg/kg orally bid	Rae (1995)
Non-steroidal anti-inflammatory agents		
Carprofen	2–4 mg/kg i.m., orally sid	Moore and Rice (1998)
Ketoprofen	2 mg/kg orally, i.m. sid	Malley (1994)
Meloxicam	0.1 mg/kg orally sid	
Psychotropic agents		
Amitriptyline	1–2 mg/kg orally sid to bid	Welle (1998)
Clomipramine	1 mg/kg orally sid for up to 6 weeks	Ramsey and Grindlinger (1994)
Delmadinone acetate	1 mg/kg i.m. once only	Lawton (1996)
Fluoxetine	0.4 mg/kg orally sid	Carpenter et al. (2001)
Haloperidol	1–2 mg/kg i.m. every 21 days, 0.15–0.20 mg/kg orally bid	Gould (1995)
Hydroxyzine	2-2.2 mg/kg orally tid As an antihistamine	Gould (1995)

35.17 (continued) An avian formulary derived from numerous sources.

Depot progestogens are contraindicated, as they may cause an unacceptable incidence of polyuria, polydipsia, diabetes, weight gain and immunosuppression (Carpenter et al., 2001).

References and further reading

Bauck L and Hoefer HL (1993) Avian antimicrobial therapy. *Seminars in Avian and Exotic Pet Medicine* 2, 17–22
Carpenter JW, Mashima TY and Rupiper DJ (2001) *Exotic Animal Formulary, 2nd edn.* WB Saunders, Philadelphia
Clyde VL and Paul-Murphy J (1999) Avian analgesia. In: *Zoo and Wildlife Medicine: Current Therapy 4,* ed. ME Fowler ME and RE Miller RE, pp. 309–314. WB Saunders, Philadelphia
Colombini S, Foil CS, Hosgood G et al. (2000) Intradermal skin testing in Hispaniolan parrots (*Amazona ventralis*). *Veterinary Dermatology* 11, 271–276
Dahlhausen R, Lindstrom JG and Radabaugh CS (2000) The use of terbinafine hydrochloride in the treatment of avian fungal disease. *Proceedings of the AAV Annual Conference,* pp. 35–39
Dorrestein GM (1993) Antimicrobial drug use in pet birds. In: *Antimicrobial Therapy in Veterinary Medicine, 2nd edn,* ed. JF Prescott and D Baggot, pp. 491–506. Iowa State University Press, Ames
Flammer K (1996) Fluconazole in psittacine birds. *Proceedings of the AAV Annual Conference,* pp. 203–204
Flammer K (1998) Common bacterial infections and antibiotic use in companion birds. *Compendium on Continuing Education for the Practicing Veterinarian* 20(suppl. 3A), 34–48
Forbes NA (1999) Birds. In: *BSAVA Manual of Small Animal Anaesthesia and Analgesia,* ed. C Seymour and R Gleed, pp. 283–293. BSAVA, Cheltenham
Forbes NA, Cooper JE and Higgins RJ (2000) Neoplasms of birds of prey. In: *Raptor Biomedicine III,* ed. JS Lumeij et al., pp. 127–146. Zoo Education Network, Florida
Forbes NA and Simpson GN (1993) Pathogenicity of ticks on aviary birds. *Veterinary Record* 133, 532
Gould WJ (1995) Caring for birds' skin and feathers. *Veterinary Medicine* (Jan) 53–63
Greenacre CB, Young DW, Behrend EN et al. (2001) Validation of a novel high-sensitivity radioimmunoassay procedure for measurement of total thyroxine concentration in psittacine birds and snakes. *American Journal of Veterinary Research* 62, 1750–1754
Harlin RW (1994) Pigeons. *Veterinary Clinics of North America: Small Animal Practice* 24, 157–173
Hawley B, Ritzman T and Edling TM (2000) Avian nutrition. In: *Manual of Avian Medicine,* ed. GH Olssen and SE Orosz, pp. 369–390. Mosby, St Louis
Johnson-Delaney C (1989) The avian immune system and its role in disease. In: *Proceedings of the Association of Avian Veterinarians,* pp. 20–27. AAV, Lake Worth, Florida
Johnson-Delaney CA and Harrison LR (1996) *Exotic Companion Medicine Handbook for Veterinarians.* Wingers Publishing, Lake Worth, FL
King AS and McLelland J (1984) Integument. In: *Birds, Their Structure and Function,* ed. AS King and J McLelland, pp. 23–42. Baillière Tindall, Philadelphia
Lawton MPC (1996) Behavioural problems. In: *BSAVA Manual of Psittacine Birds,* ed. PH Beynon et al., pp. 106–114. BSAVA, Cheltenham
Lucas AM and Stettenheim PR (1972) *Agricultural Handbook 362.* Agricultural Research Service, US Department of Agriculture, Washington DC
Macwhirter PJ and Mueller R (1998) Comparison of immediate skin test reactions in clinically normal and self-mutilating Psittaciformes. In: *Proceedings of the Association of Avian Veterinarians, Australian Committee Conference, Canberra*
Malley AD (1994) Practical therapeutics for cage and aviary birds. *Veterinary Annual* 235–246

Marshall R (1993) Avian anthelmintics and antiprotozoals. *Seminars in Avian and Exotic Pet Medicine* **2**, 33–41

McLelland J (1990) *A Colour Atlas of Avian Anatomy*. Wolfe, Aylesbury

Millam JR (1993) Leuprolide acetate can reversibly prevent egg laying in cockatiels. In: *Proceedings of the AAV Annual Conference*, pp. 46

Moore DM and Rice RL (1998) Exotic animal formulary. In: *Veterinary Values, 5th edn.*, ed. KM Holt *et al.*, pp. 159–245. Veterinary Medicine Publishing Group, Lenexa, KS

Murphy J (1992) Psittacine trichomoniasis. In: *Proceedings of the AAV Annual Conference*, pp. 165–170

Norton TM, Gaskin J, Kollias GV, *et al.* (1991) Efficacy of acyclovir against herpes virus infection in Quaker parrots. *American Journal of Veterinary Research* **52**, 2007–2009

Oglesbee BL (1992) Hypothyroidism in a scarlet macaw. *Journal of the American Veterinary Medical Association* **201**, 1599–1601

Orosz SE and Frazier DL (1995) Antifungal agents: a review of their pharmacology and therapeutic indications. *Journal of Avian Medicine and Surgery* **9**, 8–18

Orosz SE, Oliver JW and Schroeder EC (1997) TRH stimulation test for the evaluation of thyroid function in Amazon parrots. In: *Proceedings of the 4th EAAV Conference, London*, pp. 41–45. AAV, Lake Worth, Florida

Rae M (1995) Endocrine disease in pet birds. *Seminars in Avian and Exotic Pet Medicine* **4**, 32–38

Ramsay EC and Grindlinger H (1994) Use of clomipramine in the treatment of obsessive compulsive behaviour in psittacine birds. *Journal of Avian Medicine and Surgery* **8**, 9

Ritchie BW (1991) Avian polyomavirus: an overview. *Journal of Avian Medicine and Surgery* **5(3)**, 147–153

Ritchie BW and Harrison GJ (1997) Formulary. In: *Avian Medicine: Principles and Applications (abridged version)*, ed. BW Ritchie *et al.*, pp. 227–253. Wingers, Lake Worth, FL

Romagnano A and Heard DJ (2000) Avian dermatology. In: *Manual of Avian Medicine*, ed. GH Olsen and SE Orosz, pp. 95–123. Mosby, St Louis

Rupley AE (1998) Critical care of pet birds: procedures, therapeutics, and patient support. *Veterinary Clinics of North America: Exotic Animal Practice* **1**, 11–41

Schmidt RE (1993) The use of biopsies in the differential diagnosis of feather picking and avian skin disease. In: *Proceedings of the Association of Avian Veterinarians*, pp. 113–115. AAV, Lake Worth, Florida

Scott PW (1996) Nutrition. In: *BSAVA Manual of Psittacine Birds*, ed. PH Beynon *et al.*, pp. 17–26. BSAVA Publications, Cheltenham

Stadler C and Carpenter JW (1996) Parasites of backyard game birds. *Seminars in Avian and Exotic Pet Medicine* **5**, 85–96

Tully TN (1993) Chlamydiosis. *Seminars in Avian and Exotic Animal Medicine* **2**, 154–174

Welle KR (1998) A review of psychotropic drug therapy. In: *Proceedings of the AAV Annual Conference*, pp. 121–124

36

Reptiles

Mark Mitchell and Sarah Colombini

Reptile skin structure and function

The reptile integument is composed of an epidermis and a dermis. The epidermis has two primary cell layers, a superficial stratum corneum and a deeper stratum germinativum. The stratum corneum consists of six to eight cell layers and serves as an external barrier. The keratinized epidermal layers of chelonians (turtles, tortoises and terrapins) are modified into scutes. The stratum germinativum produces the cells that eventually migrate to the stratum corneum. Normal reptile skin often takes up to 4–6 weeks to heal, which is significantly longer than mammalian skin.

Reptile skin is typically dry and scaly. The scales originate in the stratum germinativum and are covered by the stratum corneum. Reptile scales may vary in size, shape, and texture from species to species. Scales may be smooth or have a keel (ridge down the centre). Reptile skin is relatively aglandular, although some reptiles have developed regionalized glands that are useful in attracting mates, marking territory (Figure 36.1) or defending against predators.

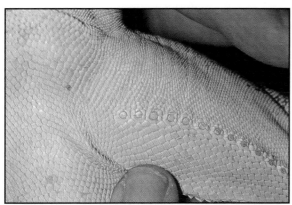

36.1 Femoral pores. The glands are pronounced in adult male green iguanas and are located on the ventral aspect of the thigh. The glands secrete a waxy substance used to mark territory.

Pigment cells, including chromatophores and melanocytes, are located in the dermis. Some reptiles can alter their colour by altering the size and shape of these pigment cells. The dermis is supported by a thick layer of connective tissue. A characteristic feature of the reptile integumentary system is the osteoderm or bony plate, which provides integumentary support and protects underlying soft tissue structures. Crocodilians possess several rows of osteoderms on their dorsum. The osteoderms of chelonians, in combination with the ribs, spine, and pelvic and pectoral girdles, form the shell. Osteoderms are metabolically active tissues, and drug dosages should be calculated based on the chelonian's total body weight.

Ecdysis

Ecdysis, or skin shedding/moulting, is a common occurrence in reptiles. Chelonians and crocodilians shed their epidermis continuously, whereas squamates (lizards and snakes) shed their epidermis periodically. Aquatic chelonians will periodically shed scutes from the carapace (top of the shell) or plastron (bottom of the shell). Snakes routinely shed their epidermis in one entire piece, though large snakes (> 2 m) typically shed their epidermis in pieces. Lizards generally shed their epidermis in small pieces.

Ecdysis can be affected by a number of factors, including age of the animal, gender, species, size, nutritional state, parasites, dermatological lesions, neurological disease, and environmental and endocrine factors. For example, juvenile reptiles may shed as frequently as every 1–2 weeks, whereas an adult reptile may only shed two to four times per year. Ecdysis is regulated by endogenous hormones produced from pituitary–thyroid interactions (Maderson, 1985).

The process of ecdysis in snakes takes approximately 14 days. Snakes preparing for an impending shed will become anorectic and avoid contact. Handling during this period can be hazardous for the animal if the underlying new epidermis is damaged. Approximately 14 days before the shed, the snake will have a dull (greyish) appearance. The spectacles become a bluish colour approximately 7–10 days before the shed and then clear 2–3 days later. The dull colour is associated with the lymphatics and enzymes that fill the space between the old and new epidermal layers. The snake should be provided with appropriate cage furniture (e.g. rock), so that it can rub its rostrum against a hard surface and facilitate the shedding process. Because they originate from the epidermis, the spectacles are normally shed during ecdysis. Retention of the spectacles has been associated with the development of subspectacular abscesses.

Approach to the case

History

A complete history is an important first step in the diagnosis of dermatological lesions in reptiles. The history should include questions detailing the exact husbandry standards provided for the reptile, including questions covering enclosure size and type, ventilation, enclosure lid, substrate, cage furniture, heat sources, temperature, humidity and nutrition.

Clinical examination

A two-step clinical examination should be performed. First, the reptile should be observed from a distance. Special attention should be given to mental state, respiration and locomotion. Secondly, a hands-on physical examination should be performed in a thorough and consistent manner. When evaluating the integumentary system, there are several specific sites that should be examined:

- The spectacles of snakes should be clear, with no apparent indications of a retained spectacle or subspectacular disease
- The nares should be clear and free of discharge or retained shed skin
- The integument should be inspected closely for ectoparasites, traumatic injuries and inflammatory responses
- The ventral surface of the reptile should be inspected for necrotic dermatitis
- Retained shed skin should be removed gently and inspected for ectoparasites
- The digits and the tail of lizards should be examined for retained shed skin and avascular necrosis
- The scutes of a chelonian should be firmly attached to the carapace and plastron
- Detached scutes and pitting of the osteoderms are suggestive of an underlying infectious agent.

Diagnosis

The diagnostic plan for dermatological disease in a reptile should follow standard protocols described for domestic species.

Blood samples: A complete blood count and plasma biochemistry analysis should be performed when systemic disease is suspected.

Radiography: Radiographs can be useful when assessing damaged osteoderms. Shell fractures are a common finding in both captive and wild-caught chelonians. Evaluating the extent of damage to the osteoderms and surrounding soft tissues is important when planning an appropriate therapeutic plan. Radiography can also be used to evaluate for the presence of underlying bone disease in deep abscesses.

Skin scrape: A skin scrape using a number 15 scalpel blade can be used to collect samples of the epidermis. Samples collected from the skin scrape should be placed on a microscopic slide and prepared for interpretation using mineral oil or the appropriate stain.

Double-sided tape or a cotton applicator soaked in mineral oil can be used to collect ectoparasites, such as mites, for identification.

Cytology: Cytology is an important but often underutilized tool in herpetological medicine. Cytological samples can be used to assess the general microflora present and the host's response to a dermatological lesion. Microbiological culture of samples collected from skin lesions should be performed when a bacterial or fungal disease is suspected. Cytological sampling should be performed prior to submitting the microbiological assay to guide the diagnostic laboratory and help the clinician to determine the relevance of culture results. Serial samples may need to be collected to confirm a diagnosis.

Biopsy: A biopsy of the affected tissue provides the best opportunity to confirm a diagnosis. Anaesthesia should be used to control pain when performing a biopsy. Lidocaine (2%) can be infiltrated in a line or regional block to provide appropriate anaesthesia. If manual restraint is insufficient to manage the reptile for the biopsy procedure, a dissociative anaesthetic, such as tiletamine and zolazepam (3–8 mg/kg i.m.) or propofol (10–15 mg/kg i.v.), can be used to provide chemical restraint. The biopsy specimen should include both healthy unaffected tissue and affected tissue. Excisional or punch biopsy samples should be full thickness with little to no preparation of the skin prior to the biopsy. Veterinary surgeons working with reptiles should establish a relationship with a pathologist familiar with the unique anatomy of reptile integument.

Husbandry-related problems

Abrasions

Skin abrasions are common in reptiles housed in glass tanks. Skin abrasions can occur anywhere on the reptile's body, although rostral abrasions are the most common. Certain species, such as the Chinese water dragon (*Physignathus cocincinus*), green iguana (*Iguana iguana*) and boa constrictor (*Constrictor constrictor*), are more prone to develop rostral abrasions because they constantly run into or rub the surfaces of an enclosure in an attempt to escape. These abrasions can progress into ulcers, abscesses and osteomyelitis if not managed properly. Placing problematic animals into enclosures with solid-coloured walls or hanging coloured paper over the sides of a glass tank may reduce the development of rostral abrasions.

Abscesses

Bacterial and fungal infections, foreign bodies and parasites have been associated with abscess formation in reptiles. Reptile abscesses tend to be well defined caseous masses (Figure 36.2).

Antimicrobials have limited value and surgical removal of the abscess/granuloma is necessary to control the infection. After the abscess is removed, a specimen should be collected for culture and impression smears made for cytological examination. Surgical debulking of the abscess is generally curative.

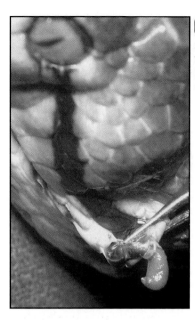

36.2 Surgical removal of a caseous abscess from a reticulated python (*Python reticulatus*).

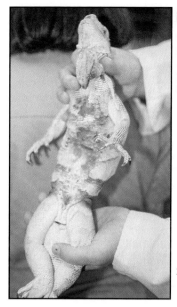

36.3 Third degree thermal burns on the ventrum of this green iguana (*Iguana iguana*) resulted from prolonged contact with a 'hot rock'.

Dysecdysis

The most common causes of dysecdysis in captive reptiles are inappropriate husbandry conditions, such as a low environmental temperature and/or humidity. Because of the diversity of habitats from which reptiles originate, clients should be directed to the literature to determine the appropriate environmental temperature and humidity ranges for their pet reptile. Environmental humidity for desert species should be 30–50%, for subtropical species 50–80% and for tropical species 70–90%. Low environmental humidity can also lead to chronic dehydration. Previous traumatic injuries, dermatological disease, neurological disease and ectoparasites have also been associated with dysecdysis. Avascular necrosis of the digits or tail may occur when the old skin constricts around these appendages.

Treatment for dysecdysis should include correcting deficiencies in the reptile's environment and removing the retained old epidermis. Soaking the reptile in a basin filled with shallow warm water (26.5–28.8°C) for 15–30 minutes will facilitate removal of the retained shed. Irrigating retained spectacles with ophthalmic eyewash can facilitate spectacle removal. Never attempt to remove a retained shed or spectacle that does not come away easily. Excessive tearing of the retained shed or spectacles can cause permanent damage to the underlying new epidermis.

Thermal burns

Thermal burns can occur when a reptile is not provided with an appropriate heat source. Reptiles typically bask in radiant light to regulate their body temperature. In captivity, 'hot rocks', heating pads, exposed incandescent light bulbs and other unnatural heating elements have been used to provide 'heat'. These heating elements can cause severe burns (Figure 36.3). Unfortunately, reptiles may not have the natural reflex to excess heat that higher vertebrates have, and they will continue to remain in contact with a heat source while being burned.

Management of a thermal burn should follow standard protocol. First degree wounds can generally be managed using cool compresses and irrigating the wounds with physiological saline. Second and third degree wounds require topical management of the wounds and systemic antimicrobials to prevent opportunistic infections. A broad-spectrum antimicrobial, such as a fluoroquinolone or third generation cephalosporin, with activity against *Pseudomonas* spp., should be empirically selected pending culture and sensitivity results.

Trauma

Injuries sustained from prey-induced trauma can be severe (Figure 36.4). Rodents are responsible for the majority of the trauma-related cases reported in reptiles, although invertebrates can also inflict biting injuries. Any prey-induced trauma should be managed as a contaminated wound and allowed to heal by second intention. Wet-to-dry bandages can be used to control wound discharge and facilitate debridement of the wound. These injuries can be prevented by instructing clients to feed pre-killed prey.

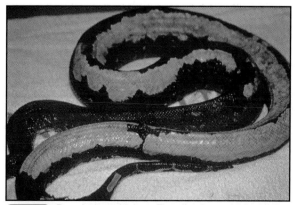

36.4 Prey-induced injury. The distal two-thirds of the dorsal integument of this boa constrictor (*Constrictor constrictor*) was eaten by a live rat offered to the snake as food.

Infectious diseases

Bacteria

Bacterial dermatitis is the most common form of infectious dermatitis in reptiles. Affected animals may develop focal or generalized vesicles, ulcers, crusts and granulomas. The majority of the infections result from inappropriate husbandry conditions. Immunosuppression is a common finding in reptiles maintained at suboptimal environmental temperature, predisposing them to chronic infections. The majority of the bacterial dermatitis cases reported in reptiles are associated with Gram-negative bacilli, including *Aeromonas*, *Citrobacter*, *Escherichia coli*, *Klebsiella*, *Proteus*, *Pseudomonas*, *Salmonella* and *Serratia*. Although less common, Gram-positive cocci (*Staphylococcus* and *Streptococcus*), Gram-negative cocci (*Neisseria*), *Dermatophilus congolensis*, *Mycobacterium*, and anaerobic bacteria have also been associated with bacterial dermatitis in reptiles.

Necrotizing dermatitis or 'blister disease'

This is commonly reported in snakes kept in enclosures with excess moisture. Affected animals develop coalescing vesicles on their ventral scales. The vesicles are typically sterile, but often become infected by an opportunistic microbe as the disease progresses. Placing the snake in an environment with optimal humidity and providing appropriate antimicrobial therapy and supportive care are usually curative. However, fatal septicaemia can occur in severe cases.

Septicaemic cutaneous ulcerative disease (SCUD)

This is a common problem in aquatic chelonians maintained in poor quality water. *Citrobacter freundii* was the first microbe described as the causative agent of SCUD; however, the authors have also isolated other species of Gram-negative microbes (Enterobacteriaceae) from shell ulcers. It is likely that any opportunistic pathogen producing exotoxins could create similar lesions in the chelonian epidermis and dermis. Aquatic chelonians, especially soft-shelled turtles (*Trionyx* spp.), fed a diet of crustaceans and maintained in water of poor quality, can develop severe ulcerative disease associated with *Benekea chitinovora* infection.

Diagnosis

Microbiological culture is required to confirm a bacterial dermatitis. Most bacterial pathogens isolated from reptiles will replicate at 37°C, although performing parallel cultures at 28°C may increase the likelihood of isolating fastidious organisms. An antimicrobial sensitivity profile should be performed on every isolate.

Therapy

Aggressive wound therapy is necessary to prevent the dissemination of a bacterial infection. Necrotic tissue should be removed and the wound irrigated with warm physiological saline. Irrigating severely infected wounds with 50% dextrose can be useful to 'kill' bacteria rapidly. The dextrose solution should be removed by irrigation with warmed physiological saline after 2–4 hours to avoid potential skin irritation. Localized infections can be managed using topical disinfectants (0.5–1% chlorhexidine diacetate), and a topical antibacterial cream, such as silver sulfadiazine. Combination therapy with silver sulfadiazine (14 g) and insulin (50 IU) has been used to manage topical wounds by reducing the glucose availability for microbes. Topical pH modulator sprays are also beneficial (but these may not be available in the UK or Europe) and can be applied to a wound to reduce the tissue pH and kill bacteria.

Systemic antimicrobials should be used only for generalized infections.

Viruses

Viral dermatitis has been reported in chelonians, crocodilians, lizards and snakes (Figure 36.5). New molecular diagnostic assays (e.g. enzyme-linked immunosorbent assay, polymerase chain reaction) and cell culture lines for isolating viruses have improved our ability to identify viral infections in reptiles.

There are relatively few options for treating viral infections in reptiles. In the case of virus-induced tumours, such as fibropapillomas and pox lesions, surgically debulking the tumour is recommended. Aciclovir has been used to eliminate viruses in reptiles with some success (Rossi, 1995).

Fungi

Fungal dermatitis has been reported in chelonians, crocodilians and squamates. *Aspergillus*, *Candida*, *Fusarium*, *Geotrichum*, *Mucor*, *Oospora*, *Paeciliomyces*, *Penicillium*, *Trichoderma* and *Trichophyton* are routinely isolated from skin lesions in reptiles. Most of these fungi are ubiquitous in the reptile's environment and are opportunistic pathogens. Inappropriate

Virus	Reptile host(s)	Clinical signs	Diagnosis
Herpesvirus	Green sea turtles (*Chelonia mydas*)	Grey patch disease: grey, coalescing papules	Histopathology: eosinophilic intranuclear inclusion bodies
Iridovirus	Soft-shelled turtles (*Trionyx sinensis*)	Erythematous epidermis in the cervical region	Viral culture, PCR
Poxvirus	Crocodilians and squamates	Grey—white epidermal pox lesions	Histopathology
Herpesvirus and/or retrovirus	Green sea turtles (*Chelonia mydas*)	Fibropapillomas: large epithelial tumours	Histopathology PCR

36.5 Common causes of viral dermatoses in reptiles.

Hyperpigmentation
Increased pigmentation via excessive deposition of melanin in the basal layer and within the epidermal cells

Hypertrichosis
Increased amount of hair, usually from increased length (hirsutism)

Intertrigo
Eroded or inflamed patches of skin on opposed surfaces, i.e. fold dermatitis

Keratinocyte
Cell of the epidermis

Leucoderma
Decreased or absent pigmentation of the skin

Leucotrichia
Decreased or absent pigmentation of the hair

Lichenification
Thickening of skin with exaggeration of normal skin markings. Consists of acanthosis, hyperkeratosis and dermal thickening

Macule
Small (<1 cm), circumscribed, flat change in skin colour. May be pale, hyperpigmented, erythematous, petechial or telangiectatic

Nodule
A circumscribed large (>0.5 cm) lesion raised above the level of the skin surface and which often extends into dermis (some authors use >1.0 cm, e.g. Scott *et al.*, 2001)

Papilloma
An exophytic, lobulated, benign, epithelial tumour, usually viral

Papule
Circumscribed, palpable elevation of skin <0.5 cm in diameter (some authors use <1.0 cm, e.g. Scott *et al.*, 2001)

Parakeratosis
Subset of hyperkeratosis with retention of nuclei in keratinized cells; clinically results in adherent hyperkeratosis

Paronychia
Inflammation of the nail fold

Patch
Macule >1 cm diameter

Pityriasis
Bran-like flaking of skin

Plaque
Raised flat-topped lesion

Poliosis
Depigmentation of the hair following various pathological conditions

Pruritus
Itching

Pustule
Small (<1 cm), circumscribed epidermal or dermal accumulation of purulent exudate

Pyoderma
Purulent dermatitis. Often implies staphylococcal infection of the skin

Scab
Common word for 'crust'

Scale
Visible flake of abnormal or compacted epithelial cells

Scar
Fibrotic area resulting from healing of a wound or lesion. Lacks hair follicles and covered with thin atrophic epidermis

Seborrhoea
Keratinization defect accompanied by a functional disturbance of sebaceous glands or of lipid metabolism of the epidermis with increased epidermal cell proliferation

Spongiosis
Intercellular epidermal oedema

Stratum basale
Innermost layer of epidermis composed of columnar cells arranged on a basement membrane. The germinative layer of the skin

Stratum acanthosum
Middle viable layer(s) of epidermis with prominent intercellular bridges. Metabolically active epidermis. Also called stratum spinosum

Stratum corneum
Outermost layer of epidermis composed of dead keratinized epidermal cells

Stratum granulosum
Layer of epidermis composed of flattened cells with pyknotic nuclei and keratin granules

Subcorneal
Below stratum corneum, as in subcorneal pustule

Tumour
Swelling or enlargement. Usually, but not always, neoplastic

Ulcer
Loss of skin tissue exposing dermis and/or subcutis

Urticaria
Superficial dermal oedema and erythema; circumscribed and multiple; eruption of wheals

Vesicle
A circumscribed elevation of epidermis caused by accumulation of clear fluid within or beneath the epidermis, <1 cm

Verrucous
Wart-like

Vitiligo
Patchy loss of skin pigmentation

Wheal
Sharply circumscribed skin elevation produced by oedema of the superficial dermis

Index

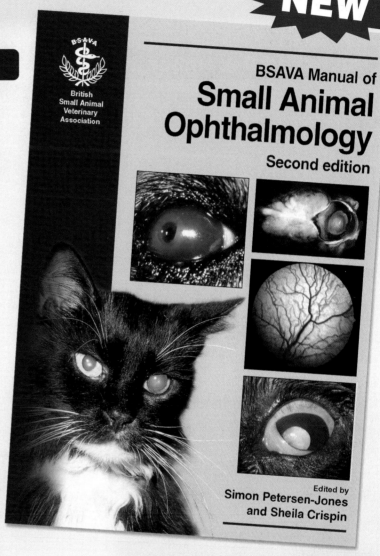
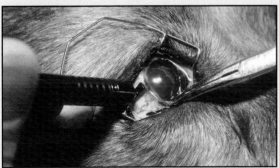
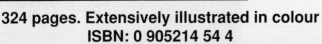
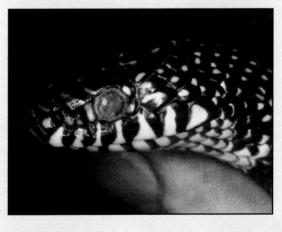

BSAVA Manual of
Ornamental Fish
Second Edition

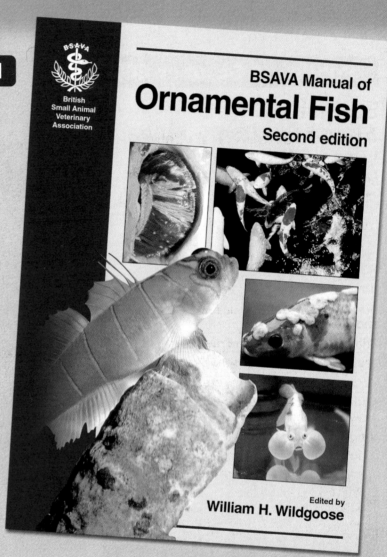
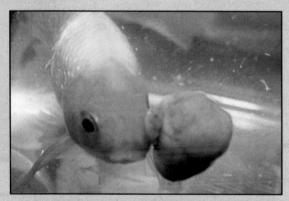
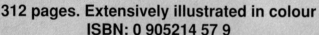
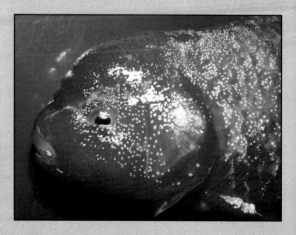
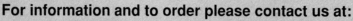